Conflicts of Interest and the Future of Medicine

Conflicts of Interest and the Future of Medicine

The United States, France, and Japan

Marc A. Rodwin

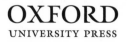

OXFORD
UNIVERSITY PRESS

OXFORD
UNIVERSITY PRESS

Oxford University Press, Inc., publishes works that further
Oxford University's objective of excellence
in research, scholarship, and education.

Oxford   New York
Auckland   Cape Town   Dar es Salaam   Hong Kong   Karachi
Kuala Lumpur   Madrid   Melbourne   Mexico City   Nairobi
New Delhi   Shanghai   Taipei   Toronto

With offices in
Argentina   Austria   Brazil   Chile   Czech Republic   France   Greece
Guatemala   Hungary   Italy   Japan   Poland   Portugal   Singapore
South Korea   Switzerland   Thailand   Turkey   Ukraine   Vietnam

Copyright © 2011 by Marc A. Rodwin

Published by Oxford University Press, Inc.
198 Madison Avenue, New York, NY 10016

www.oup.com

Oxford is a registered trademark of Oxford University Press

Library of Congress Cataloging-in-Publication Data
Rodwin, Marc A.
Conflicts of interest and the future of medicine : the United States,
France, and Japan / Marc A. Rodwin.
    p.   cm.
Includes bibliographical references and index.
ISBN 978-0-19-975548-6
1. Medical economics—United States. 2. Medical economics—Japan.
3. Medical economics—France. 4. Conflict of interests—United States.
5. Conflict of interests—Japan. 6. Conflict of interests—France. I. Title.
[DNLM: 1. Conflict of Interest—France. 2. Conflict of Interest—Japan.
3. Conflict of Interest—United States. 4. Physicians—France.
5. Physicians—Japan. 6. Physicians—United States. 7. Ethics, Medical—France.
8. Ethics, Medical—Japan. 9. Ethics, Medical—United States. 10. Morals—France.
11. Morals—Japan. 12. Morals—United States. W 50 R697m 1993]
RA410.53.R627   2010
338.4'73621—dc22   2010046033

9 8 7 6 5 4 3 2

Printed in the United States of America
on acid-free paper

For
Wendy,
Nina,
and
Benjamin

Contents

PART V   IMPLICATIONS

Foreword

Concern over conflicts of interest first caught my attention in the early 1990s, when I was editor-in-chief of the *New England Journal of Medicine*. During the White House deliberations on the design of the Clinton health care plan, doctors were more or less excluded from the discussions based on the presumption that they were just another interest group. How could a profession on which health care so critically depends be so undervalued, I wondered?

I soon found the answer when the *Journal* published Douglas Waud's "Pharmaceutical promotions—a free lunch?" and Dennis Thompson's "Understanding financial conflicts of interest," and I read Marc Rodwin's path-breaking book, *Medicine, Money, and Morals: Physicians' Conflicts of Interest.*[1] These analyses explained that professionalism had been steadily eroded by complex financial ties between practicing physicians and academic physicians on the one hand and the pharmaceutical, medical device, and biotechnology industries on the other. These financial ties were deep and wide: they threatened to bias the clinical research on which physicians relied to care for the sick, and they permeated nearly every aspect of medical care. Physicians were accepting gifts, taking free trips, serving on companies' speakers' bureaus, signing their names to articles written for them by industry-paid ghostwriters, and engaging in research that endangered patient care.

What had been a covert issue, occasionally brought to the surface by reporters who stumbled on a story, soon morphed into a national concern. Revelations soon surfaced that some Food and Drug Administration and clinical practice guideline panels were tainted by the participation of physicians with financial ties to companies that marketed the drugs and devices under scrutiny, that leaders of some professional physician organizations had inappropriate financial ties to industry, and that some editors were using their own journals to call attention to products in which they had a financial stake.

Slowly the public became more and more aware. People who had sat in their doctors' offices surrounded by drug company materials and forced to wait while drug reps brought lunch for the doctor's staff began to complain. Although when polled, patients claimed that they trusted their own doctor, they expressed skepticism about the motives of the profession and began to ask what the profession was doing about these financial conflicts. The answers they received were not reassuring. Most major medical institutions and professional organizations had no policies against financial arrangements with industry, or they set limits on gifts that were exceptionally lenient. When organizations did develop guidelines, they had no enforcement mechanisms.

How much clinical research is tainted by financial conflicts of interest is difficult to assess. More money is now spent on clinical research by industry than by the National Institutes of Health, and many researchers depend on industry support to keep their laboratories operating. Although many of these researchers do not personally receive funds from industry, they nonetheless are under pressure to find outcomes favorable to their study's sponsor, and some are intimidated in describing the class of drugs they study as anything but the top choice in fear of losing research funding. The pressure to get positive results is strong. Researchers are well advised to insist that they retain control of the data, are able to publish their results no matter what the outcome, and have full authority over the manuscripts submitted for publication. Unfortunately, some are willing to compromise if their research program is in jeopardy.

Eventually, position papers by the Association of American Medical Colleges and the Institute of Medicine of the National Academy of Sciences, two influential organizations, set new standards, at least for academic institutions and physicians. One by one, universities and medical schools developed or revised their conflict of interest policies. True, many of the policies were not overly restrictive and "picked off the low-hanging fruit," such as eliminating "free" lunches sponsored by drug companies. Yet they failed to eliminate more egregious practices, such as paid participation in speakers' bureaus and industry-sponsored continuing medical education.

Many of the solutions to financial conflicts of interest rely on disclosing the nature and amount of the conflict. Disclosure, as Rodwin pointed out twenty years ago in a "Sounding Board" piece in the *New England Journal of Medicine*, is a weak solution or a nonsolution.[2] The patient who receives a statement of the physician's conflict of interest is in a quandary. Knowing that an individual has such a conflict does not enable the patient to interpret his or her remarks or written material about a product from a company with which the physician has financial ties. Some physicians believe that disclosing a conflict allows them to say whatever they wish: the disclosure makes them feel absolved of any bias. Needless to say, the ideal solution to financial conflicts of interest is not disclosure but to have no conflict at all. Financial arrangements are, after all, optional. A physician who is recruited by a company can accept or reject the arrangements the company offers.

Critics of physicians' financial ties to industry generally do not seek to eliminate collaborations between academic physicians and industry scientists: such collaborations can result in new drugs, new uses for old drugs, refinements in medical devices, and other breakthroughs. But the discussion about what constitutes appropriate and inappropriate collaborations has become polarized. In general, the greater the social value of a physician's relation with industry, the greater should be our willingness to bear the risk of financial conflicts of interest. Yet identifying these boundaries is difficult and as yet there is no universally accepted guideline.

The lack of a nuanced approach has been problematic. Some highly placed scientists have interpreted criticism of their collaborations with industry as personal attacks. Others have launched a backlash, using irrational arguments to try to avoid rules that might inhibit their relations with industry and personal gains from these arrangements.

Given the lack of an accepted approach by the profession, legislators have launched their own creative attempts to address the issue. A few states have required companies to report their payments to physicians, and the revelations from these requirements have been interesting and useful. By far the most potent legislative action, however, has been taken by the staff of Senator Chuck Grassley (R-IA), which has the power to subpoena records from industry, universities, and individuals. These initiatives have shone the light on physicians' financial conflicts, and in some instances have uncovered vast sums of money that academic physicians have received from industry but failed to report even to their own universities. In addition, a "Sunshine Act" Grassley and Herb Kohl (D-WI) introduced in the U.S. Senate and attached to health reform legislation sets up a searchable Web site of physicians who have received even minimal payments from industry.

Finding effective approaches to deal with financial conflicts of interest in medicine is a continuing challenge. Until now, little has been known about how other countries approach this problem. Marc Rodwin has added immeasurably to this fund of knowledge. As he points out, France and Japan use very different strategies to handle the issue, and their efforts should certainly inform the debate in the United States. Rodwin's book also analyzes how the American medical economy and physician' conflicts of interest evolved and gave rise to policies to cope with conflicts of interest. He turns a critical eye to the current proposals to address conflicts of interest and suggests new directions for reform. His book offers important advice that policy makers must heed if we are to restore trust in our profession.

Jerome P. Kassirer, M.D.

Distinguished Professor, Tufts University School of Medicine

Visiting Professor, Stanford University

Editor-in-Chief Emeritus, *New England Journal of Medicine*

Part I

FRAMING THE ISSUES

Introduction: Patient Stories

In the introduction to his 1906 play, *The Doctor's Dilemma*, George Bernard Shaw wrote:

> And what other men dare pretend to be impartial where they have a strong pecuniary interest on one side? Nobody supposes that doctors are less virtuous than judges; but a judge whose salary and reputation depended on whether the verdict was for plaintiff or defendant, prosecutor or prisoner, would be as little trusted as a general in the pay of the enemy.
>
> That any sane nation, having observed that you could provide for the supply of bread by giving bakers a pecuniary interest in baking for you should go on to give a surgeon a pecuniary interest in cutting off your leg, is enough to make one despair for political humanity.[1]

Shaw suggests that patients and the public should worry about physician payment. More generally, they should consider what sort of financial incentives compromise good medical care. Three stories of contemporary patients illustrate his point.

When Tom Jones felt his chest tightening again, he decided to play it safe. He consulted a cardiologist in a private group practice in Boston. Dr. Nilufar Sharif asked Tom some questions about his symptoms, reviewed his medical history, listened to his heart, checked his blood pressure, and had her assistant draw blood for testing and take an electrocardiogram. After reviewing the results, she recommended further tests. First, Tom had a stress test to check his cardiac output. While he walked on an exercise treadmill set on an uphill slope, a physician monitored his heart with an electrocardiogram. Then Tom had an angiogram. Dr. Sharif inserted a catheter into an artery near his groin, extended it to his heart, and checked Tom's arteries. Informing Tom that plaque had reduced the blood flow to his heart, she recommended that he have coronary artery bypass graft surgery performed by the surgeon in her group practice and scheduled the surgery for the next week. The surgeon removed a piece of blood vessel from Tom's leg and grafted it into the heart muscle so that blood would flow through it and around the blocked artery. He also implanted a pacemaker to regulate Tom's cardiac rhythms.

In the weeks after his surgery, Tom kept meeting people who also had been treated for arteriosclerosis. To his surprise, their treatment was different. Esperance Garcia's physician, Dr. Sean Carroll, performed a stress test and electrocardiogram but did not recommend an angiogram. Dr. Carroll prescribed calcium channel blockers to increase blood flow to her heart and control her blood pressure, beta blockers to slow her heart rate and lower her blood pressure, and ACE (angiotensin converting enzyme) inhibitors to increase blood flow. Dr. Carroll also prescribed statins to help lower her cholesterol and slow the progression of her coronary artery disease. In addition, Dr. Carroll told Esperance to change her diet, exercise, and lose weight. Esperance also received training in managing her medications and in biofeedback to reduce her stress.

After an initial exam, Kang Li's physician, Dr. Rachel Feldman, told him that she found no signs of a heart attack and that several ailments could cause his symptoms. Most likely, she thought, the culprit might be his long-standing hiatal hernia. But it might be angina, caused by coronary artery disease restricting blood flow to his heart. Dr. Feldman referred Kang to a colleague for the same stress test that Tom received and then for an angiogram. After reviewing the results, Dr. Feldman informed Kang that plaque was reducing blood flow to his heart and recommended angioplasty. Dr. Feldman explained that she would insert a catheter into his artery and a balloon at the end would inflate to push away the plaque and widen the artery. Dr. Feldman performed the procedure two weeks later at a separate cardiac facility. Afterwards, she told Kang that one artery was narrow even after she removed the plaque, so she had inserted a wire stent to hold the artery walls apart and reduce future plaque buildup.

Tom, Esperance, and Kang initially thought that differences in the extent of plaque in their coronary arteries accounted for their differing treatment. As they compared notes, however, they found that factors other than their clinical condition might have caused their different treatment. Tom speculated that having different insurers affected their treatment. His interest was also piqued when he read the front-page *New York Times* article on financial ties between cardiologists and drug companies and stent and pacemaker manufacturers.[2] The article suggested that these ties affected physician prescribing and clinical choices and could cause inappropriate medical care and higher costs. When Tom shared the article with Esperance and Kang, they discussed whether their doctors' practice settings and payment arrangements affected their treatment.

These factors might well have influenced their medical care. Tom's physician was in private group practice and earned income from the tests and from the surgery. Esperance's physician, on the other hand, worked in a group practice that had a contract with the insurer, and their compensation varied with the cost of their treating all their patients. If the cost of hospital care and tests exceed a target, physician income declined. Esperance's physician needed to get her insurer's approval for any invasive medical procedures. Moreover, if Esperance's insurer became dissatisfied with the group practice's performance, it could remove the group from the network. Kang's physician was employed by a Health Maintenance Organization and received a set salary. Other ties might also affect their physicians' choices. Dr. Carroll had his expenses for attending the American Cardiology Association annual meeting paid by a drug company that made the drug he prescribed for Esperance. Dr. Feldman inserted a stent from a company that paid her to serve on its advisory board and to lecture other physicians about its stents as part of their promotion.

In Paris, François Fort experienced symptoms similar to Tom. François consulted a general practitioner in private practice, Dr. Claude Pascal, who examined him and prescribed blood tests and an electrocardiogram. But French private practitioners are not allowed to be paid for these tests, so Dr. Pascal referred François to an independent testing center. After seeing the results, Dr. Pascal referred François to a cardiologist who worked at a private hospital. The cardiologist performed the angiogram and then discussed with François whether he should be treated by angioplasty or coronary artery bypass graft surgery. François was treated with angioplasty and a stent implant. However, his cardiologist used a stent without drug coating of the kind Tom had received. Dr. Pascal said he thought the drug-coated stents presented greater risk. Dr. Pascal also prescribed medication for François to reduce the risk of future cardiac problems, including Enalapril (Vasotec) manufactured by Merck, Sharpe and Dome.

François was pleased with his care but found that some of his colleagues had received different treatment for similar cardiac problems. He was disturbed when a colleague told him that to promote their new cardiology drugs, Merck, Sharpe and Dome invited nearly all French cardiologists and their spouses to attend a meeting on their new drug in Beijing, China, with all expenses paid.[3] François wondered if Dr. Pascal had accepted the invitation to Beijing and if so, whether it influenced his choice of medication. Later, François was reading Le Canard Enchaîné, a newspaper known for its exposés and satirical commentary, when he spied an article exposing hip prosthesis manufacturers paying kickbacks to physicians to choose their product.[4]

In Tokyo, Hideo Tanaka also felt chest pain. He consulted Dr. Tatsuo Watanabe, who owned a small, well-equipped clinic near his home. Dr. Watanabe drew Hideo's blood for tests and arranged for one of his colleagues to perform an electrocardiogram and stress test. Then Dr. Watanabe prescribed eight medications, which he dispensed to Hideo immediately, and scheduled a follow-up visit to perform an angiogram. Before the follow-up visit, however, Hideo spoke to a neighbor about his cardiac treatment. The neighbor suggested that he would be better off seeking care at the prestigious Tokyo University Hospital. He pointed out that the university hospital employed elite physicians and that, as public servants, they did not need to prescribe medication to ensure their livelihood. So Hideo consulted Dr. Naoko Sakae at the Tokyo University Hospital. Dr. Sakae performed new tests, told Hideo that he needed a pacemaker to control his cardiac arrhythmias, and implanted one. Hideo learned that some fellow workers also had coronary artery disease and were treated with different regimes. A month later, when reading the *Mainichi Daily News*, Hideo learned that the head of the Tokyo University Metropolitan Hospital was prosecuted for taking kickbacks from an American pacemaker manufacturer in return for using their model rather than a competitor's.[5]

The hypothetical patients in these stories all fared well, but their treatment might have resulted in injury or death, and the main effects of their treatment are in the future. Because their treatment varied, these patients have different risks of complications and of future cardiac problems. Variations in these patients' medical condition or their physicians' training might explain their differing treatment. But financial incentives also affect clinical care.

Conflicts of interest are endemic in private practice in countries with very different medical, legal, and political systems. Yet there are also big differences among countries in the extent and kind of conflicts of interest that exist in private practice, the measures used to cope with them, and the alternatives to private practice that are available. Each country's laws, insurance, and medical institutions shape medical practice; and within each country, different forms of practice affect clinical choices. Consider just a few differences relevant to these patients.

Francois Fort's physician referred him to an independent testing facility because France prohibits nearly all physicians from earning income by prescribing ancillary services they supply. Private practitioners cannot be paid to dispense drugs or medical products, perform clinical or diagnostic tests, or supply ancillary services, although they can own or invest in private hospitals that do. Physicians cannot even dispense vaccines; patients obtain a prescription for a vaccine, purchase it from a pharmacy, and then bring it to their physician to perform the inoculation.

Tom's, Esperance's, and Kang's American physicians could legally provide stress tests, electrocardiograms, and blood tests. They could also have dispensed medication because they did not reside in the only five states that prohibit physician drug dispensing. But Esperance's insurer requires physicians to obtain their approval before performing an angiogram, while Tom's and Kang's insurers do not. Moreover, when ordering more tests, Tom's physician earns more money, while Esperance's physician's income declines and Kang's physician's income is unaffected.

Dr. Watanabe provided all tests for Hideo Tanaka. In Japan, there are no prohibitions on private practitioners dispensing drugs, performing clinical and diagnostic tests, or supplying ancillary services. Physician drug dispensing in Japan began with ancient Chinese medicine, when physicians were compensated not for their services but only for supplying drugs. Until very recently, drug dispensing and laboratory testing were a major source of physician income. However, in public hospitals in Japan, as in France and the United States, physicians are paid a fixed salary and have no incentive to make particular clinical choices.

In Japan, as in the United States and France, medical suppliers sometimes pay physicians kickbacks to induce sales. The temptation is not greater for publicly employed physicians than for those in private practice, but often laws are stricter for public employees. Hideo Tanaka read a story about the prosecution of the Tokyo University Hospital physician for switching pacemakers in return for kickbacks. Publicly employed Japanese physicians can be criminally prosecuted for accepting kickbacks, but their colleagues in private practice cannot. In France private practitioners can be prosecuted for accepting kickbacks; in the United States federal law prohibits kickbacks for private practitioners only for patients insured by Medicare or Medicaid.

In all three countries, drug firms and other medical suppliers use gifts and grants to influence physician choices and boost sales. A drug firm paid for Esperance's physician to attend a professional meeting. Merck, Sharpe and Dome invited French cardiologists to Beijing. A stent manufacturer cultivated Tom's physician by hiring her as a consultant and speaker. Each of these countries regulates gifts to doctors differently, with varying results.

Patients are not usually familiar with the details of medical organization and finance. As a result, they typically believe that practice arrangements do not affect what is most important in medicine—the patient-doctor relationship. As we shall see, nothing could be further from the truth.

1

The Heart of the Matter

The patient-doctor relationship lies at the heart of medicine. Patients rely on physicians to advise them about their medical needs, to supply medical treatment and services, and to act in their interest. Society expects that medical norms will induce physicians to act on behalf of patients. Yet, physicians earn their living through their medical work and so may practice in ways that enhance their income rather than the interests of patients. Moreover, when physicians prescribe drugs, devices, and treatments and choose who supplies these or refer patients to other providers, they affect the fortunes of third parties. As a result, providers, suppliers, and insurers try to influence physicians' clinical decisions for their own benefit. Thus, at the core of doctoring lies tension between self-interest and faithful service to patients and the public. The prevailing powerful medical ethos does influence physicians. Still, there is conflict between professional ethics and financial incentives. Consequently, patients have reason to ask: "Is my physician's judgment biased by her economic interests? Will she serve me loyally?"

In part to address this tension, society often arranges medical care differently from the way it does many other services. The institutions that supply medical services and the manner in which medical practice is organized shape how these conflicts unfold and sometimes contain them. The state grants the medical profession a monopoly over medical practice and allows physicians to set standards for entry into medical practice, to judge their work performance, and to a high degree, to regulate themselves.[1] Physicians and others justify this arrangement on the grounds that physicians have expert knowledge and that medicine is a profession, not merely an occupation. Professional values embody important ideals, they say, and medical practice should be governed by them, rather than by business and bureaucratic values, which are very different. In sum, they claim that *medical professionalism* has a moral core that both justifies physician authority over medical practice and regulates these conflicts.

In the last four decades of the twentieth century, however, new thinking challenged the authority of physicians and the value of professionalism.[2]

Market proponents argued that organized medicine created an oligopoly that advanced physicians' interests over those of patients. Professionals masked their self-interest, they maintained, and markets would better serve the public. Other critics championed patients' rights and individual autonomy. They claimed that physicians used their authority to usurp value-laden choices that patients ought to make. Still others believed that medical organizations should be subject to democratic processes and have to listen to the voices of patients and consumers to be held accountable.[3] A common theme unites these and other critiques: that physicians' conflicts of interest compromise medical practice. This concern spurs efforts to reform the organization and financing of medicine and to increase legal oversight. Failure to cope effectively with conflicts of interest undermines the credibility of physicians and professionalism.

THE MEDICAL PROFESSION AND THE MEDICAL ECONOMY

The future of the medical profession will be shaped largely by how society answers these key questions: In what context can physicians be trusted to act in their patients' interests? How can medical practice be organized to minimize physicians' conflicts of interest? How can society promote what is best in medical professionalism? What roles should physicians and organized medicine play in the medical economy? What roles should insurers, the state, and markets play in medical care?

This book explores these questions by examining the political economy of medicine in the United States, France, and Japan—all postindustrial democratic societies. They illustrate how differences in the roles of organized medicine, markets, and the state affect the existence and resolution of physicians' conflicts of interest.

In each country the state assumes major responsibility for financing medicine, allows private practice and physician ownership of medical facilities, and operates public hospitals. In each, most citizens receive medical insurance through their employer. In the United States and Japan, private insurers cover much of the public. France and Japan have universal coverage and national health insurance (NHI), but the United States does not.

These countries initially supplied medical care through unregulated markets. However, charities, the state, and mutual aid societies created alternatives. Their efforts were driven by religious missions, political revolutions, efforts to Westernize society, wartime necessity, and in peacetime by movements to enhance social solidarity and economic security. The alternatives were at first designed for the poor but later were extended to the general public. Over time, several arrangements were used to supply medical care. They were sometimes symbiotic, but at other times they clashed, and their boundaries overlapped, blurred, and shifted. Practice now occurs in four main forms:

- under physician ownership and direction
- through lay-directed charities and not-for-profit organizations
- under state sponsorship, usually through public institutions
- through investor-owned firms

How do these alternative ways of supplying medical care affect the tension at the core of doctoring? An unregulated medical market—one that does not even require training or certification—exhibits the greatest tension between provider self-interest and patients' interest. Yet, even with state licensing, private practitioners confront this tension because they are entrepreneurs who accrue profit or loss from their practice. In contrast, medical care supplied as a public service using publicly employed physicians typically precludes physician entrepreneurship. These physicians do not earn profits or risk loss and have employment security, so profit seeking does not affect their advice or clinical choices.

Supplying medical services through lay-directed charities and not-for-profit organizations presents an ambiguous alternative between private practice and public employment. When not-for-profit organizations employ physicians, they can preclude physician entrepreneurship. However, they sometime choose to compensate physicians in ways that reward practicing medicine in an entrepreneurial manner, particularly when they seek to generate income to expand, or when they need to be frugal to stay solvent. Investor-owned firms that employ physicians are likely to compensate them in ways that call forth entrepreneurial behavior that influences clinical choices. These four forms of practice are not mutually exclusive. For-profit firms sometimes form joint ventures with physicians or not-for-profit organizations, and both not-for-profit and for-profit entities can intermingle with private practitioners.

In addition, several factors affect medical practice. Organized medicine can influence practice standards, professional norms, professional discipline, and medical institutions. Physician compensation, ties to third parties, and other aspects of the economy also affect physicians and medical institutions. The state and insurers may regulate all four forms of medical practice. This book examines the interaction of the four basic forms of practice with

- organized medicine's influence over private practice;
- professional self-regulation;

- market competition;
- the role of the state and insurers.

These shape the presence of conflicts of interest and how nations address them. Each country's experience offers evidence about what helps cope with these conflicts and what does not work well.

NATIONAL PROFILES

This book takes the reader on a journey across three continents spanning several centuries, so bear in mind some key points of each nation's experience.

France

France illustrates the effects of professional control and self-regulation on physicians' conflicts of interest. Organized medicine has had long-standing, strong influence over France's medical economy. The medical profession regulates itself and the state grants it an official legal role. Since World War II, organized medicine has exercised authority through the Order of Physicians and physician trade unions. The Order of Physicians oversees the organization of private practice. It drafts a legal code and uses it to supervise the finances of private practice, physician contracts, and professional licensing and discipline. The code also affects the behavior of private firms and insurers. Physician unions negotiate accords on fees and other matters with national health insurance funds (NHI funds) and influence the policies of state and NHI funds through strikes, lobbying, and other political activities.

Organized medicine has restricted physicians from engaging in certain entrepreneurial activities, but it has tolerated many more. In the nineteenth and early twentieth centuries it opposed public hospitals and the public employment of physicians except to serve the poor. In the early twentieth century, France developed not-for-profit medical practice overseen by lay-directed insurers that own medical facilities and employ physicians, but this model did not thrive because of organized medicine's opposition. Since 1930, organized medicine blocked state and NHI efforts to monitor private practitioners, oversee their practice, set practice guidelines, or use alternatives to fee-for-service to pay physicians. Starting in 2004, however, the state began reforms that may give it the tools necessary to manage private practice.

To control compromising ties between physicians and firms that sell drugs, medical devices, and other medical products, in 1993 the state assigned to the Order of Physicians responsibility to oversee financial ties between commercial firms and physicians. It only prohibited grants unrelated to professional activities and kickbacks. Rather than stop commercial interests from developing financial ties that compromise physicians, the Order of Physicians joined with industry trade associations to ensure continued funding. Pharmaceutical and other medical supply firms still pick up the tab for physician registration fees, travel and related expenses to attend conferences, continuing medical education (CME), and other professional activities. Commercial interests also supply most of the funds to develop CME, conduct clinical research, and publish medical journals, all of which are powerful means to influence practice norms and individual clinical choices.

State direction is a distinctive feature of France's medical economy. The state operates a prestigious public hospital system that employs about 28 percent of physicians and owns 75 percent of hospital beds. The state restricts the scope of entrepreneurship within private practice. It prohibits most private practitioners from being paid to dispense drugs or provide tests or ancillary services, and from having financial ties with facilities that do. State regulation restricts the growth of physician-owned hospitals and medical facilities. Yet, the state neglects many physicians' conflicts of interest. It allows public hospital physicians to spend 20 percent of their time in private practice, to accept funds from commercial interests to cover their professional expenses, and to consult for commercial firms.

The United States

The American medical economy is distinguished by the dominance of markets and the private sector. Its experience reveals that promoting markets for medical services and insurance increases the variety and scope of physicians' conflicts of interest. However, markets also supply some means to help cope with them. In overseeing contemporary markets, public authorities have not imposed broad, clear limits on the scope of physician entrepreneurship as France has. Market freedom has created conditions that led the government to regulate particular practices. Detailed rules have had only minimal effect, however, because the remarkable adaptability of entrepreneurs and markets quickly makes regulations obsolete.

American medicine arose without the restrictions of medieval guilds, monopolies, or strict state licensing. Only in the early twentieth century did organized medicine become a significant political force and secure state licensing laws that allowed it to create a protected medical market.

As a protected medical market replaced an unregulated one in the United States, professional control yielded consequences somewhat different from those in France. During this phase, organized medicine assumed many responsibilities that were exercised by the state in other developed countries, including oversight of hospitals, medical education, and drug marketing. Professional control allowed the American Medical Association (AMA) to secure for physicians roles as intermediaries between their patients and hospitals, insurers, and drug companies. As gatekeepers, physicians influenced these third parties and were influenced by them.

Meanwhile, the AMA blocked alternatives to private practice with fewer conflicts of interest and resisted oversight by insurers and the state. Then, in the 1950s, the AMA relaxed its ethical restrictions to allow greater physician entrepreneurship. It also deepened its financial ties with the drug industry, which created conflicts of interest for the AMA and its journals and for private practitioners. Professional self-regulation addressed certain conflicts of interest but neglected many others. The inadequacy of self-regulation set the stage, in the 1970s, for the state to chip away at organized medicine's control. It increased its oversight role and promoted market competition. Nevertheless, the state sets comparatively few restrictions on the medical economy's development and operates relatively few public hospitals.

The promotion of markets allowed private insurers to become countervailing powers to organized medicine. Some insurers ended fee-for-service payment and certain entrepreneurial aspects of private practice. Staff-model health maintenance organizations (HMOs) employed physicians. Other HMOs oversaw self-employed physicians and countered entrepreneurial incentives. To manage private practitioners, HMOs changed physician payment, monitored their practice, and oversaw, or even restricted, their clinical options. In this way insurers helped cope with many physicians' conflicts of interest. However, they often rewarded physicians when they reduced services, creating new conflicts of interest.

Not-for-profit organizations, which are more prominent in the United States than in France of Japan, played an ambiguous role. Charities became the dominant owners of hospitals and, along with public hospitals, supplied some medical care to the poor through the mid-twentieth century. Subsidized by the state, not-for-profit hospitals performed a public service, but they also supported the entrepreneurial practice of self-employed physicians. Not-for-profit insurers also performed dual roles. Prepaid group practice and staff-model HMOs created alternatives to entrepreneurial practice. However, Blue Cross and Blue Shield insurance and independent practice association HMOs promoted private practice rather than alternatives to it.

Investor-owned insurers and medical facilities control a much larger market share in the United States than in France or Japan. They promoted the logic of markets, which affected the behavior of physicians and not-for-profit entities. They sometimes formed joint ventures with physicians and not-for-profit organizations, which also reduced the differences among these sectors.

Japan

Japan's medical economy is characterized by physicians who dispense drugs, supply ancillary services, and own most hospitals and clinics. The law virtually precludes investor-owned hospitals and clinics. Japan enables us to explore whether physicians' conflicts of interest exist in the absence of for-profit firms when physicians own medical facilities. In fact, they thrive— even though Japan traditionally considered medicine a humane art in which physicians did not charge fees for specific services but accepted voluntary contributions to defray their expenses.

Japan has relatively few lay-directed not-for-profit hospitals and insurers compared to France and the United States. This difference is due, in large part, to the fact that Japan had no equivalents to the religious medical charities that in Europe have operated hospitals since the medieval era. Although Japan developed medical co-ops in the late nineteenth and early twentieth centuries, they never dominated the medical economy in the way that France's mutual insurers or the U.S.'s Blue Cross insurers once did. The comparatively weak role of independent not-for-profit hospitals and insurers reduces the alternatives to physician entrepreneurship.

Organized medicine in Japan concentrates on the protection of private practice. After World War II, the Japan Medical Association neglected to develop standards for ethical conduct; relations between physicians and drug firms; clinical practice, competency, and education; quality assurance; hospital accreditation; physician certification; and continuing medical education. It focused on raising fees and blocking government and insurer oversight of physicians.

The state plays a prominent role in Japanese medicine. It introduced Western-style practice, hospitals, and medical schools. Today, state-operated medical schools and public hospitals employ 30 percent of physicians and own about one-third of hospital beds. The state also leads in promoting hospital accreditation and physician certification, and raising standards for practice and CME.

Until recently the state regulated private practice mainly by capping physician fees and drug prices. That controlled spending but did not mitigate physicians' conflicts of interest. In the early twenty-first century, the state began to curb physician entrepreneurship. It modified or replaced fee-for-service payment; it disallowed new physician-owned medical corporations through which physician groups own hospitals; it promoted a new kind of not-for-profit hospital by reorganizing state-funded university hospitals into independent not-for-profit organizations; and it offered physician-owned medical facilities tax incentives to reorganize into entities that resemble American-style not-for-profit hospitals.

Japan oversees relations between drug firms and private practitioners using laws that promote fair trade practices. Since 1993, Japan has restricted *individual* drug firms from granting funds to physicians or medical societies. Pharmaceutical firms now pool money and collectively grant funds for medical activities through two drug industry foundations. This approach precludes direct links between individual drug firms and individual recipients, which still exist in the United States and France.

Collective industry funding makes it more difficult for individual firms to influence physicians. But it still allows the industry to decide what to fund and to promote activities that highlight drug therapy rather than other important medical practice issues. Japan's reform points toward the ultimate solution to this problem: severing the link between drug firms and physicians entirely and replacing it with alternative funding through a tax on medical suppliers and insurers.

SOURCES OF CONFLICTS OF INTEREST

Before assessing the relative effectiveness of alternative strategies that address physicians' conflicts of interest and proposed reforms, it is helpful to lay some groundwork.

Medical ethics, law, and social norms require that physicians act in their patients' interests. Many writers describe this as a fiduciary obligation.[4] Physicians have conflicts of interest when they have incentives to act in ways that breach their obligations to their patients or when their loyalties are divided between their patients and other parties.[5] Conflicts of interest compromise physicians' loyalty to their patients and their independent judgment. They increase the risk that physicians will not fulfill their obligations, but they are not themselves a breach of duty. The law can regulate conflicts of interest or supply remedies when there is misconduct or harm to patients.

Two main kinds of conflicts of interest exist. Financial conflicts of interest arise from incentives that bias physicians. Incentives that reward physicians for increasing or decreasing services, or providing one kind of service rather than others, encourage treatment that is not based on the patient's circumstances or criteria of good medical practice. Instead, they encourage physicians to make medical choices for their own financial benefit. Incentives to refer to particular providers or to prescribe particular tests and therapies also bias their choices. The risk of misconduct increases as the incentive grows larger and the link grows closer between the physicians' actions and their reward. But not all financial incentives create conflicts of interest. Incentives that reward excellent medical outcomes, quality, or patient satisfaction are unequivocally in patients' interests. Bonuses for working longer than average hours or night shifts do not bias clinical choices or advice.

Divided loyalty conflicts of interest occur when physicians perform roles that interfere with their acting in their patients' interest or when their loyalty is split between patients and a third party. Physicians often engage in activities that are fine in themselves, yet compromise their ability to act in their patients' interest, for example, by conducting experiments to assess a new drug while simultaneously treating patients. Patients and doctors can easily confuse these two roles despite efforts to ensure the patient's informed consent. For example, patient care and research are at odds when a physician enrolls one of his patients in a drug trial because the aim of research is not to benefit the research subject but to advance science. True, the experimental drug may help the patient who volunteers as a research subject; but whether it is safe or effective is unknown, and the patient might fare much worse than otherwise.

Conflicts of interest arising from financial incentives and those that arise from divided loyalty or dual roles often overlap. Physicians who prescribe and supply services perform two roles: (1) they diagnose medical problems and prescribe treatment; and (2) they supply therapies. Performing the second role can interfere with the first because it creates an incentive for the physician to prescribe therapies she can supply. That perverse incentive disappears when an independent provider supplies these services.

Certain aspects of medical practice affect key sources of conflicts of interest, including these five salient features:

- which services physicians perform
- whether physicians or other parties own medical facilities
- whether physicians are self-employed or employed by others
- how physicians are paid
- what financial ties exist between physicians and third parties

Providing Services

Self-employed physicians are entrepreneurs in the sense that they earn profits by selling services and bear the risk of any financial loss or debt. The entrepreneurial aspect of private practice calls forth self-interested behavior, which compromises the ability of physicians to give patients disinterested advice regarding what services they need. However, private practice can be more or less entrepreneurial depending on the type of services that physicians supply. First, they can perform basic services: examine patients, diagnose problems, prescribe therapies, advise patients, and refer them to others. Second, physicians can perform medical procedures or treatments. Third, they can supply ancillary services, such as laboratory or diagnostic tests. Finally, physicians can sell medications, medical devices, and other products.

Consider a continuum of practice arrangements from the least to most entrepreneurial. Start with traditional solo practitioners who are paid on a fee-for-service basis. The main way they can boost their income is to raise fees or supply more services. If they have time available, they might persuade their patients to obtain more services than they sought, or than are desirable. In addition, they can market their services, solicit business, and seek referrals, or negotiate reciprocal referral arrangements with other practitioners.

Physicians increase their entrepreneurial opportunities when they offer more than basic services or develop their practice so that it can produce a higher volume of services. They can broaden the kind of services they offer by learning new skills and procedures or developing practice specialties. They can increase their volume of services by employing assistants, allied health professionals, or other physicians.

In addition, physicians can add ancillary services such as laboratory and diagnostic tests, or sell medication and medical products. When they provide more than basic services, physicians can leverage their diagnoses, prescriptions, and advice to generate income. They have an incentive to prescribe tests, therapies, procedures, and medicines that they supply. By forming group practices, physicians facilitate supplying ancillary services because they share the cost of the necessary equipment and personnel. Physicians in groups can refer patients within the group and share practice income.

Owning Medical Facilities

Physician ownership or investment in medical facilities extends the range of entrepreneurial opportunities. It expands the variety of services physicians sell and their opportunity to generate income through their prescriptions and referrals. Groups of physicians, or physicians jointly with not-for-profit organizations or for-profit firms, can own clinical laboratories, centers for diagnostic imaging and other testing, clinics, ambulatory care surgical centers, hospitals, and nursing homes. Legal rules and the economics of practice, not medical requirements, limit what services physicians can supply in their practice and whether they can invest in medical facilities.

Employment

When not self-employed, physicians can be employed by public authorities, not-for-profit organizations, for-profit firms, or physician-owned practices. Employers can influence physicians' clinical choices through compensation or supervision so physicians might promote their employers' rather than their patients' interests. Whether employers do compromise medical choices depends on their authority and practice arrangements.

Consider physicians employed as public servants in public hospitals. Typically, they receive a fixed salary set by rank, enjoy tenure, and have clinical discretion. As a result, they lack financial incentives that bias their choices and have clinical freedom. Such arrangements preclude employment conflicts of interest. But relax some of these conditions and employers can compromise medical practice. Physicians who lack job security are more likely to take account of their employer's interests. When employers can vary physician compensation they acquire another tool to sway medical decisions.

Furthermore, employers can manage physicians to promote the organization's goals. As a result, employed physicians might practice in ways that promote their employer's over their patients' interests. If employed physicians practice with the aim of increasing their employer's profits, typically, they will increase services or choose expensive services over inexpensive ones. However, if the employer is compensated with a fixed payment or with some form of financial risk sharing, then employed physicians may reduce the volume of services or reduce other practice expenses.

The conventional wisdom holds that physicians have greater conflicts of interest when employed by a for-profit firm than a not-for-profit organization. This conclusion presupposes that physicians will help their for-profit employer generate profit, even when compensated by salary, and that not-for-profit employers lack a profit motive and so will not offer physicians compromising incentives. However, not-for-profit employers face pressures to remain solvent and can offer financial incentives for physicians to reduce costs or generate revenue in ways that are detrimental to patients' welfare. Similarly, many physicians suppose that employment by lay-owned firms creates conflicts of interest while employment by physician-owned firms does not. However, both might offer physician employees compromising financial incentives.

Physician Payment that Biases Clinical Choices

Payment can encourage physicians to supply more, less, or different kinds of services, or to refer to particular providers. Each form of payment has some bias, but some compromise clinical decisions more than others do.

Fee-for-service rewards increasing services regardless of whether they are beneficial. Depending on how fees are set, it may also encourage physicians to choose some services over others and skew their choices. As George Bernard Shaw remarked in the quotation that begins the Introduction, it can perversely encourage physicians to perform procedures that harm their patients rather than heal them.

In contrast, salary is relatively neutral because it does not typically link physician income to particular clinical choices or reward them for increasing, decreasing, or providing particular services. But it has other drawbacks; it does not reward physicians for extra work, productivity, or efficiency. It may engender what its critics pejoratively call a *civil-service mentality*. Moreover, employers can adjust salary yearly to reward performance. In theory, they can increase or decrease salary to reward physicians who generate revenue, reduce costs, or both, encouraging financially driven medical choices. Employers can also set salary to reflect the organization's financial performance, another incentive to practice in ways that promote the employer's interest. Still, annual salary adjustments are less sensitive to individual clinical choices than physician income that is fee-for-service.

Some insurers employ *capitation* payment and *risk sharing* to create incentives for physicians to control spending. Capitation is a fixed payment per patient for a set period. Typically, physicians receive capitation payment in return for their labor, not other medical services that patients may need. Frequently, payers adjust capitation rates for the age and gender of the patient to account for differences in expected medical needs. Often used to pay primary care physicians, capitation provides physicians a fixed monthly income that varies with the number of patients under their care, but not with the volume of patient visits, services supplied, time spent, or referrals. When a primary care physician has a full practice, capitation payment resembles a salary.

Sometimes insurers modify capitation to make physicians responsible for part of the resources used to care for their patients. They increase the capitation rate but make the primary care physician responsible for the cost of certain services, such as laboratory or diagnostic tests, medication, or treatment by specialists. This arrangement encourages physicians to change their clinical choices to reduce expenditures. They can order fewer or different tests, prescribe fewer or different drugs and services, and make fewer or different referrals.

Modified capitation payment and other arrangements that make physicians bear certain medical costs are called *risk sharing*, because physician compensation is at risk based on how they manage their patients' medical care. Payers can also modify fee-for-service and salary so that physicians bear a portion of the financial risk, making part of the physician's fee or salary contingent on the cost of their patients' treatment. For example, the payer can set aside 20 percent of physician fees or salary and pay the amount withheld only if medical spending for their patients does not exceed a threshold. Risk sharing creates conflicts of interest. It rewards physicians for reducing services, regardless of whether it is in their patients' interest. Still, risk sharing is not the exact opposite of fee-for-service. Rather, physicians' income increases or decreases based on the total volume of services that they provide for a group of patients over time.

Typically, insurers have a group practice share financial risk for its physicians' patients. Spreading the risk over the physician group reduces the effects of any individual physician's decisions or a particular patient's medical condition. Yet payers can make individual physicians bear financial risk. Payers who do that often limit physician risk with so-called stop-loss protection, which ends physician responsibility for any individual patient's expenses after they exceed a set amount.

Payers sometimes combine different compensation methods. They may pay physicians by salary or capitation but add fees for specified services. Alternatively, they can pay physicians fee-for-service or salary while placing part of this compensation at risk. In short, they blend different types of payment to create more nuanced incentives. In recent years, some payers have introduced *pay for performance*, which supplements compensation based on several measures of performance. It usually includes incentives that reward quality or patient satisfaction and do not create conflicts of interest.

Financial Ties to Third Parties

Insurers may not only share financial risk with physicians but also monitor physicians' practice and restrict the services that physicians provide by limiting what they reimburse. They may require that patients and physicians receive their authorization before paying for certain services, referrals, and elective hospitalizations. In this way, they can influence physicians' clinical choices and oversee their practice.

Physicians affect other providers' income through their prescriptions and referrals. These providers sometimes offer physicians financial incentives for referrals. For example, hospitals sometimes subsidize the practices of affiliated self-employed physicians. Some guarantee practice income to recruit physicians to relocate near their hospital and be affiliated with it;

others provide free or subsidized office space, or assistance with office management. Hospitals, clinical laboratories, diagnostic testing centers, and other providers sometimes pay physicians kickbacks to refer patients or medical work. They may pay cash, or in-kind benefits, such as medical equipment, or personal goods and services or gifts, such as wine, art work, or trips to vacation resorts. Today, many physicians' activities rely on discretionary funding from pharma and other commercial interests that also creates conflicts of interest. These activities include CME, medical research, and testing drugs and medical devices to ensure they are effective and safe.

Even physicians employed in public or not-for-profit organizations can have ties with third parties. They may receive funding, gifts, or kickbacks from drug and medical device firms and other medical suppliers. They may consult for private firms on a part-time basis. The risk is clearer when the quid pro quo for the payment is explicit and direct, as occurs when firms pay physicians kickbacks. However, more subtle arrangements also place patients at risk. Gifts beget indebtedness and generate reciprocity. Even though most physicians do not believe gifts influence their conduct, studies show they do.

REFORMS

The experiences of the United States, France, and Japan highlight the inadequacy of six common remedies for physicians' conflicts of interest. One proposal attributes the problem to investor-owned firms and would replace them with physician-owned or physician-directed organizations, or with not-for-profit organizations. Yet physicians' conflicts of interest exist even with physician ownership and not-for profit organizations. A second attributes the problem to external influences on physicians and would grant the organized medical profession greater authority to oversee medical practice. Yet, when organized medicine controlled or significantly shaped the medical economy in all three countries, it often tolerated or even spawned serious conflicts of interest. A third approach attributes the problem to professional monopoly and promotes markets instead. Yet, far from eliminating conflicts of interest, market competition increases their variety.

The problems with markets prompt proposals to eliminate any profit motive by employing all physicians as public servants. That would eliminate a great many conflicts of interest, but not necessarily those arising from ties to third parties. It also makes physicians dependent on the state, which can be a source of other conflicts of interest. A fifth idea is to make physicians legally accountable as fiduciaries through court oversight. Yet judicial oversight has enormous practical limitations. A sixth approach sees disclosure of

conflicts of interest as a panacea. But, disclosure neither eliminates conflicts
of interest nor provides adequate safeguards or remedies.

No magic bullet can eliminate or cure physicians' conflicts of interest.
Yet the collective experience of these countries yields evidence that several
strategies help to cope with them. It suggests that regulation of the market
is necessary, but a market under professional control is not the answer. Increasing the supply of medical care outside of physician-owned private practice, either through public hospitals or carefully structured and regulated
not-for-profit organizations, creates a setting that avoids entrepreneurial
conflicts of interest. Similarly, restricting entrepreneurial opportunities in
private practice—for example, by not allowing physicians to supply ancillary
services or dispense medication, or to invest in facilities that do—reduces
the presence of conflicts of interest.

When private practitioners have incentives to increase services, then
insurers, the state, or others can oversee medical practice to make it more
difficult for physicians to supply unneeded services or the wrong kind
of therapy. Furthermore, regulation of physician payment can minimize
incentives to increase or decrease services for self-employed physicians and
physician employees. Finally, rules can protect physicians who exercise professional judgment from interference by third parties that attempt to over-
ride physicians without adequate evidence or grounds to do so.

State control and employment can also create physicians' conflicts of
interests, so it is wise to preserve options to receive medical care outside of
public medical facilities. Physician employment in carefully structured
not-for-profit entities can offer an alternative to entrepreneurial practice.
The state and private sector can each supply checks and balances to conflict-
of-interest problems caused by the other, yet independently neither is sufficient to cope with them all effectively.

Physicians often have financial ties to drug firms and other commercial
interests through grants, gifts, and consulting. The varied approaches of
France, the United States, and Japan demonstrate why most current regulation fails and suggest that the solution is to eliminate these financial ties.
I offer examples of alternative ways to finance activities now funded by the
pharmaceutical and medical device industries.

Changing the organization of practice and financial incentives can reduce
the scope of conflicts of interest and mitigate the harm caused by those that
remain. But we need to allow physicians a measure of clinical discretion and
to rely on their medical judgment. That makes it important to foster medical
professionalism.

The conventional wisdom holds that in order for professionalism to
thrive, physicians must be insulated from the state and the market, both of
which promote antithetical values. But this study reveals that this thesis

oversimplifies the relation of professionalism to the market and the state. Both the state and the market have in different ways promoted key professional values, such as public service over profit, fidelity to patients, and the development of knowledge and expertise. Although both the state and the market sometimes undermine professionalism and professional values, both have also fostered what is most valuable about professionalism. Robust professionalism requires the countervailing power of the state and markets, but limits on both as well.

In the future, public policy must also address the conflicts of interest of investor-owned firms, not-for-profit organizations, third-party payers, and government organizations. If there are controls on physicians' conflicts of interest the medical profession can help oversee the conflicts of interests of these actors and hold them accountable.[6]

As the twenty-first century began, the United States, France, and Japan all sought to control spending and promote efficiency; to improve quality of care, service, and public health; and to rationalize the organization of medicine. Policy makers, however, neglected to consider how alternative measures to promote these objectives affect physicians' conflicts of interest. That was a major oversight, because reforms that set up conflicts of interests or fail to resolve those that exist often undermine those policy goals.

Following President Barak Obama's lead, the U.S. Congress debated several health reform proposals in 2009 and in 2010 passed Patient Protection and Affordable Care Act.[7] The law (1) extends Medicaid coverage to all individuals earning less than 133 percent of the federal poverty level; (2) provides subsidies to help individuals with low income purchase private insurance; (3) lowers the price of insurance purchased individually or through small groups by creating a federally regulated health insurance exchange where firms sell policies; (4) encourages employers to offer health benefits to employees and individuals to purchase insurance by levying modest penalties on employers and individuals if they do not; and (5) prohibits private insurers from denying coverage to individuals based on their individual medical risk or to limit coverage based on an individual's preexisting medical conditions.

Some critics argued that a public program modeled on Medicare would be less expensive than subsidies for private insurance, because it would eliminate the 15–20 percent of premiums that private insurers typically spend on marketing, underwriting, administration, and profit. Moreover, a public program could also lower spending by controlling provider reimbursement. However, many insurers and private firms opposed the creation of a public insurance program, believing that it was detrimental to their interests.

The law enacted will not resolve the conflicts of interests that plague U.S. medical practice and it will have only a minor impact on medical quality and spending.[8] Nor would the alternative proposals debated cope with physicians' conflicts of interest much better. Even a Medicare-style program would leave intact entrepreneurial private practice and the other key sources of physicians' conflicts of interest. The United States needs more fundamental reform. Self-styled realists may claim that the political obstacles are so large that we should abandon efforts to reduce physicians' conflicts of interest. But this book shows that each of these three countries have made reforms that reduced the severity and effects of conflicts of interest. The future of medicine is at stake; we should not remain prisoners of the past.

THE PLAN OF THE BOOK

The core of this book is the case studies of France, the United States, and Japan. Each one includes two parts. The first part traces the history of the nation's medical political economy through the interaction between organized medicine, the market, and the state. It chronicles the rise of organized medicine, changes in medical markets, the growth of national legal and organizational frameworks, the origins of private and social medical insurance, and changes in the relations between physicians and the pharmaceutical industry. Struggles between organized physicians, the state, and various groups shaped the political economy that gave rise to physicians' conflicts of interest and sometimes helped tame them. The second part of each case study focuses on strategies used to respond to physicians' conflicts of interest.

Following the case studies three chapters reflect on the experience of these countries. One chapter draws lessons from common reform efforts that are inadequate and reveals several measures that have proved effective. A second chapter draws inferences for medical professionalism. A conclusion sets forth the direction in which I propose we move. An appendix traces the origin and spread of law related to conflicts of interest.

Part II

FRANCE

2

The Evolution of French Medicine

France has national health insurance (NHI) funded by contributions from employers, employees, and the self-employed and general tax revenue for the unemployed. The state finances insurance for individuals with low income, including their private supplemental insurance for items not included in NHI. The state operates public hospitals that own over three-quarters of hospital beds and employ 28 percent of physicians. Public hospitals supply an alternative to private practice with its conflicts of interest. The private sector includes physician-owned and lay-owned for-profit hospitals, with about 19 percent of beds, and independent not-for-profit hospitals with 5 percent of beds. The state controls the growth and operation of private hospitals through licensing, planning, and regulation.[1]

Private practitioners have conflicts of interests that arise from entrepreneurship, fee-for-service payment, and financial ties to commercial interests, particularly drug and medical device firms. However, the state restricts entrepreneurial opportunities within private practice. Self-employed practitioners cannot generally earn income from dispensing drugs or performing laboratory and diagnostic tests, nor have a financial interest in facilities that supply those services.

Organized medicine has greater authority over the medical economy in France than it does in most countries. The physician-elected Order of Physicians sets rules for the private sector with a Code of Medical Deontology (Medical Deontology) and reviews physician contracts to ensure that they comply. Publicly employed physicians are also bound by Medical Deontology and the state and NHI insurers respect Medical Deontology. Multiple physician trade unions represent self-employed physicians and negotiate accords over fees and terms of practice with NHI insurers. They also influence policy through lobbying, electoral politics, lawsuits, and strikes. Organized medicine has exercised its authority to thwart competition and oversight of private practice. It blocked effective use of practice guidelines and utilization review, thereby hampering state and insurer controls on physicians' conflicts of interest. It restricted the growth of

not-for-profit medical facilities as an alternative to physician-owned private practice. It preserved financial ties between pharma and physicians
and tolerated many other physicians' conflicts of interest.[2]

Today's medical political economy emerged from very different earlier
arrangements: medieval guilds, church charity, and corporatism, that is
organized bodies that represent different economic sectors and perform
social welfare functions. Class position, charity, markets, and organized
groups determined access to medical care and practice arrangements, but
revolutionary social change created a system that guarantees universal coverage and empowers physicians as organized professionals. That history
illuminates contemporary physicians' conflicts of interest and responses
to them.

THE OLD RÉGIME

In the medieval era, two medical sectors emerged. In one, physicians
practiced in a protected market and supplied services to those with means.
As private practitioners they experienced entrepreneurial conflicts of
interest. In the other sector, medical care was part of church charity which
had a public service mission. This division influenced the subsequent
development of medicine, including its relation to the national interest,
its financing, and physicians' role in the medical economy.

Early medieval France had no formal system for training healers, and
the work of various types of practitioners overlapped. Over time, universities became centers to train physicians. Surgeons, on the other hand,
trained through apprenticeships. They treated wounds (including venereal
and skin lesions), performed lancing and bleeding, and healed fractures
and dislocations. Apothecaries prepared and dispensed remedies, often at
a physician's request. Other healers included midwives, bonesetters, and
herbalists.[3]

In cities and large towns, self-employed practitioners formed guilds
and sought royal charters, which conferred a corporate status, a regional
monopoly, control over training and membership, and privileges.[4] The
historian William Sewell has shown that medieval corporations had a
moral and spiritual dimension. They developed fraternity and an *esprit de
corps* modeled on the church or the state. This was linked to their self regulation.[5]

By the seventeenth century, the royal government had granted corporate
charters to between thirty-six and forty-three medical schools and about
300 corporations for surgeons and apothecaries. Still, poaching led to lawsuits over practice jurisdiction. Moreover, approximately 85 percent of the

population lived in rural areas without corporate charters and practice restrictions.[6] Practitioners other than physicians cared for most people who sought treatment for illness. The rural poor often consulted folk healers, monks, nuns, and charitable women.

A 1777 royal decree granted apothecaries a charter and a monopoly on drug sales.[7] However, surgeons could dispense medicine for lesions they treated, and in towns lacking an apothecary, physicians and surgeons could dispense medicine. Abbeys, convent nurses, and parish priests continued to sell medicine. Selling drugs became a sideline for herbalists, distillers, beverage retailers, confectionaries, wigmakers, old-clothes dealers, tallow chandlers, and executioners. Physicians frequently sold proprietary remedies, the equivalent of patented drugs.[8] A few physicians received royal patents for remedies and became wealthy. Others sold proprietary medicines and mineral waters, supervised by a royal commission. Lay healers also sold secret remedies.

From the sixteenth through the eighteenth centuries, physicians' compensation and their payment conflicts of interest varied with their patients' class position.[9] Physicians employed by royal courts or nobility were generously compensated with money or land and housing. The pay of physicians employed by households varied with their patron's economic fortunes. Most physicians served urban elites and were well off. Some corporate orders of physicians set fees. In 1754, the Nîmes physician fee schedule was graduated based on the patient's status. Visits cost 40 sous for nobles, the bourgeois, and wholesalers, and 30 sous for well-off artisans and farmers.[10]

Medical practitioners also engaged in other entrepreneurial practices. They began to advertise with posters on walls and notice boards in the sixteenth century. By the end of the seventeenth century, bills, posters, business cards, and announcements in newspapers were common in urban centers.

Small-town physicians competed with surgeons and folk healers. In the 1770s, surgeons' fees were typically the daily wage of an agricultural worker or artisan, while physicians charged three times as much, plus travel time, which in rural areas could be more than the fee. Most rural residents paid with foodstuffs or services. Physicians usually collected payment seasonally or annually and had to write off one-fifth of their bills. Rural residents typically consulted a physician only in dire circumstances. A folk saying declared, "Wounds heal themselves but money cannot be renewed."[11]

The market failed to supply medical care for most people because they lacked money. Sometimes third parties paid physicians to treat those who could not afford it. Masters might pay for their servants; mutual aid associations and guilds sometimes employed physicians for their members. Some towns paid physicians stipends to supplement patient fees. Municipalities, abbeys, and charities occasionally employed physicians to tend to the poor, paying them annually in cash or in kind and sometimes providing them with housing.[12]

The Catholic Church—the center of moral authority in pre–Revolutionary France—played a key role in medicine's development and was the source of public service values we now attribute to medical professionalism. In the early Middle Ages, many physicians were clerics and the church influenced the universities that trained physicians. Even more important, the church created hospitals as part of its charitable mission. Unlike private practitioners, who supplied medicine for profit, it provided medicine in not-for-profit institutions. Hospitals did not originate as medical facilities, however. They were custodial institutions that offered refuge for those who no one else cared for: infants, the insane, the aged, and people with physical disabilities or incurable diseases. The state also used these institutions as asylums for able-bodied beggars, vagabonds, and criminals.[13] As part of their custodial responsibility, hospitals supplied medical care.

Enlightenment thinkers wrote articles in Denis Diderot's 1765 Encyclopedia that suggested placing hospitals under state control and reorganizing them to heal the sick using science, rather than to supply charity. They also proposed that the state supply medical care for the public and alleviate poverty.[14] These ideas sparked reform efforts. In 1774, Jacques Turgot, the minister of finance, created a commission on poverty that distinguished between the *deserving poor*—the sick, insane, blind, and disabled—and others that were poor, the able-bodied, vagabonds, and criminals.[15] However, church officials who controlled hospital operations blocked government reforms intended to make them centers for the ill rather than charitable institutions for the poor.

The Revolution

The French Revolution attempted to make medicine a public responsibility. Although unsuccessful in the short run, it nevertheless inspired future reforms.

When the French Revolution created a republic and modern French law, the state assumed the Catholic Church's moral authority. In the Old Régime the church had clothed monarchy with a moral mission by advancing the idea that rulers should govern for the public good. Jean-Jacques Rousseau's 1762 book, *The Social Contract*, conceived of the public interest as distinct from the sum of individual interests. Influenced by this idea, the state defined the public interest as the good of the nation.[16] Later, policies on conflict of interest sought to ensure that public employees served the state's mission rather than private interests. This conception differs from that of the liberal state model exemplified by the United States, which views the public interest as the sum of individual interests reconciled through competition and negotiation among interest groups.[17]

Revolutionary leaders believed that the state should alleviate poverty by ending restrictions on employment. In the name of freedom to work, the 1791 Decree d'Allarde abolished corporations, monopolies, guilds, and privileged associations. From 1791 to 1801, no medical schools conferred degrees and anyone could practice medicine. Then, in 1803, after Napoléon became Consul, the state took charge of medical education, authorized universities to train physicians, and established license requirements. It created public health officers with training similar to Old Régime surgeons to practice in towns with fewer than 2,000 people in the department that licensed them. Moreover, while the state abolished guilds and corporations, it created a state supervised system for occupational groups and oversaw them to further its conception of the public interest. Unlike in other countries, state supervision of occupational groupings has continued in contemporary France.[18]

The state assumed the Catholic Church's responsibilities and public service mission. It developed the idea that medicine should be supplied publicly rather than by religious charity or through commerce. In 1794, the state nationalized church property, including hospitals. It raised the physician's status, refocused hospitals on medical care for the poor, used hospitals to train physicians, improved their sanitation, and ended custodial care, which unfortunately evicted many destitute hospital residents.[19]

Revolutionary leaders believed the state should supply medical care for the ill so they could work. As early as 1789, reformers proposed funding state-appointed physicians and surgeons in each canton to treat all citizens, but the state lacked funds for the program. By around 1810, however, Alsace had each canton employ a physician to serve the indigent. The *cantonal system* spread to four other provinces by 1859.[20]

Still, a physician's care remained beyond most people's means and medical entrepreneurship continued. Some physicians sold secret remedies, advertised, and split fees for referrals.[21] By the restoration of the monarchy in 1830, medical charity resembled that of the Old Régime. Religious orders of monks and nuns cared for the destitute sick. Legislation in 1816 allowed only apothecaries to dispense drugs from pharmacopeia of authorized medicine, but allowed patented medicine, and nonpharmacists continued to dispense drugs and sell secret remedies. The state also allowed religious orders to dispense medicine, and religious dispensaries outnumbered pharmacies in some regions.[22]

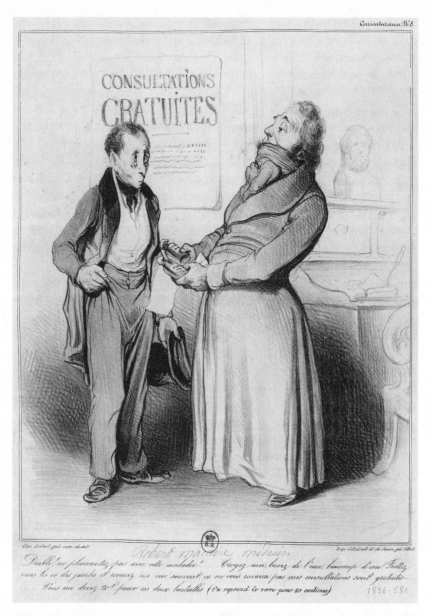

Daumier: Free Consultations. Doctor says: "For Heaven's sake, don't take this sickness lightly . . . believe me, drink water, lots of water. Rub the bones of your legs . . . and come to see me often . . . that won't impoverish you . . . my consultations are free. Now, you owe me 20 francs for these two bottles (this includes 10 centimes deposit on each container)."

Bibliothèque nationale de France. D. 361, Consultations Gruatuites, le Charivari, 16 Octobre 1836.

UNIONS, MUTUAL AID, AND THE STATE DURING
THE NINETEENTH CENTURY

In response to growing labor unrest, in 1813 the state mandated that employers provide medical care for employees injured at work. It required medical benefits for miners in 1894 and for industrial workers in 1898. The mining, railroad, and metallurgy industries supplied on-site occupational medical services and opened hospitals. Industrial firms also employed physicians. The state increased access to medicine through public facilities. It removed restrictions that required hospitals to serve only local residents in 1851, and starting in 1901, created dispensaries that supplied free medicine and ambulatory care, treated venereal diseases and tuberculosis, and promoted public health.[23]

Even more important, during the early 1850s, the state rescinded the Revolution's ban on private associations, until then considered a legacy of the Old Régime contrary to the public interest. This reform allowed the middle class to form mutual aid societies, typically organized by occupational groups. They became a means to medical care that was more affordable, but they also permitted physicians to organize unions that defended entrepreneurial private practice.[24]

The emergence of these solidarity groups precipitated a struggle over the role of physicians and set the stage for the transformation of the medical economy. Previously, most people could not afford medical care, which limited physicians' entrepreneurial opportunities. Mutual aid societies removed this budget constraint; but they also challenged physician control by negotiating with private practitioners for lower fees and offered an alternative to private practice by creating hospitals with physician employees.

The Birth of Mutual Aid and Physician Unions

In the mid-nineteenth century, the state was neither philosophically inclined nor financially able to fund medical care for citizens who were not indigent. According to laissez-faire liberal thought, assisting individuals undermined their initiative and dignity so the state should aid only those unable to care for themselves: children, women, the disabled, and the destitute. All others should exercise prudence, that is, obtain security through insurance.

However, the 1810 penal code and 1834 legislation had banned associations, so the state made exceptions for mutual aid societies through decrees between 1813 and 1843. Initially, these not-for-profit associations, most of which were small, served shopkeepers, artisans, and the petite bourgeoisie. They excluded individuals considered high risk: manual laborers, women, and "unclean" migrants. Many people lacked funds to pay membership fees. Still, the number of mutual aid societies grew from 2,438 in 1852 to 6,169 in 1869.[25]

France industrialized rapidly during the reign of Louis-Napoléon Bonaparte.[26] As Emperor Napoléon III, he promoted mutual aid for laborers to reduce the pauperism that resulted when illness prevented them from working. The expansion of mutual insurance continued under the Third Republic, which deposed Napoléon III in 1870. In 1898, legislation established a Mutual Charter that required insurers to grant members the same benefits unless based on different premiums or risks. In 1902, insurers formed the National Federation of French Mutual Insurers (FNMF), which later developed its own pharmacies, dispensaries, hospitals, and public health facilities. Mutual insurance covered 2.5 million individuals by 1900, about 6 percent of the population, and 3.5 million, about 9 percent of the population, by 1910.[27]

Physicians created mutual aid societies and used them as professional associations to represent self-employed physicians. By the first National Congress of Physicians in 1845, fifty-eight physician mutual aid societies existed outside Paris. Over time, they began to perform union functions such as setting fee schedules. There were seventy-four physician associations by 1884, when they formed their first alliance named the Union of French Physician Syndicates (USMF).[28]

In 1892, acknowledging the growth of organized medicine, the Chevandier Act legalized physician unions and created a protected medical market. It set fines for unlicensed practitioners and allowed unions to sue unlicensed practitioners. It restricted midwives' practice and stopped licensing new public health officers—then 12 percent of practitioners—whom physicians viewed as unfair competition. It allowed physicians more time to sue for nonpayment and to collect debts from deceased patients' heirs. Physician unions set fee schedules and negotiated fees with mutual insurers. By 1910, 58 percent of physicians were union members, a higher rate than among manual laborers.[29]

Physician Unions' Struggles with Mutual Aid Societies and Public Insurance

Physicians' unions perceived both the state and private firms as potential threats because they offered medical services that competed with those offered by self-employed physicians and tried to control physician payment. In 1910, one physician lamented, "The employer wants to make the physician a salaried employee. The state wants to turn the physician into a bureaucrat."[30] Physician unions struggled against both.

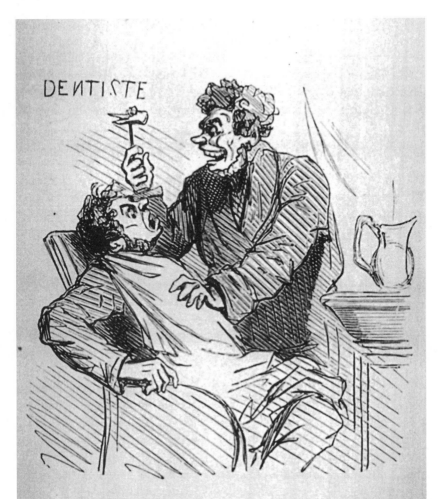

ART. 1110. — L'erreur n'est pas une cause de nullité de la convention.

— Sapristi! je me suis trompé! je vous en ai arraché une bonne, et elle tenait fièrement; mais ça ne fait rien, vous ne payerez pas plus cher que si je vous en avais ôté une mauvaise.

Article 1110—Mistakes are not grounds to nullify the contract. "Darn it! I made a mistake! I pulled out a good one, and it held on fiercely; but it doesn't matter, you won't pay more than if I extracted a rotten tooth."

Artist: Cham [i.e., Amédée Noé]. One of four vignettes from articles of the Civil Code by Cham, this being Art. 1110 U.S. National Library of Medicine, History of Medicine Collection.

Rural patients had often paid physicians at year's end or quarterly. Physician unions insisted on payment at time of service and set fees, which sometimes varied based on five categories of patients' status and income and on three categories of physicians' status and training. They held that physicians who charged less than the fee schedule competed unfairly.[31] Mutual aid societies, however, used their collective purchasing power to bargain over fees and sometimes negotiated contracts with selected practitioners, excluding other physicians from treating their members.

In the early nineteenth century, many physician unions tolerated mutual aid societies employing physicians if patients could choose physicians within the insurance network; they also accepted capitation payment. In Bordeaux, a group of physicians provided services to forty mutual insurers for per capita payments for each member. In Lyon, in 1873, a mutual insurer made per capita payments to a medical society, which apportioned income based on each physician's consultations. Mutual insurers also were accommodating. In 1860, the Société du Faubourg St. Denis allowed patients to use their own physician if they did so from the start and the physician supplied all medical care for a fixed annual fee.[32]

Conflicts between physician unions and mutual aid societies intensified in the mid-nineteenth century. In 1858, the General Association of French Physicians (AGMF) opposed insurers who sought information to verify bills, claiming that they could not divulge medical secrets/confidentiality. Napoléon III supported the AGMF.[33] In Marseille, mutual insurers imposed a fee schedule in 1861 so physicians formed their own insurance plan. When pharmacies did not grant a 35 percent discount, mutual insurers opened a pharmacy that fifty-three mutual insurers used in 1865. In 1900, the USMF said insurers must allow members to choose their physician and not set fees.[34]

During this period, the Radical Party—a coalition that advocated a graduated income tax, social insurance, and the separation of church and state—proposed public support for the poor. In the early 1890s, it backed legislation for state-funded medical care for the rural poor. Parliament endorsed medical assistance rather than food, shelter, or income support, because physician unions backed the legislation as a means to subsidize rural practitioners. Physicians harnessed social solidarity into the service of physician entrepreneurs.

By then, most cities employed physicians in public hospitals, dispensaries, and Bureaus of Good Work. However, in 1888 over half the indigent lived in rural areas without them. Only forty-four of 100 departments assisted the rural poor. Most of them used Alsace's cantonal system, employing one or two physicians to serve the indigent, vaccinate needy children, and perform other public health work.[35]

The initial bill only required local governments that did not supply medical care for the poor to do so. Physician unions secured changes to allow rural local governments to use private practitioners instead of publicly employed physicians and to permit sending patients to public hospitals only if private practitioners could not treat patients outside hospitals. In 1893, Parliament enacted the Law on Free Medical Assistance. Then physician unions lobbied local officials to replace their long-standing cantonal systems with private practitioners chosen by each patient.[36] Physician unions supported similar legislation to fund private practitioners to supply medical services to people with disabilities or incurable diseases in 1905 and to the rural elderly in 1910.

MUTUAL INSURANCE, ORGANIZED MEDICINE, AND THE STATE, WORLD WAR I–WORLD WAR II

Between the two world wars, four competing medical sectors expanded access to medical care: public hospitals, and hospitals owned by mutual insurers, physicians, and employers. Labor unions, employers, and mutual aid associations offered competing proposals for mandatory insurance. Parliament passed mutual insurance legislation in 1928. However, physicians secured amendments in 1930 that promoted private entrepreneurial practice and shielded it from insurer or state oversight. Later, the state created the Order of Physicians, which set rules for medical practice and markets.

Before World War I, physicians had treated paying patients at home and public hospitals treated the poor. Advances in aseptic practice and improvements in medical technology made it preferable to perform surgery in hospitals, so during the war a few surgeons and obstetricians started private hospitals, referred to as clinics, to support their practice. They allowed other physicians to treat patients there and earned income from hospital services. Some entrepreneurial physicians combined hospitals with resorts that offered spas and thermal baths, especially in the Mediterranean region. They frequently split fees with physicians who referred patients.

Clinical laboratories also emerged during this time, with tests for tuberculosis and syphilis. Some physicians performed tests or owned laboratories. Hospitals, pharmacists, and firms also supplied tests, competing with physicians.

The growth of medical commerce and physicians' conflicts of interest inspired Jules Romains' 1925 satirical play, *Knock: The Triumph of Medicine*.[37] Dr. Parpalaid has a fledgling practice in a town where patients pay physicians seasonally or annually. He dupes Dr. Knock, an inexperienced physician,

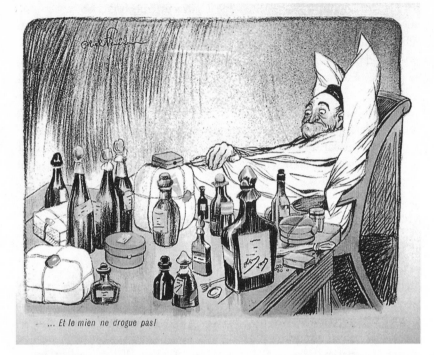

... Et le mien ne drogue pas!

**L'assiette au beure: Les Médecins, 51. ". . . and mine doesn't drug me!" says an
elderly invalid in a chair next to a table filled with pills and potions.**
  *Artist: Abel Faivre, 1867–1945. Publication: 22 Mars 1902. U.S. Library of Medicine,
History of Medicine Collection.*

into purchasing his medical practice and patient list for a high price. Return-
ing less than three months later, Dr. Parpalaid is startled at how Knock
changed his practice. Rather than bill seasonally, Dr. Knock charges fee-for-
service. Knock pays kickbacks to the pharmacist and others to refer patients
to him and to tell patients that they agree with his diagnosis. He gives free
consultations to generate business and enlists the help of teachers and
others to *educate* the public about health problems. In this way, Dr. Knock
has turned almost everyone into a patient who needs constant attention and
transformed the local hotel into his infirmary to treat them. Dr. Parpalaid
also falls under Knock's spell and seeks medical treatment. Dr. Knock then
reveals his visions of a brave new world in which everyone becomes a patient.

   After the Great War, local public hospitals were insolvent, so to raise
funds, Parliament allowed them to serve "half-paying patients," individuals
who could not pay the full cost but were not indigent. These included the
working class and pensioners. Later, public hospitals added maternity wards
and other services to attract the middle class.[38] As public hospitals treated

more paying patients, they competed with physician-owned hospitals. Still, patients with means perceived public hospitals as old and unsanitary and preferred private hospitals. In 1941, the Vichy régime opened public hospitals to all citizens.[39]

The expansion of mutual aid societies increased the number of paying patients for physician-owned hospitals. However, these societies sometimes built their own hospitals, which competed with self-employed physicians. The FNMF established its first hospital in 1909 and four others between 1930 and 1935.[40] Typically, they employed physicians, but some used self-employed physicians. Mutual aid societies also contracted with public hospitals to treat their patients. Some large employers built medical facilities for their employees. Physician unions usually opposed employer provision of medical care.[41]

Solidarity and Mutual Insurance

Léon Bourgeois had championed social solidarity, linking *solidarism* to mutual aid. He transformed mutual insurance from a mode of individual prudence and responsibility into a means of fulfilling the Revolution's promise of fraternity. The Radical Party formally adopted this idea in its 1908 platform, after it joined the ruling coalition.[42]

After the Great War, in the name of solidarity, Parliament awarded over three million wounded veterans pensions and medical care. However, physician unions objected that the public insurance required private practitioners to treat veterans for state-set fees and restricted patients' choice of physician. The USMF went on strike, forcing the state to raise fees.[43]

Solidarism also shaped policy as France reintegrated Alsace and Lorraine, which had been under German rule since 1871 and had social insurance initiated by Chancellor Otto Von Bismarck. The government could have allowed these provinces to keep social insurance, which the rest of the country lacked, or ended their social insurance. But by then, social insurance seemed more acceptable than the alternatives proposed by socialist and communist parties. So Parliament invoked social solidarity and extended mutual insurance to all of France's industrial employees.[44]

The French debated the terms for social insurance until 1930. Labor unions and the communist and socialist parties wanted independent unions to control insurance. Employers wanted pension and medical benefits to promote employee loyalty and forestall unionization. They argued that employers who contributed money should control insurance. Others preferred state-sponsored, publicly administered insurance.[45]

In 1923, Édouard Grinda proposed the compromise that Parliament passed in 1928: state-organized social insurance for employees in industry and commerce whose incomes were below a specified level. Funded by obligatory contributions, mutual insurance could be managed by mutual aid associations, labor unions, or employers. Mutual health insurance, however, took effect only after amendments in 1930. Initially it covered one-third of salaried workers and by 1939 more than half the population.[46] It served as the model for the social security statute enacted after World War II that created NHI.

Organized Medicine's Charter

As Parliament considered proposals for mutual insurance, most physicians supported it under certain conditions. There were two main camps. The largest union, the USMF, argued that every physician union should negotiate its own arrangement with mutual insurers and even be able to accept alternatives to fee-for-service payment. A small union led by Paul Cibrié wanted each physician to individually set his or her fees. It insisted that patients pay physicians directly and then be reimbursed by insurers, calling this arrangement a *direct relationship*. Conflict between these two camps precipitated a schism in 1927 and the creation of a new union, the Confederation of French Medical Unions (CSMF). It became the dominant union and enshrined its views in a Medical Charter *(Charte de la Médicine Libérale)* that included seven principles.[47]

- Patients must have free choice of physicians.
- All parties must respect professional secrecy/ confidentiality.
- Physicians have a right to receive "honoraria" for all patients treated.
- Patients must have a direct relationship with physicians; namely, patients must pay physicians directly using union fee schedules as a minimum payment.
- Physicians must be free to choose therapies and prescribe medicine and treatment.
- The medical profession regulates the conduct of its members.
- Physician unions must be represented on insurance fund commissions.

The demand for a direct relationship was new, unlike the other provisions. It precluded insurers from being intermediaries between physicians and patients. Later, ethical and legal codes incorporated these principles, but restated the direct relationship principle as two separate points: physicians must set their fees without intervention by insurers; and patients must pay physicians directly.

The 1928 mutual insurance law did not conform to the Medical Charter. Physician unions threatened a boycott. In 1929, CSMF president Paul Cibrié explained to the minister of labor why he insisted on a direct physician-patient relationship. Insurers, he warned, will "want to impose allowable charges and third-party payments. . . . We have great difficulty identifying an impartial institution capable of arbitrating between the opposing positions of the medical profession and . . . insurance funds."[48]

Parliament amended the law to meet physician union demands in 1930. It required patients to pay physicians directly. Insurers could not set fees, restrict choice of physicians, or set up medical facilities that employed physicians without approval of local physician unions. In the name of protecting medical secrets/confidentiality, billing codes did not specify what services physicians performed or the patients' diagnosis, so insurers could not monitor physicians practice.[49]

Physician unions and mutual insurers continued their struggle after the law's enactment. The law anticipated that insurers and unions would reach fee accords, or that insurers would set their fee schedule giving due regard to the local physician union's fee scale. However, writing in 1937, American economist Alvin Millis explained that "some . . . physicians increased their charges . . . owing to the greater capacity of the insured to pay medical bills. Greater disparities appeared between the doctors' scales and the fund scales adopted for . . . reimbursement for medical bills."[50]

In theory, insurers could fine or exclude physicians for inappropriate medical care or fraud, but physicians claimed that patient secrecy precluded their reporting any information regarding their diagnosis or services.[51] So insurers hired physicians to examine and test patients in order to determine whether medical bills and certifications of incapacity were correct. This cumbersome oversight was ineffective. Isadore Falk's 1936 study noted that mutual insurance sickness funds "engaged on a large scale in checking the work of the individual private practitioners . . . [and] led to the most extensive system of supervision. . . . In Paris . . . about 50 percent of the cases are investigated, and in about 60 percent of these, the patient is examined by . . . physicians of the [mutual insurers]."[52]

To counter overuse of services, some mutual insurers opened their own hospitals and dispensaries or steered members to affiliated pharmacies and physicians. Angry physician unions insisted that this violated the Medical Charter. In a 1932 report to the Ministry of Health (MH), Romain Lavielle, a mutual insurance leader, said that surgeons formed their own mutual insurance societies and routinely split fees with referring physicians and that the practice sometimes spread to traditional mutual insurers.[53]

In 1937, a mutual aid society–owned hospital, Pavillon Bordelais de la Mutualité, hired four physicians to work in its dispensary. A medical society expelled one physician, claiming that physician employment was illegal since it interfered with the patients' right to choose their physician.[54] The physician and insurer argued that the physician association could not terminate the physician's right to practice. A court held that patients did have a free choice of physicians because membership in the mutual insurance society was voluntary. Nonetheless, it fined the union only a symbolic single franc.

From Medical Charter to Medical Deontology

Today, the French term *liberal professions* is equivalent to the English *free professions* and refers to self-employed professionals in contrast to *professions of office*, those employed by the state as civil servants.[55] The term *liberal medicine* refers to private practitioners as opposed to publicly employed hospital physicians. However, *liberal medicine* also invokes the doctrines of the Medical Charter, which became organized medicine's creed and was enshrined in ethical principles and law. This transformation reveals the close connection between physician unions and the other major organ of organized medicine created in 1940, the Order of Physicians.

Physicians had long suggested the creation of an institution for professional ethics and discipline, following the legal profession, which had created an Order of Attorneys in 1810.[56] 1929, the CSMF and Action Française, an extreme right-wing, anti-republican group, proposed the creation of a medical order to license and discipline physicians. In 1932, the government introduced a bill to create an Order of Physicians. In 1934, the Senate and Chamber of Deputies each passed bills but they were not reconciled.[57]

Meanwhile, the Academy of Medicine had adopted ethical rules in 1929, but physician unions never put them into effect. Instead, the CSMF drew on the Medical Charter as the starting point for its 1936 Rules of Medical Deontology and used these in its *family councils* that resolved patient complaints against physicians and disputes between physicians.[58] The term *deontology* refers to general principles to guide action. However, in France today most professions have codes of deontology that have the force of law, so deontology also means authoritative rules used to regulate conduct.

After Germany occupied France in 1940, the state suppressed physician and other unions. Provider group representation fit with the Vichy régime's corporatist philosophy, so it established the Order of Physicians to represent and govern physicians and appointed its officers. The Order of Physicians developed a Code of Medical Deontology based on the CSMF's 1936 Rules of Medical Deontology, incorporating the 1927 Medical Charter. Medical Deontology included key physician union policies, namely, that physicians should not discount fees for the state or mutual insurers. It also prohibited kickbacks, fee splitting, commissions, and other financial ties. The Order of Physicians used Medical Deontology to oversee private practice and discipline physicians.

LIBERAL MEDICINE UNDER NATIONAL HEALTH INSURANCE, 1944–1970

After the liberation of France in 1944, the transitional military authority legalized physician unions, reconstituted the Order of Physicians as a democratic organization, and affirmed the Vichy régime's opening public hospitals to all citizens, since it was consistent with social solidarity.[59] As France emerged from the war, the government promulgated a social security ordinance and planned for NHI.[60]

The postwar medical system continued existing institutions and payment arrangements with increased coverage. When NHI began, mutual insurers covered agricultural workers, sold supplemental insurance, and operated hospitals, but national health insurance funds (NHI funds) assumed most functions previously performed by mutual insurers. However, public authorities, mutual insurers, and physicians struggled over who would control the terms of medical practice. Organized medicine opposed state and insurer oversight of private practice and alternatives to it.[61]

Medical Deontology as a Means of Professional Control

The government promulgated a revised Code of Medical Deontology by decree in 1945 that highlighted key provisions of the Medical Charter under the heading *general principles*. Since then, the Order of Physicians has revised Medical Deontology seven times. It submits its draft to the MH, which can negotiate over the final text. When they reach agreement, the MH submits the text to the Council of State, which can modify it if it does not conform to legislation or legal principles that take precedence. Then the government issues a decree making the code an administrative regulation.[62]

The Order of Physicians writes and interprets Medical Deontology, which the legislature cannot amend.[63] Courts have the final word in interpreting Medical Deontology and review disciplinary decisions for legal errors when physicians appeal. However, neither French nor European antitrust law curbs the Order of Physicians' authority over medical markets. In 1993, the European Court of Justice (ECJ) held that the Treaty of Rome—adopted to reduce national competitive barriers within the European Community (EC)—allows deontological codes that restrict competition.[64]

Medical Deontology exempts physicians from oversight by third parties and affects patients, other professionals, and the public. Its rules govern insurers, hospitals, and patients in relations with physicians in both the public and private sectors. Courts invoke Medical Deontology to resolve disputes between physicians and others.[65] Furthermore, the Order of Physicians uses Medical Deontology to regulate medical practice. It reviews all proposed physician contracts except those negotiated with NHI funds, and advises physicians as to whether they comply. It can suspend or revoke medical licenses when a physician violates Medical Deontology or social norms, or is drug or alcohol impaired.

Struggles to Shape Medical Practice under NHI

After the war, the National Federation of French Mutual Insurers (FNMF) sought to expand its hospitals, but the Order of Physicians, soon dominated by physician union activists, blocked it by sanctioning FNMF physicians.[66] Initially, the Order charged that the FNMF violated Medical Deontology by depriving patients of physician choice because only FNMF physicians treated patients. In 1947, the Council of State held that since patients voluntarily subscribed to the FNMF's supplemental insurance, the FNMF did not interfere with their choice. It added that Medical Deontology states that the normal functioning of social insurance takes precedence over liberal medicine when the two conflict.[67] In later cases, the Order of Physicians alleged that being an employee precludes independent physician judgment, which Medical Deontology requires. The Council of State overturned that ruling in 1949, explaining that the law sanctions employers who interfere with physicians' clinical choices.[68]

The Order of Physicians continued to sanction employed physicians. It lodged three distinct charges. First, salary interfered with direct patient-physician relations. Second, salary payment constituted fee splitting because physicians did not receive all patient fees. Third, salary was incompatible with fee-for-service payment rates established by NHI accords with physician unions. In appeals from 1950 to 1954, the Council of State found these charges lacked merit and ordered the Order of Physicians to pay the FNMF damages for persistent interference in violation of its rulings.[69]

Even then, the Order of Physicians did not approve mutual insurance employment contracts, which Medical Deontology required physicians to obtain. Until 1956 it ignored the FNMF's request for model contracts that did not require individual approval. It also sought legislation to restrict mutual insurers from supplying services. Since then, not-for-profit hospitals have been able to employ physicians, although the Order of Physicians' continued opposition stunted their growth.

Meanwhile, about sixty for-profit hospitals per year were started between 1945 and 1962. Most were physician owned.[70] Many physicians worked half-time in public hospitals, which paid poorly, and half-time in private hospitals. They used their public position to become better known and to recruit patients for their private practice.

Organized medicine frustrated the efforts of the state and NHI funds to control spending. Initially, local trade unions and employers controlled the

NHI funds, which negotiated fee accords with local physicians' unions. As with the 1930 mutual insurance law, NHI indemnified expenses up to 80 percent of its fee schedule, but physicians set their own fees. Many physicians accepted the NHI fee schedules, but elite physicians and specialists, particularly in Paris and on the Côte d'Azur, charged more. Patients paid expenses not reimbursed by NHI, sometimes with supplemental insurance.

In 1952, the National Federation of Social Security Organizations (FNOSS) sought to have the government set fees, or sign contracts with individual physicians in departments where physician unions and NHI funds reached no accord. It also tried to create NHI fund diagnostic and treatment centers as an alternative to physician-owned facilities. Both efforts failed. In 1956, Albert Gazier, the minister of social affairs, tried to get physician unions to agree to a national fee schedule and to permit only 15 percent of physicians to charge more. That effort also failed, and the stalemate between organized medicine and the state continued.

In 1958, France founded the Fifth Republic with a constitution that granted its president, Charles de Gaulle, strong enough executive powers to break political deadlocks. Health policy changed rapidly thereafter. Prime Minister Michel Debré made public hospital employment a full-time career and started to expand and modernize public hospitals. In 1960, President de Gaulle implemented Gazier's 1956 plan by decree. In the absence of an accord between the physician unions and NHI funds, individual physicians could accept the government fee schedule, and their patients would receive higher reimbursement than other patients would. Initially, the CSMF resisted, contending that "medical fees will become an affair of the state, and . . . [physicians] will . . . cease . . . to be a liberal profession."[71] Eventually it accepted a negotiated fee schedule that capped physician payment. Dissident physicians formed a separate union, but by 1964, 80 percent of physicians accepted NHI fee schedules.

Henri Hatzfeld titled his 1963 history of the conflict between the physician unions and NHI *The Great Turnaround of French Liberal Medicine* (*Le Grand Tournant de la Médecine Libérale*), which suggests that organized physicians were turned away from liberal medicine.[72] However, although unions accept fee schedules, they still lobby and strike to raise fees. Since 1963, the state has allowed some physicians to charge more than the fee schedule, and today other physicians do so without permission.[73] Physician unions still champion other aspects of the Medical Charter: they resist insurer and state oversight and alternatives to physician-owned practice.

In 1967, Parliament reorganized the NHI to promote fiscal control over social democracy. National NHI funds gained control over local affiliates. The NHI Fund for Salaried Workers then covered 80 percent of the population and became the dominant payer and a countervailing power to physician unions, which feared that it would start medical centers, employ physicians, and compete with private practitioners.[74]

COMPROMISE AND CONSOLIDATION, 1970–1995

In 1971, the NHI Fund for Salaried Workers (CNAMTS), the Ministry of Health, and key physician unions forged a historic compromise. Physician unions agreed to negotiate national fee schedules with CNAMTS and allow only one and a half percent of physicians to charge more. In return, CNAMTS promised to pay physicians fee-for-service, to respect the Medical Charter, and not to operate or subsidize medical or diagnostic centers without permission of departmental unions. The MH introduced legislation that amended the Social Security Code by including "fundamental principles of medical deontology" drawn from the Medical Charter: direct patient payment to physicians, no limits on physician prescribing or practice or on patients' choice of physicians, and medical secrecy.[75] The agreement protected private practitioners from competition or oversight from CNAMTS and thereby reinforced their entrepreneurial and payment conflicts of interest.

Since then, physician unions and NHI funds have regularly negotiated accords on fees and other matters. Starting with the 1980 accords, physicians could choose to practice in sector II, where they can set their own fees if done with "tact and moderation" as Medical Deontology requires; they are typically 50 percent higher than the schedule. Patients are responsible for paying the balance not reimbursed by NHI. The proportion of physicians in sector II grew from 7.5 percent in 1980 to 30 percent in 1990, but fell to 24 percent by 2003 due to government restrictions.[76]

Nevertheless, NHI funds and the state clamped down on physician entrepreneurship. Social security and public health legislation in 1975 precluded NHI from paying for laboratory and diagnostic tests performed by physicians or in physician-owned facilities. Physicians are not paid for dispensing drugs or vaccines. Other legislation prohibited physicians from owning or having other financial ties to pharmacies or clinical and diagnostic laboratories. Today, independent centers perform nearly all tests.[77] Physicians can own facilities that provide diagnostic imaging, but very few physicians do because planning agencies limit permits. Hospitals and radiologists own most capital-intensive diagnostic imaging equipment.

After these reforms, private hospitals were the main area for physician entrepreneurship. However, that sector has also changed. Starting around 1970, hospital planning agencies regulated expansion of for-profit hospitals. Ironically, restricting growth boosted the economic value of existing facilities. Capped licenses granted existing hospitals a limited opportunity to generate income. Physician owners could practice with little competition or sell their hospitals to lay investors.

As founders of small physician-owned hospitals retired, hospitals needed new capital to refurbish aging facilities. Many small hospitals merged. Others were purchased by lay-owned firms, privately held insurance companies, and publicly traded corporations. Investors started Parly 2, the first private multicenter hospital chain, in 1970.[78] In the 1980s, other hospital chains grew and then consolidated. Between 1988 and 1996, 292 hospitals merged. However, in 1992, legislation virtually stopped new private hospitals, and licensing disallowed purchasing of capital-intensive imaging equipment without approval. The state began to absorb most not-for-profit hospitals into the publicly funded hospital system around 1970, but granted them administrative autonomy.

At the turn of the twenty-first century, for-profit hospitals included three broad categories. Slightly more than a dozen were high-tech hospitals with over 250 beds, most of which were part of investor-owned, multihospital firms. The main investor-owned firms in 2009 were Générale de Santé, VITALIA, and Capio; other chains included Vedici and Medipartenaire. The second, and by far the largest, category was comprised of general service facilities with between 150 and 180 beds, usually owned by physician groups. Third, individual physicians or their families owned numerous older hospitals; typically, they focused on the physician's specialty. About 80 percent of for-profit hospitals were at least partly physician-owned as of 1996. For-profit hospitals handle about 20 percent of all hospitalizations and perform nearly half of all minor surgery. They own between 30 percent and 40 percent of expensive imaging equipment.[79]

REFORMS, 1995–2010

Conflicts of interest led private practitioners to supply more services than beneficial and to prescribe and supply inappropriate service. Since 1995, the state and NHI funds have tried to oversee private practice to control spending and improve medical care. Organized medicine maintained that these efforts undermine principles of the Medical Charter.

The Juppé Plan

In 1995, Prime Minister Alain Juppé initiated major health reforms, but implementation stopped when his party lost the 1997 election. Nevertheless, his plan influenced future reform efforts. Its major features were (1) caps on spending for private practitioners; (2) compulsory practice guidelines

(3) reform of hospital payment; (4) an agency to accredit hospitals and evaluate medical therapies; and (5) experiments with provider networks.[80]

The 1997 social security finance law created goals to control spending on physician services. If spending exceeded the budget, the law reduced physician fees retrospectively, or for the next year. Physician unions sued and courts overturned several versions of budget caps. In 1998, the Council of State refused to enforce the spending caps agreed to by the CNAMTS and specialists because only one small union signed the accord. In addition, the Constitutional Council struck down CNAMTS's accord with general practitioners because it reduced fees based on regional norms rather than on each physician's conduct. In 1999, the Constitutional Council struck down similar caps because they reduced fees the following year when services were not overused.

In 2000, the social security finance law adjusted fees as much as 20 percent based on the level of spending. But the government did not implement it and in 2002, rather than cutting spending, NHI cut benefits. In 2003, the law raised fees despite the fact that expenditures for physician services had exceeded spending goals in 2002. Indeed, expenditures have exceeded goals every year since 1997. In 2000, Parliament began to use the previous year's spending as a baseline in setting new spending goals.[81]

The Juppé plan proposed sanctions for physicians who failed to follow compulsory practice guidelines. Although the guidelines specified only dangerous practices to avoid, physician unions sued, arguing that the Medical Charter precludes any interference with clinical decisions. In 1999, the Council of State struck down the fines, holding they were disproportionate and applied collectively rather than to individual violators.

In 1996, the MH created committees to determine whether physicians who prescribe much more than usual drugs lack justification and if NHI should stop payment. Physician unions refused to participate on the committees, and the government terminated them in 2003. In 2000, CSMF lobbying blocked a bill that would have sanctioned individual physicians for abusive medical practices. It opposed similar provisions in the proposed 2002 social security finance law, arguing that NHI funds lack this authority.

In 1991, the government began reforms to rationalize hospital reimbursement, create payment parity between public and private hospitals, and facilitate management. The government had funded public hospitals with annual budgets since 1983. National health insurance funds had paid private hospitals a per diem for boarding and nursing expenses, fixed amounts for supplies and drugs, and fees for surgical suites. To initiate the reform, the government developed a medical information system to track the services used for patients with specific illnesses. From 1996 through 2007, all hospitals reported data used to calculate relative resource use by type of service, employing a point system. In 2002, the government paid fixed fees per patient based on their diagnoses in sixty public hospitals. This step set the stage for using the new payment method to pay both public and private hospitals, called T2A payment.[82] By 2009, the government reimbursed about 11 percent of public hospital expenditures by T2A payment.[83] It plans to pay all hospitals by T2A by 2012. Public hospitals that perform public functions (medical education, research, and public health work) will receive supplemental grants; so will hospitals that provide emergency care or organ transplants.

Previously, public hospitals complained that fixed budgets did not reward them for increasing services and private hospitals claimed their payment was inadequate. Both public and private hospitals support payment reforms and payment parity in principle. However, public hospitals worry that the government may not adequately compensate them to perform public functions, while private hospitals fear that the government may unfairly subsidize public hospitals with such payments.

State-Led Managed Care

Health policy scholars Victor Rodwin and Claude Le Pen characterize recent reforms as state-led managed care, by which they mean the coordination and finance of medical practice to control spending and promote effective treatment. The reforms draw on practices developed in the United States, including physician gatekeepers who coordinate care, provider networks, incentives to control spending, and utilization review. Such reforms had been discussed since the 1980s and policy makers attempted to implement some of them.[84] So far, though, organized medicine has blocked incentives for physicians to follow practice guidelines, and providers have lacked incentives to coordinate activities or take full responsibility for their patients.

The 2004 Health Insurance Reform Act encourages all patients to choose a treating physician, called the *médecin traitant*, who coordinates their care and acts as a gatekeeper to specialists. This reform is based on an earlier experiment called the *médecin referent*. Only one physician union, MG France, took part in the earlier experiment, which required a yearly contract between the patient, doctor, and CNAMT. Patients had an incentive to participate because they paid lower co-payment but in return had to consult their coordinating physician before accessing a specialist. The coordinating physician had to create medical records to follow their patients, participate in continuing medical education organized by social security, and in return, received additional payment.

In contrast, the *médecin traitant* system that replaced the *médecin referent* does not require a commitment between the patient and doctor to work together. Patients consult their coordinating physician to avoid paying higher specialist fees and higher copayments.[85] Coordinating doctors serve as gatekeepers, but if patients do not like their advice they can choose a new doctor to act as the *médecin traitant* which encourages doctors to allow all referrals that patients request. *Médecins traitant* receive a fixed yearly payment for care of chronic care patients but not more income for coordinating routine patient care. It is not clear how many patients will obtain referrals from their treating physician since they are used to consulting specialists directly, and 86 percent have supplemental insurance, which often covers copayments. The 2004 law grants insurers certain benefits if they offer policies that do not reimburse all copayments. Mutual insurers approve of physician gatekeepers. For-profit insurers do not, and they may market insurance that covers the additional copayments.[86]

In 2004, the government also reformed physician billing. Previously, due to physician union demands, bills did not specify what services patients received or their diagnosis, and included only twenty-eight categories of service combined with coefficients to indicate the fee. For example, consultations with a general practitioner and specialist were coded C and CS, respectively. Surgery was coded K or KC. Since 2004, bills use the newly created Common Classification of Medical Procedures, which assigns a unique code for 7,200 services. National health insurance funds assign fees for each billing code using a resource-based relative value scale. The new billing system makes detailed utilization review possible. Physicians will eventually have to record information in electronic medical records to receive payment. In the future, bills will also indicate the patient's diagnosis.

From 1997 until 2004, the National Agency for Accreditation and Evaluation of Health assessed the effectiveness of medical treatments, but its conclusions did not affect reimbursement. The 2004 health insurance reforms replaced it with a High Authority on Health (HAS) that evaluates the efficacy of medical procedures, drugs, and devices and creates practice guidelines. The law authorizes NHI funds to exclude coverage of services the HAS deems ineffective.

In the future, supplemental insurers might manage some medical care, reclaiming a role they performed in the past.[87] Juppé suggested allowing NHI to fund local provider networks and coordinate reimbursement. When the universal insurance law of 2000 financed supplemental insurance for the poor, the FNMF offered to do so using a limited provider network, but its proposal was not adopted. In 2002, however, legislation made funding available for experiments with provider networks.

In 2009, President Nicolas Sarkozy ushered through Parliament the law on Hospitals, Patients, Health and Regions that increase centralized state control. The law transformed hospital planning agencies into regional health agencies with greater power over hospitals and new authority over ambulatory care. Individual public hospital administrators lost their administrative autonomy and hospitals will be subject to increased internal controls and supervisions by the MH through regional health agencies. The law also authorizes regional health agencies to oversee private hospitals and when necessary, even control their contracts with private practitioners.[88]

At the same time, the law includes provisions that could promote liberalization of the medical economy. It uses subsidies to promote the growth of multidisciplinary private practices and coordinated networks that include physicians, pharmacists, and nurses. For self-employed practitioners willing to work in groups and meet certain conditions, the Ministry of Health will supply office space, equipment, and administrative personnel for office management. The MH will give highest priority for funding practices in areas where there is a need for more primary care providers. The implementing rules, not yet issued, will define how these new medical centers will operate. For the moment, practitioners will still be paid fee-for-service, but there might be new financial incentives that could affect their referrals and prescribing. The law anticipates an expanded role for pharmacists in educating patients, renewing prescriptions, and perhaps even prescribing certain drugs. As a result, this reform might introduce new entrepreneurial conflicts of interest for physicians and allied health professionals.[89]

EMERGING ISSUES: SUPPLEMENTAL INSURANCE, MARKETS, AND THE EUROPEAN COMMUNITY

Changes in supplemental insurance might also promote markets. Currently, NHI pays for 73 percent of medical spending; supplemental insurers cover another 12 percent, and patients pay the remaining 15 percent. About 92 percent of the population has supplemental insurance.[90] Some market proponents support universal publicly funded coverage for *basic* medical benefits but want individuals to finance other services themselves without subsidies, either by purchasing private supplemental insurance or paying out of pocket. A 2003 report commissioned by the MH, conducted by Jean-François Chadelat, a senior civil servant with expertise in insurance, proposed changing supplemental insurance in line with this view.

The Chadelat report proposed dividing supplemental insurance into two parts. The first would cover basic services, and the state would fund insurance for those with low incomes. Providers that offered services covered by basic supplemental insurance could not *balance bill* (i.e., charge more than the NHI reimbursement rate) low-income individuals, but they could balance bill all others. The second part would cover optional services. The state would not subsidize this optional supplemental insurance; insurers would choose which services to cover and set their premiums.[91] If in the future the state adopts this model, NHI funds could limit their financial responsibility by shifting services they now cover to optional private supplemental insurance paid by patients. That would move France toward tiered coverage and a more market-oriented system, which clashes with its ethos of social solidarity.[92]

European law affects medical care even though medical policy is in principle beyond the prerogative of the EC.[93] For example, France exempted mutual insurers from a 7 percent premium tax because they promoted social solidarity. However, EC law requires that governments treat all insurers the same way. The French Federation of Insurers challenged France's differential taxation in the ECJ, which in 2002 held that for-profit insurers that do not use medical status or risk to exclude individuals or charge different premiums must receive the same tax exemption.[94]

In addition, the ECJ held that NHI must reimburse individuals when they receive medical treatment in the EC outside their country of affiliation. Providers of goods and services can also cross national borders, which will influence the production and distribution of medical services. European integration is likely to create pressures for controlling social benefits and health spending while encouraging patient cost-sharing and the introduction of financial incentives in medical facilities.[95]

3

Coping with Physicians' Conflicts of Interest in France

As we have seen, during the French Revolution, the state assumed the Catholic Church's moral authority and charitable functions and enshrined the idea of the common good in secular public law.[1] It also replaced occupational guilds and corporations with state supervision of public professions and private occupational groups.[2] Today, the state attempts to regulate individual pursuit of private interests that conflict with its conception of the public interest. This approach shapes French ideas about conflicts of interest and the state's response.

THE STATE ROLE IN PUBLIC, FOR-PROFIT AND NOT-FOR-PROFIT MEDICAL PRACTICE

Yves Mény, a French scholar who writes about corruption, points to French public figures holding several offices as evidence that the Anglo-Saxon idea of conflict of interest has not fully developed in France.[3] Nevertheless, France first developed conflict of interest rules to prevent public servants (and private actors serving public functions) from using their power or position to further their private interests or those of other parties. Ideas about conflicts of interest for private actors developed later, often as a result of the importation of conflict of interest rules from Anglo-American law.

The state serves the public interest in medicine by operating public hospitals that employ physicians. It thereby increases access to medical care, controls medical costs and quality, and eliminates many conflicts of interest that arise from physician entrepreneurialism, fee-for-service payment, and ties between physicians and third parties. The state also organizes public medical schools, funds medical research, and licenses physicians. National health insurance (NHI) ensures access to medical care but does not preclude conflicts of interest that arise in private practice. To address these conflicts, the state oversees and limits the scope of physician entrepreneurship much more than do the United States or Japan. At the same time, the state gave a role to NHI insurance funds (NHI funds) in overseeing private practice and to the Order of Physicians in professional self-regulation.

Creating and Overseeing the Public Medical Sector

After World War II, the state expanded public hospitals and made them centers for research and innovation. Prime Minister Michel Debré's 1958 reforms ended the practice of physicians working half-time as public hospital employees and half-time as self-employed practitioners in private hospitals. Since then, physicians in public hospitals have been paid a salary set by rank and are eligible for tenure. They lack conflicts of interest arising from physician entrepreneurship, fee-for-service payment, and indirect incentives to control costs or further management goals. Medical school faculty members are also public employees paid a salary set by rank. Rules restrict certain outside paid activities that conflict with their employment.[4]

However, to retain prominent physicians who might otherwise choose private practice to earn more, the Debré reforms allowed chiefs of medical service to devote two half-days a week to private consultations and to reserve 8 percent of hospital beds for their use. Physicians could charge patients seeking private consultations sector II fees, which are typically about 50 percent more than the NHI fee schedule. In return, physicians received a 20 percent lower salary and paid the hospital a user fee for services the hospital supplied for their private work. In 1987, the Ministry of Health (MH) set user fees as a percentage of the physician's fee, ranging from 15 percent for office visits to 60 percent for certain surgeries.[5]

Private consultations created conflicts of interest arising from fee-for-service payment and led physicians to favor private over public patients. Some physicians promoted their private practice at the public's expense. They instructed receptionists to tell patients that they could choose a particular physician only by obtaining a private consultation, or had receptionists schedule private consultations immediately and make public patients wait longer for appointments. Reserved beds created bottlenecks. An investigation by the government oversight agency qua court, the Council of Accounts, confirmed that many hospital physicians exceeded the legal limits on private consultations.

In 1989, under Socialist president François Mitterrand, legislation ended reserved private beds and began to phase out private consultations.[6] To ensure that physicians did not underpay user fees or engage in too many private consultations, patients seeking private consultations were supposed to pay the hospital, which would subtract their user fee and then pay the physician. But administrators never strictly enforced that rule.

When the center right party won the election in 1995 and Jacques Chirac became president, he continued the ban on reserved beds but introduced legislation to allow *all* physicians two half-days for private consultations or other remunerated work in return for a 20 percent lower salary. The government did not issue rules to implement the requirement that patients pay hospitals until 2001, and in 2002 the new center-right government repealed them. Since then, administrators have accepted physicians' reports on their income and time spent.[7] Hospital administrators guesstimate that 90 percent of physicians bill private patients directly, which precludes oversight.

Most not-for-profit hospitals voluntarily joined the publicly funded hospital system after 1970. They are subject to rules different from those that govern public hospitals. Their physicians cannot engage in private consultations and so lack conflicts of interest arising from fee-for-service payment. However, they are not eligible for tenure and have yearly contracts.[8] In theory, hospital managers can choose not to renew a physician's contract. Not-for-profit hospital managers typically need to control spending on pharmacy, diagnostic tests, and other resources to stay within their budgets. Therefore, these physicians have indirect incentives to cut resource use, a conflict of interest.

In practice, these indirect incentives for physicians to cut services do not change clinical behavior, because several policies limit their effect. French employees have strong job protection, and employers pay high unemployment insurance charges if they terminate an employee. Furthermore, not-for-profit hospitals can cut costs without skimping on services to individual patients; they can close a medical service near the year's end, treat fewer patients, or refer patients to private or public hospitals. Moreover, the Code of Medical Deontology (Medical Deontology) prohibits direct financial incentives based on physicians' clinical choices or productivity.[9]

Physician Experts Serving on Government Commissions

French law distinguishes the duties of public officials or agencies involved in government purchasing and planning from the interests of private actors. Rules often require that public employees have no conflicts of interest.[10]

The state has also attempted to address the conflicts of interest of physicians who influence policy by serving on government commissions and advisory boards. Statutes regulate publicly employed physicians and employees of the Drug and Medical Product Safety Agency (AFSSAPS) and the agency that sets insurance reimbursement for drugs. Other rules oversee individuals who serve on government commissions or as experts for the government, such as medical school faculty who may also have consulted for pharmaceutical firms.[11]

The Drug and Medical Product Safety Agency's predecessor, the Medication Agency, developed conflict of interest policies for experts in 1983. Decrees then precluded individuals serving as experts when they have a personal interest in the issue.[12] In 1994, AFSSAPS required all experts serving on advisory panels to disclose their financial ties to firms that sell products regulated by the agency. But AFSSAPS rarely requires experts with conflicts of interest to recuse themselves.[13] In commenting on these policies, the peer review journal *Prescrire* (which accepts no commercial funds or advertisements) published a cartoon in which the protagonist says "Conflict disclosed, conflict disposed."[14] This succinctly summarizes the problem of relying on disclosure of financial ties rather than eliminating them or creating some means of effective oversight.

A 2004 evaluation of how government agencies oversee experts' conflicts of interest highlighted a key problem.[15] AFSSAPS relies on physicians who consult for pharmaceutical firms to serve as experts without compensation. They are unlikely to forego consulting income in order to perform public service. Agencies have little leverage over experts who fail to disclose their financial interests. In addition, AFSSAPS has not developed its own independent expertise. The report recommends that France secure independent experts by paying competitive fees, as Finland does.

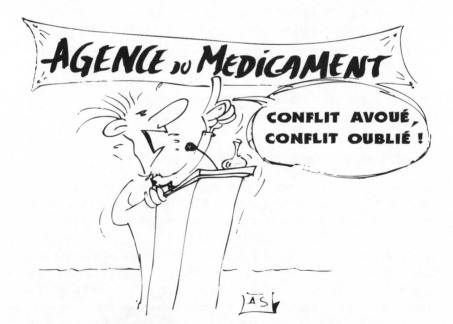

"Conflict Disclosed, Conflict Disposed! Or Conflict Confessed, Conflict Forgotten!"

Artist: Alain Savino. Source: La Revue Prescrir 16, no. 168 (1996): 891.

The activities of the High Authority on Health (HAS) highlight problems that occur when agencies delegate decision making to conflicted physicians. HAS guidelines are used to determine best practices and check medical practices that are distorted by conflicts of interest. The guidelines are used by NHI to determine whether to reimburse drugs and therapies and by others to teach medical students, for continuing medical education (CME), and for quality improvement programs. Yet some HAS guidelines are compromised by conflicts of interest, according to *Formindep*, a physician organization that advocates eliminating financial ties between pharma and practicing physicians.

In 2009, it asked the Council of State to enjoin HAS from issuing guidelines that don't comply with conflict of interest rules and to overturn HAS's guidelines for treatment of patients with type 2 diabetes and for care of Alzheimer's patients. Formindep charged that several individuals on these two HAS guideline panels, including its director, had major financial ties to drug firms, violating HAS conflict-of-interest rules. It alleged that other panel members violated conflict-of-interest rules by not disclosing their conflicts of interest and that HAS had not made public what information it had on the conflicts of interest of individuals who developed the guidelines.[16] Formindep and the journal *Prescrire* charged that the guidelines were not based on solid evidence of efficacy and safety.[17] The Council of State has not yet decided the case, but in response to the suit, in 2010 the HAS revised the way it chooses expert panels. It will use physicians who are not research experts in the area under consideration to direct panels when that is necessary in order to avoid physicians with conflicts of interest.[18]

Restricting the Scope of the Private Sector

The state and NHI funds have capped the size of the private sector and entrepreneurial opportunities within it, but have refrained from promoting not-for-profit alternatives to physician-owned practice.

Starting in the 1970s, the state regulated expansion of private hospitals; after 1990, it stopped licensing new private hospital beds. Government regulation curbed permits for diagnostic imaging and capital-intensive equipment used in ambulatory settings. Other policies check physicians' entrepreneurial opportunities. Since World War II, the law prohibited physicians from dispensing drugs except for a few rural physicians when no nearby pharmacy exists. In 1975, Social Security Code amendments ended payment for diagnostic, clinical, or laboratory tests in most physician practices or physician-owned testing facilities.[19] Today, independent testing centers supply virtually all these services, and physicians lack financial incentives to prescribe tests or ancillary services. Through these means,

France restricts the entrepreneurial conflicts of interest of self-employed physicians much more than the United States or Japan do.

Nonetheless, some entrepreneurial conflicts of interest persist from physician ownership of medical facilities. A few physicians own hospitals and profit from diagnostic imaging, tests and ancillary services used for ambulatory and hospitalized patients. Radiologists typically own radiology equipment and can prescribe studies. Some other physicians own diagnostic imaging facilities through a professional corporation and refer patients to them. However, licensing and planning authorities regulate the growth of these facilities and the percentage of physician-owned hospitals has declined as lay-owned firms have purchased them. Observers report that very few physicians own imaging equipment, but I am aware of no hard data.

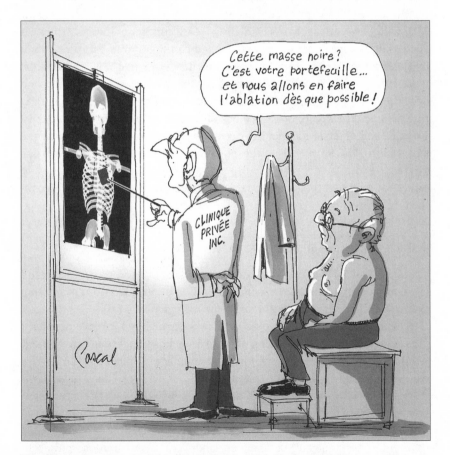

The doctor who owns a private hospital says, "This black mass? It's your wallet . . . and we will remove it as soon as possible."

Artist: Pascal Elie; Publication: Le Plateau; *www.leplateau.com.*

National Health Insurance funds and the state have not fostered independent not-for-profit alternatives to private practice because of organized medicine's concerted opposition. After World War II, the Order of Physicians
blocked mutual insurer hospitals from employing physicians by sanctioning
physicians who accepted such employment. By the mid-1950s, multiple court
decisions upheld the right of mutual insurers to employ physicians, but their
centers remained a small part of the medical system.[20]

NHI funds assumed many roles that mutual insurers had performed
before the war, so they might have developed medical facilities or
employed physicians. However, in 1971, the dominant payer, the NHI
Fund for Salaried Workers (CNAMTS) agreed not to create medical centers or employ physicians without physician unions' permission, in return
for physician unions agreeing to negotiate accords with binding fee
schedules.[21]

In the future, public policy could reverse course and allow mutual insurers to develop limited provider networks. In 2000, the National Federation of French Mutual Insurers (FNMF) proposed creating a limited provider network for individuals covered under the new program for individuals
not insured. In 2003, the Chadelat report proposed dividing supplemental
insurance into two parts (one of which would not receive state subsidies),
and allowing insurers to supply unsubsidized supplemental insurance
using their own clinics or provider networks.[22]

Overseeing Private Practice

France lags behind the United States in monitoring private practitioners.
Mutual insurers, the state, and NHI funds have tried, without success, to
employ utilization review to ensure that physicians only supply appropriate
services. After World War II, the Order of Physicians reasserted the position
that physician unions had previously taken: that medical secrecy/
confidentially prohibits bills from specifying the patient's diagnosis or medical condition or the services that physicians perform. A study by law professor Dominique Thouvenin has shown that medical secrecy in France
protects physicians more than it does patients.[23]

Only in 2004 did reform legislation require physicians to use billing
codes that specify 7,200 procedures or services. Soon bills will have to note
the patient's diagnosis as well. These codes make utilization review possible. As yet, however, NHI funds have been unable to deny payment for
unnecessary services. Physician unions have blocked the use of compulsory
practice guidelines and sanctions against individual physicians.[24] Since
2004, however, HAS has adopted Good Medical Practice Guidelines that
make it difficult to justify practices that do not conform. The MH and NHI

funds now promote the evaluation of medical practices, evidence-based medicine, and norms that constrain abusive practices.

Other reforms initiated state-led managed care. Since 2005, patients pay more if they consult specialists without a referral from their treating physician. However, primary care physicians lack incentives to take full responsibility for their patients, and medical facilities do not bear financial responsibility for all their patients' care and costs.

French law has strict rules that prohibit physicians from splitting fees or sharing practice income. However, legal changes have allowed financial ties that can create similar conflicts of interest. When Parliament revised corporation law in 1966 drawing on American law, it permitted groups of up to ten physicians to form one of two types of professional corporations. The *Société civile de moyens* allows sharing practice expenses; the *Société civile professionnelle* allows sharing practice income and expenses.[25] Group practices can use professional corporations to coordinate their financial interests. Through professional corporations, group practices have incentives to refer patients to their colleagues and to manage costs. The Order of Physicians opposed professional corporations and delayed their growth for several decades. Even today, most physicians in private ambulatory care practice are solo practitioners.

Financial ties between physicians and hospitals that create conflicts of interest have proven hard to regulate. As a matter of law, private hospitals and physicians are financially independent. Each bills patients for the services it provides. The hospital receives fees for distinct services, including operating room use, lodging and meals, and inpatient nursing, fees for computed tomography (CT), magnetic resonance imaging (MRI) and other tests performed for ambulatory patients.

To promote the financial independence of hospitals and physicians, the law requires self-employed physicians to pay a user fee to hospitals in which they practice to cover the cost of services the hospital supplies them, such as surgical assistants, examining rooms, office space and equipment, and secretarial and billing assistance. Hospitals that charge physicians a user fee greater or less than the cost of services they provide risk sanctions for violating laws against kickbacks, fee splitting, and gifts. They may also violate tax law since different tax rules apply to hospitals and physicians.

Typically, contracts between hospitals and physicians estimate the user fee as a percentage of practice revenue—frequently between 5 percent and 15 percent—and stipulate that at the end of each year the physician will adjust the payment to correspond to the actual expenses the hospital incurred.[26] Physicians, hospital administrators, and lawyers acknowledge that in the past, hospitals liberally adjusted their user fee payments from zero to 25 percent. Many say that now they follow the rules.

However, interviews suggest that physicians and hospitals are not financially independent.[27] Hospitals do not charge physicians the actual cost for their services in part because of the difficulty in determining individual physician-related costs objectively. Most hospitals lack sophisticated cost accounting and cannot calculate the true cost of services they supply individual physicians. Moreover, hospitals can choose among various methods to allocate costs, and different methods yield starkly different results. For example, they can divide total costs equally among physicians, or on a pro-rata basis corresponding to the volume of surgery each physician performs. At best, user fees only roughly approximate costs.

More important, varying user fees functions like a kickback, gift, or other financial tie through which the hospital subsidizes physicians. Private hospitals are eager to recruit and retain physicians who generate high income for the hospital through attracting and admitting high numbers of patients, or by prescribing ancillary services. Subsidizing their practice is one way to reward them.

In interviews, several physicians reported that their hospital waived the user fee to recruit them. Others said that they negotiated the size of the user fee rather than setting it based on the estimated cost of hospital services. Still others revealed that they never adjust payments at the end of year to correspond to actual costs. One physician explained that contracts specify a typical user fee, but the hospital often provides services that are not typical. Thus, inspectors find no evidence of impropriety in the contract or payments, but the user fee does not correspond to cost of services.[28]

Hospitals are particularly likely to reduce user fees when they are financially stressed, not well known, or located in settings where it is difficult to attract patients or physicians. When a physician practices in more than one hospital, a hospital may lower its user fee to encourage the physician to admit patients there rather than the other hospital. The reverse situation also occurs: some physicians relinquish part of their income by paying high user fees to be affiliated with a hospital because its reputation, location, or loyal clientele will generate patients for their practice, or because there are no alternative hospitals nearby.

To avoid illegal payments but harmonize the financial interests of physicians and the hospital, some for-profit hospitals contract with physician group practices through professional corporations that allow physicians to pool their expenses and income. Group practices then supply services that hospitals customarily provide physicians in return for a user fee. In assuming this responsibility, the group practice physicians bear some financial risk for hospital costs. They have an interest in managing these services in ways that lower the cost of these services or that increase their practice revenue.

In a similar vein, lay-owned firms can jointly own a hospital with the self-employed physicians who practice in it. Typically, the lay-owned firm is the majority owner and the physicians' professional corporation owns a minority share.[29] The lay-owned firm controls management and incurs most of the profit or loss. Physician investors, however, have incentives to practice in ways that increase their hospital's revenue and reduce its resource use.

PROFESSIONAL SELF-REGULATION

Medical Deontology's status as law distinguishes France from the United States and Japan, where medical associations' ethical codes are voluntary and aspirational. In contrast, the Order of Physicians may suspend or revoke the license of physicians who violate Medical Deontology.

Medical Deontology requires that physicians be loyal to patients and remain independent and unconstrained by third parties when they prescribe and make medical decisions.[30] It does not permit physicians to:

- split fees, pay or accept commissions, kickbacks, or payment for prescriptions;
- share fees within a group practice or employ a physician;
- profit from dispensing medical products, prescriptions or advice;
- accept remuneration based on productivity;
- advertise or perform public roles to attract patients;
- practice in a commercial manner or commercial setting;
- practice in a setting that sells drugs or medical products;
- review insurance claims regarding or assess damages regarding their patient;
- open a second office without the Order of Physicians' approval.[31]

Other provisions of Medical Deontology govern the relations among physicians and between physicians and third parties; they restrict competition among physicians and impede insurer oversight.

Physicians must seek the Order of Physicians' advice regarding whether proposed contracts comply with Medical Deontology and its opinions constitute administrative law decisions.[32] The Order of Physicians publishes model contracts, which lawyers use in negotiating agreements. Local chapters of the Order of Physicians review proposed contracts and, in doing so, oversee relations between self-employed physicians, hospitals, and insurers, and among physicians in group practice. The Order of Physicians has used contract oversight to inhibit the development of alternatives to fee-for-service payment. Other provisions of Medical Deontology govern the relations among physicians and third parties; they restrict competition among physicians and impede insurer oversight.

Physician Discipline

The Order of Physicians can sanction physicians for breach of Medical Deontology with a warning, censure, license suspension ranging from one week to three years, or license revocation; but it does not disclose the names of physicians disciplined. This secrecy undermines its most frequently used sanctions, censure and warning, because it precludes negative publicity from deterring misconduct. It also prevents the public from knowing about physicians who engage in dubious conduct.[33]

The Order of Physicians lacks the means to monitor compliance with Medical Deontology. It typically does not initiate discipline, but waits until it receives complaints from patients, other physicians, or physician unions. In 2002 and 2005, legislation reformed the administrative structure of the Order of Physicians to separate its administrative from its disciplinary functions and to ensure that its disciplinary hearings conform to standards set by the European Court of Justice.[34]

A report on professional discipline by legal scholar Joël Moret-Bailly sheds light on this secret world.[35] In 2000, when nearly 200,000 physicians practiced in France, the Order of Physicians decided 446 appeals of departmental decisions for violating Medical Deontology. Only fifty-eight physicians received suspensions for two months or more. Among these, the appeals board revoked five physicians' licenses and suspended fifty-three physicians' licenses for two months to three years.[36] The Order of Physicians overturned 95 complaints on the merits and dismissed 128 for procedural errors. Forty-eight physicians had licenses suspended from eight days to a month; five were censured, and thirty–two received warnings.

My own review of disciplinary decisions in 2000 reveals infrequent sanctions for violations of Medical Deontology that compromised professional independence or involved conflicts of interest. Initial disciplinary decisions made by departmental chapters were unavailable, but knowledgeable observers report that physicians nearly always appeal sanctions that suspend their license. I reviewed all such appeals.

The most serious sanctions for violating Medical Deontology were for physicians who were drug or alcohol impaired, or who sexually abused or defrauded patients. This is striking because the Order of Physicians holds administrative hearings to restrict practice to ensure public safety when physicians are drug or alcohol impaired or pose other dangers.[37] The five physicians who had licenses revoked were accused of raping, sexually exploiting, or defrauding patients. The less severe sanctions were for malpractice, incompetence, improper issuance of certificates of disability, breach of con-fidentiality, and business disputes between physicians.

Thirty-seven physicians had their licenses suspended from three months to three years.[38] Of these, only eight were for issues related to financial conflicts of interest, or for practicing medicine as commerce. Four were disciplined for accepting kickbacks or commissions, two for practicing in a commercial location, and another two for advertising.[39] Of the 138 physi-cians with licenses suspended for less than three months, eight offenses involved commercial practices and two involved kickbacks.

What accounts for the paucity of sanctions for code violations that con-cern conflicts of interest? A low level of physician misconduct, perhaps. But a more likely reason is the lack of means to monitor physician conduct and obstacles to patients and the public bringing complaints. Moreover, the Order of Physicians is more interested in other goals, especially promoting physician-owned medical practice and limiting oversight by insurers and the state. The Order of Physicians serves physicians and is accountable to them, which constrains it from taking measures to counter their conflicts of interest when that would reduce their income.

PHARMACEUTICAL FIRMS, ORGANIZED MEDICINE, AND THE STATE: GIFTS AND FUNDING

Physicians and pharma are linked by a web of gifts and financial ties. Drug and medical device firms and other medical suppliers offer perks to publicly and privately employed physicians. They reimburse expenses of physicians who participate in professional meetings and CME and supply most of the income for CME providers. In addition, they organize promotional meet-ings and provide extensive hospitality.[40] Drug firms fund the overwhelming share of clinical research and evaluation, and they pay many physicians for each patient using their drug as part of post-marketing clinical trials, called phase IV trials. They directly support most medical journals for general practitioners. They hire opinion leaders to market their products and employ influential physicians as consultants. They used to make sumptuous gifts—cases of wine, works of art, travel, and entertainment—to influence pre-scribing; and they sometimes pay illegal kickbacks to physicians who pre-scribe their products.

The regulation of gifts and funding reveals struggles among the state, the Order of Physicians, and the pharmaceutical and medical device industries. Since 1953, Public Health Law has prohibited physicians from receiving commissions or having other interests in prescribing, as well as fee split-ting. However, enforcement proved difficult. Firms and physicians found ways to bypass prohibitions, often with gifts. Two scandals galvanized public attention, leading to a 1987 decree that prohibited pharmaceutical firms from tendering certain gifts, rewards, or in-kind benefits to physicians (except to aid teaching or research), and to similar legislation in 1993.[41]

To promote their new cardiac drug Enalapril (vasotec) in 1984, Merck & Co. reportedly offered an all-expense-paid trip, with extensive sightseeing, to Beijing, China, for virtually all French cardiologists and their companions.[42] Drug firms had a tradition of inviting physicians to resorts; however, the cost of this trip stood out and led to the 1987 decree. In 1992 and again in 1994, the satirical newspaper, *Le Canard Enchaîné*, and the leading newspaper, *Le Monde*, reported that prosthesis manufacturers paid kickbacks (disguised as consulting fees or patent royalties) to physicians who used their hip or knee prosthesis. The newspapers published documents revealing that manufacturers routinely made such payments. *Le Canard Enchaîné* published a manufacturer's list of physicians it paid.[43] The practice continues according to a few physicians whom I interviewed in 1999.[44]

In January 1993, in an effort to "moralize professional relations," the Bureau of Competition, Anti-Fraud and Consumer Affairs (DGCCRF) attached an amendment to legislation titled "Diverse Measures for Social Matters." Parliament passed the legislation popularly referred to as the Anti-Gift Law without discussion. It regulated payments and in-kind benefits to physicians from firms that sold products reimbursed by NHI. However, the law permitted commercial interests to fund physician participation in professional meetings and CME, and their research and evaluations of drugs. Both funders and physicians had to submit a proposal that specified the financial arrangement to the Order of Physicians, which would advise them as to whether it complied with the law.[45]

The Order of Physicians complained that the government had not consulted it and that the law might stop industry funding for conferences, CME, and research. The trade press reported that physicians were canceling participation in professional conferences because they could not obtain funds from their usual sponsors and did not want to pay the costs themselves. Other articles stated the law caused drops in income for luxury restaurants, airlines, and other travel business.[46]

Interpretation and Implementation

In less than two months, the Order of Physicians, the Order of Pharmacists, and the Pharmaceutical Manufacturers Association (SNIP, renamed LEEM in 2003) issued a joint interpretation of the statute. Then they formed a commission, along with the Medical Device Manufacturer's Trade Association (SNITM), to implement the law.[47]

This alliance is ironic: the Anti-Gift Law appointed the Order of Physicians to oversee commercial funding, not to partner with the industries that offer the funds. Yet, the alliance defended the right of medical suppliers to promote products in ways that compromise physician independence and impartial evaluation of drugs and devices, a violation of key tenets of Medical Deontology. In defense of its actions the Order of Physicians' president wrote, "It is because doctors can no longer assume the

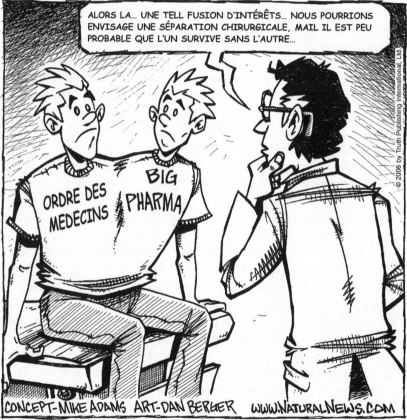

"We could attempt a surgical separation, but it's doubtful that either one of you would survive alone."

Original Concept, Mike Adams; Art, Dan Berger, February 3, 2007. From Naturalnews. com, reprinted with permission. The French version appeared in Pharmacritique, http:// pharmacritique.20minutes-blogs.fr/archive/2008/08/11/rapports-fusionnels-entre-l-ordre-des-medecins-et-l-industri.html

cost of participating in professional and scientific meetings that a sort of partnership and assistance was organized between the pharmaceutical industry and physicians."[48]

The Order of Physicians-LEEM-SNITM joint commission said that the Anti-Gift Law was ambiguous and that public officials might incorrectly construe it to prohibit medical suppliers from offering any funds for CME, professional meetings, not-for-profit associations, post-marketing drug trials, or from paying the personal expenses incurred by physicians to attend professional meetings. It also claimed that a European Community (EC) directive on promotion of medical products allowed such funding, so France could not restrict it.[49] However, the EC directive prohibited firms from promoting their products by offering financial incentives, unless the incentives were too small to matter. Rather than restricting the state's authority to regulate funding, it curbed certain marketing practices. Merely because the EC did not ban firms from funding conferences does not prevent member states from doing so.

A month after the socialist government enacted the Anti-Gift Law, the center-right won legislative elections. The new government issued an administrative circular similar to the position of the joint commission.[50] It pledged not to prosecute commercial interests that fund professional activities approved by the Order of Physicians. In 1994, the legislature amended the Anti-Gift Law to confirm the circular. The medical press still maintained that the law was too strict. However, the Order of Physicians disagreed. Its Web page asserted, "Contrary to what has been said, it leaves great latitude to firms and doctors so long as they disclose their financial relations to the Order of Physicians and respect certain limits, notably the EC directive, and limit their hospitality to what is reasonable."[51]

Everyone wanted to prevent kickbacks, which I call *pure corruption*, but tolerated *normal corruption*, that is, influence through funding.[52] The Order of Physicians wanted to stop pure corruption because that tarnished its public image. Pharma and medical device firms wanted to stop pure corruption because they did not want physicians to extort kickbacks by threatening to steer business to competitors. No one wanted to restrict commercial interests from funding physicians and medical activities. The state, physicians, and the medical industry all benefited. The state and physicians avoided incurring costs.[53] Pharma and other commercial medical interests found these expenses a prudent marketing investment.

The Anti-Gift Law mandated unfunded administrative work for the Order of Physicians. In order to employ people to perform the work, it charged firms to review their proposals. But drug firms refused to pay. As a result, reviews of proposed funding backed up, and most physicians accepted financial support and attended conferences prior to receiving approval. Later, the

Order of Physicians ended delays by performing cursory reviews. In 2000, its national office and departmental chapters each reviewed nearly 24,000 travel and lodging funding proposals. The national office approved all but 1,778 funding requests.

Since 2000, the Order of Physicians has allowed virtually all proposals for commercial support to attend professional meetings, but it does not allow funds for activities that extend beyond the meeting's duration or for a physician's partner. It presumes that the costs of meals and accommodations are reasonable. Restaurants now bill conference organizers for rental of dining halls and rooms to subsidize meals so they do not appear expensive. Sumptuous dining continues. The Order of Physicians allows support to attend professionally sponsored international conferences, but it presumes that industry-organized meetings can occur in France.

Loopholes and Limitations

The law had significant flaws. It had no sanctions for firms, which weakened enforcement because it is harder to prosecute many physicians than a few firms. It allowed commercial support for professional associations, which can launder funds for physicians using what are called Law of 1901 associations, which are tax-exempt and can hold funds from grants, contracts, and other nongovernmental sources without bureaucratic oversight.[54] The Order of Physicians does not forward its negative advisory opinions to prosecutors or the DGCCRF, both of which could investigate and prosecute misconduct under civil and criminal laws. The law did not prohibit donations of medical equipment to hospitals that benefit physicians who use it, even if they do not own the hospital. It is, in fact, common for medical equipment firms to lend or donate items to for-profit and not-for profit hospitals. These gifts promote hospital and physician loyalty to the donor and often spur purchase of related supplies and services.

The Order of Physicians accepts most proposals for industry funding without probing. It turns a blind eye to abuses such as post-marketing clinical trials in which a drug company pays physicians who prescribe their drug. Supposedly, the payment compensates physicians for recording data on the drug's effects; however, it also rewards physicians each time they prescribe the drug. One official at the Drug and Medical Safety Agency reports that, since the Anti-Gift Law, pharmaceutical firms have significantly increased the number of physicians they pay to conduct such studies.[55] However, when the Order of Physicians reviews contracts for phase IV trials, it does not examine whether the study is a means to disguise kickbacks. It issues a favorable opinion on proposed contracts as long as the amount paid follows industry norms.[56]

In 2002, amendments extended the Anti-Gift Law to pharmacists and other medical professionals and added penalties for firms, even those not reimbursed by NHI.[57] But they also weakened oversight. The joint commission had proposed that the Order of Physicians only issue negative advisory opinions. The MH adopted a similar rule: if the Order of Physicians does not issue an opinion within a designated time, the funding proposal is approved. The Council of State set the time period for approval by default at one month for professional meetings and at two month for research funding.[58] With no funds to conduct reviews and an increased workload, the Order of Physicians is unlikely to issue many negative opinions.

Amendments in 2007 required associations that receive funds to obtain advisory opinions only when they distribute funds to physicians and for payment to conduct post-marketing clinical trials.[59] In 2009, the Order of Physicians announced it would approve all industry fixed reimbursement to physicians up to €300 ($417) to cover one night's lodging and two meals while attending an event lasting more than 5 hours, and additional payment for the transportation.[60] Today, commercial interests eagerly contribute funds, physicians and professional associations graciously accept the money, and the state willingly obliges them both.

PHARMACEUTICAL FIRMS, ORGANIZED MEDICINE, AND THE STATE: CONTINUING MEDICAL EDUCATION

Continuing Medical Education as a Response to Conflicts of Interest

Physicians in France rely heavily on the information supplied by pharmaceutical representatives, who numbered over 23,000 in 2006, nearly one for every ten practicing physicians, and closer to one for every six physicians in a position to prescribe drugs. A study by the journal *Prescrire*, based on reports after their visits between 1991 and 2005, found that pharmaceutical representatives supplied biased information. They continued to supply incorrect or poor quality information following an EC directive on drug marketing in 1992 and French legislation in 1994 and 1996 that tried to reform marketing, and even after LEEM revised its marketing code of conduct.[61]

In 2004, an accord between LEEM, physician unions, HAS, and the Committee on the Economics of Health Products created a Charter for Pharmaceutical Representatives that purported to ensure accurate information.[62] Nevertheless, in 2005, over a third of physicians reported that medical representatives indicated drug uses that differed from what the official résumé of drug characteristics stated. Most medical representatives failed to provide crucial information: only 16 percent reported drug contraindications; 13 percent discussed drug interactions; 14 percent discussed precautions on use; 15 percent reported undesirable side effects.[63]

The lack of required specialty credentialing for physicians amplifies the influence of industry marketing. Furthermore, most general medical journals have close ties with pharmaceutical and medical supply firms, and most general practitioners lack the proficiency needed to use English-language journals, which are typically the leading journals in the field and considered more independent from commercial interests than French medical journals.

The Ministry of Health and NHI funds have promoted continuing medical education to counter commercial influences. Prime Minister Alain Juppé's 1996 ordinance mandated that physicians participate in CME. However, it created no mechanism to monitor, let alone enforce, compliance and offered physicians no incentives to enroll. Participation in CME remained low, by some estimates less than 20 percent in 2005. Since then, the MH has renewed efforts to develop CME, in part to train the growing number of physicians with medical degrees from outside the EC.[64]

Public hospitals are supposed to devote a fixed proportion of doctors' wages to CME but they usually spend less than the specified amount. Since 1984, public hospital physicians can take up to fifteen days off from work, with pay, to participate in CME. Hospitals sometimes pay the expenses physicians incur. More often, commercial interests supply the funds.

Legislation in 2004 created the National Councils for Continuing Medical Education (CNFMC) to oversee and accredit CME. One council oversees CME for physicians in private practice, a second for salaried physicians outside of hospitals, and a third for publicly funded hospital physicians. Legislation in 2006 required physicians to obtain CME credits and credits for performance improvement.[65] However, it offered neither incentives for physicians to engage in CME nor sanctions for those who did not.

The 2004/2006 CME legislation was only partly implemented in 2009, when parliamentary health reforms scrapped the system of CME courses for credits. The new system will promote professional development through peer review group activities and also promote control of health care spending.[66] A new entity, jointly managed by the government and NHI funds, will oversee professional development. This new approach does not mesh with the rest of Europe, which has a European Accreditation Council for Continuing Medical Education. French physicians have opposed the reform. Like the

previous law, there are no financial incentives for professionals to participate in professional development.

Conflicts of Interest within Continuing Medical Education

Until 2001, drug and medical device firms funded and developed nearly all
CME for private practitioners. It was as much promotion as education, even
though local medical societies sponsored programs. Most drug companies'
marketing departments distributed funds for CME providers. Typically one
firm supported each CME program, which encouraged slanting it toward
the sponsor's products. When soliciting funds, CME providers usually

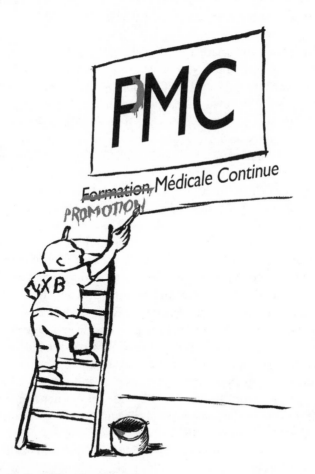

Continuing Medical Education Promotion.

Drawn by Gilles Tricoire. http://www.formindep.org

specified the topic and suggested potential speakers while soliciting the funder's advice on the faculty.

Around 2001, the NHI Fund for Salaried Workers (CNAMTS) began to fund CME for private practitioners as part of accords on fees and other matters that it negotiates with physician unions. Between one-third and one-half of the money compensated physicians for practice income lost while participating in CME; the remainder went to physician unions. In principle, the funds pay for CME costs and unions receive minor administrative compensation. However, physician union membership had declined to 29 percent of general practitioners in 2004, leaving unions financially strapped. In practice, unions use the funds for general operations and rely on volunteers to teach CME.[67] The CME funding serves as an inducement for unions to agree to accords with CNAMTS. Most people consider the CME high quality, but some doctors say it advances CNAMTS's interests in controlling costs.

The NHI Fund for Salaried Workers initially paid the Organization for Management of CME under Negotiated Accords (OGC) €12 million ($10.76 million) for CME; by 2008 it paid €70 million ($103 million). The €70 million CNAMTS spent constituted a small share of all CME funding. A report in 2006 by the Inspector General for Social Affairs (IGAS), a Ministry of Health investigative agency, estimated that commercial interests spent between €300 million ($376.86 million) and €600 million ($753.73 million) for accredited CME in 2006. Industry observers believe they still spend similar amounts for unaccredited CME. In 2005, the government spent about €112 million ($139.48 million) on CME and evaluation of medical practices.[68]

The Inspector General's 2006 report warned that an "omnipresence of conflicts of interest" clouds CME financing and administration. It complained that neither public authorities nor experts control curriculum or course content, and that CME promotes sales and supports unions. IGAS charged that the CNFMC had abandoned the principle that CME remain independent from commercial interests because it had rejected two proposals: one would have disallowed CME providers from receiving more than 40 percent of their revenue from drug firms; the second would have required several firms to support each program as a means of minimizing bias toward any one firm's products. It proposed taxing medical firms to raise funds for government-sponsored CME. The MH did not support the proposal but some physician unions did, believing that the government would then pay them to organize CME.

The National Councils for Continuing Medical Education neither restricts individuals with conflicts of interest from being CME faculty or organizers nor requires peer review of their written materials. It does not require commercial firms to report the amount of funds they contribute to each provider and CME program. Nor does it require providers to report the amount of income or proportion of revenue they receive from drug firm, which would help in evaluating whether commercial support biases their programs.

Since the start of CME accreditation in 2006, the Pharmaceutical Manufacturers Association (LEEM) pledged to the Ministry of Health that drug firms would follow Best Practice Guidelines, which hold that commercial interests will respect the educational aims of CME and the independence of CME providers; finances will be transparent; and CME providers and physician faculty will disclose conflicts of interest.[69] Yet, faculty members rarely disclose their conflicts of interest in writing; it is difficult to monitor whether they do orally.

CONCLUSION

Medicine's public service ideals originated in Catholic Church charitable hospitals. The state developed this mission when it nationalized hospitals and supplied medical care to the poor, and later when it created a public hospital system and employed physicians to serve the whole population. Publicly employed physicians lack conflicts of interest arising from entrepreneurship, payment, and most ties to third parties. But the state has allowed these physicians some private consultations, introducing the conflicts of interest that characterize private practice. The state's unwillingness to pay sufficiently high salaries to compete with private practice led it to create a loophole that compromises the benefit of publicly employing physicians.

France thwarted the growth of not-for-profit alternatives to private practice that would avoid many physicians' conflicts of interest. The French Revolution suppressed charities and delayed the growth of a not-for-profit medical sector until the state allowed the formation of mutual aid societies in the mid-nineteenth century. In the early twentieth century, mutual aid societies established not-for-profit medical centers with employed physicians, but organized medicine blocked their growth. After World War II, NHI funds assumed the insurance function of mutual aid societies but did not operate not-for-profit hospitals, unlike the United States where some not-for-profit insurers did so. In the 1970s, the state absorbed most not-for-profit hospitals into the publicly financed hospital system. France should consider enlarging the role of mutual insurers as not-for-profit providers.

Organized medicine exercises unusually strong authority over France's medical economy. It helped curb certain physicians' conflicts of interest but allowed physicians to perform laboratory and diagnostic tests. It fought vigorously to protect fee-for-service payment and invoked medical secrecy/

confidentiality to prevent utilization review, shielding physicians from oversight that can mitigate conflicts of interest.

It required NHI funds and state action in the mid-1970s to preclude nearly all private practitioners from performing laboratory and diagnostic tests and dispensing drugs, vaccines, and other ancillary services. Their intervention greatly reduced the scope of conflicts of interest in private practice. However, a few physicians still own or invest in hospitals or diagnostic imaging equipment, which create incentives to prescribe these services. State reforms in 2004 required physicians to use billing codes that reveal the services they supply. It remains to be seen whether France will develop effective utilization review.

The Order of Physicians not only tolerates physicians' ties to drug companies and other commercial interests but encourages them, although those ties compromise physicians' judgment. The Order of Physicians and the state still permit commercial firms to fund travel and professional activities of all physicians and to fund CME. The state and NHI funds could easily eliminate conflicts of interest from physician ties to pharma and other commercial interests by financing all professional activities.

To raise funds, the state could tax commercial firms and private hospitals and dedicate the revenue for independent CME and professional development. The cost of services sold by these firms would rise, but the increase in total medical spending would be small. In light of the state's major role in the medical economy, it should be politically feasible for it to assume this responsibility. Eliminating commercial influences on medical practice would foster key goals: the reduction of inappropriate prescribing and overuse of medical services, and the improvement of medical quality. The reduction in overuse of medical services, particularly of prescription drugs, would recoup part of the increased public spending.

The state has had little success in coping with physicians' conflicts of interest through oversight of medical practice, mainly because of organized medicine's resistance. Yet the state instituted effective reforms when it changed the financing, organization, and scope of entrepreneurship in private practice. But such changes engender political conflicts because they affect physician income, professional power, the fortunes of third parties, and other public policies.

Taming conflicts of interest often requires changing the balance of power between the state, NHI funds, and organized physicians. Today, however, the state and NHI funds seldom make coping with conflicts of interest a priority and rarely assess the impact of health policy options on physicians' conflicts of interest. Even more important, conflicts of interest that arise from the structure of private practice are often invisible to the public.

Part III

UNITED STATES

4

The Rise of a Protected Medical Market

The United States before 1950

The United States' market-oriented medical economy creates a wider variety of physicians' conflicts of interest than exist in France or Japan. Most physicians are self-employed in group or solo practice and can engage in a broad range of entrepreneurial activities. They can supply ancillary services such as clinical and laboratory tests, or dispense medicine. They can often co-own freestanding medical facilities that supply diagnostic imaging or other medical services that they prescribe. Private practitioners also often have conflicts of interest that arise from payment, and financial ties to third-party payers, hospitals, drug firms, and other providers. However, they often compete with not-for-profit hospitals and for-profit firms in providing these services. Other physicians work as employees of private firms, group practices, and private and public hospitals.

The United States lacks universal health insurance. Federal law does not require employers to insure their employees, but most large firms do so for full-time employees, with the employer deciding the share of premiums employees pay.[1] More than half of covered employees receive health benefits through employer self-funded plans that are not regulated by state insurance law and can include as few benefits as the employer chooses. The rest receive health insurance regulated by state laws that typically set minimum benefits covered and other terms. Employer-sponsored health benefits and insurance are heavily subsidized by tax deductions. This results in increased financial support for individuals with higher incomes. Both for-profit and not-for-profit firms sell private insurance. Currently, private insurers typically vary premiums based on the pooled risk of the employee group and, for individually purchased policies, based on individual health status or risk. They can refuse to sell insurance to high-risk individuals.

Insurers often permit—and sometimes encourage—physician entrepreneurship. Some insurers make physicians share financial risk, thus creating incentives to reduce services and conflicts of interest. Some insurers also help cope with physicians' conflicts of interest by overseeing medical practice and reviewing the appropriateness of medical services. They can refuse to supply services they do not deem appropriate, or deny payment for inappropriate services already supplied. They can restrict patients to a network of providers or impose higher copayments if patients go outside the network.

The federal government operates *Medicare*, which supplies medical benefits to individuals sixty-five and older, the permanently disabled, and patients with end-stage renal disease two years after onset. The federal government and the states jointly fund *Medicaid*, which is directed toward those traditionally considered the *deserving poor*. In 2007, Medicaid covered less than half of those with income below the federal poverty level and less than 28 percent of poor adults.[2] In recent years, private and government insurance programs left about 17 percent of the public uninsured at any time, and about a quarter uninsured at some point during a two-year period. Many more were underinsured, with inadequate benefits to cover chronic or catastrophic medical conditions.

The federal government regulates the practice and fees of institutions and practitioners for services paid by Medicare, but there is little other federal regulation of medicine or insurance. Each state sets physician and hospital fees for treating Medicaid patients. States regulate health insurance, medical facilities, and medical schools and license physicians. Providers generally set their own fees, sometimes through negotiation with the over 1,000 private insurers that operate nationwide. They can often balance bill, that is, charge patients more than the private insurer or Medicare reimburses. Americans pay much higher copayments and deductibles than patients in France, Japan, and other countries in the Organization for Economic Cooperation and Development.

Starting in 2014, the Patient Protection and Affordable Care Act of 2010 will regulate insurance outside the employer-sponsored market to prevent insurers from denying coverage or varying premiums based on preexisting medical conditions or individual medical risk.[3] However, insurers will still be able to vary premiums threefold based on an individual's age, gender, family composition, and whether or not he or she smokes. The new law sets minimum benefits for insurance policies that will be sold to individuals in this new regulated market. It also imposes fines on individuals who do not purchase insurance and provides subsidies for low-income individuals who are not eligible for insurance through an employer-sponsored plan. It expands Medicaid eligibility so that it will cover all those with incomes below 133 percent of the federal poverty level, many of whom who are not currently included.

DEVELOPMENT OF THE AMERICAN POLITICAL ECONOMY

Contemporary conflicts of interest were shaped by the American political economy as it evolved through four stages.[4] In each stage, the effects of conflict of interest and the manner used to cope with them varied. From the American colonies until the last decades of the nineteenth century, physicians were entrepreneurs who sold services and medicine in an unprotected and undeveloped market. During the second period, roughly from 1890 through the mid-twentieth century, organized medicine created a protected market, which exacerbated physicians' conflicts of interest.

In the third period, from 1950 through 1980, the medical economy underwent a commercial transformation. Organized medicine relaxed its restraints on physician entrepreneurship. Then public policy ended professional control over medical markets through regulation and the promotion of health maintenance organizations (HMOs) and market competition. The fourth period, beginning in 1980, is characterized by the logic of markets. Physicians were unencumbered by organized medicine's earlier ethical restrictions. However, they competed with lay-owned firms and were subject to oversight from third-party payers and, in part, by government.

This chapter focuses on the first two phases. In the early colonial period, most health care was provided informally within the household, not as part of the market economy. Later, physicians competed with other types of healers, and there were few barriers to entering practice. Physicians were self-employed, selling their services and medications. As they do today, they had conflicts of interest arising from entrepreneurship, fee-for-service payment, and drug dispensing. Although medical practice was no less commercial than it is today, entrepreneurial opportunities were sparse. Physicians had few services to sell, and most people had little money to pay. The underdeveloped market economy partially checked conflicts of interest that were inherent in physician entrepreneurship.

During the second phase, between 1870 and 1950, the value of physicians' services increased because of the growth of medical knowledge and the development of new technologies. Physician entrepreneurship became profitable as more people could purchase medical services because of the rise of insurance and increased individual income. Organized medicine promoted a physician-controlled market sheltered from competition and oversight.

Between 1870 and 1930, organized medicine convinced states to license physicians setting the framework for a protected market. Hospitals became the center of medical practice; private practitioners became intermediaries between patients and hospitals and used their intermediary role to promote their private practice. The American Medical Association (AMA) regulated drug marketing and directed it toward physicians. Physicians became inter-mediaries between drug firms and patients, who consulted physicians to obtain information about, or access to, drugs. Physicians also became inter-mediaries between patients and other providers. Many physicians used their control over prescriptions and referrals to increase their income, either by prescribing services that they supplied or by obtaining income from pro-viders who depended on them for referrals and prescriptions. The AMA's ethical codes recognized conflicts of interest that arose from physician entrepreneurship, but did not regulate them effectively.

Between 1920 and 1950, two developments jeopardized organized medi-cine's control. Some lay-owned firms employed physicians. Then, move-ments for prepaid group practice (PPGP) and national health insurance (NHI) threatened to shift authority to government, insurers, and lay-controlled organizations, making them intermediaries between patients and physicians. Organized medicine resisted this trend. In the process, it curbed conflicts of interest that arose through physician employment, but blocked oversight of those in private practice and alternative arrangements with fewer conflicts of interest.

THE RISE OF ORGANIZATIONS: MEDICAL SCHOOLS, HOSPITALS, AND MEDICAL SOCIETIES, 1750–1870

During the colonial period and in the early republic, medical practice gradually became distinct from the noncommercial, informal healing that women provided based on advice from those with experience and from books, and an unregulated medical market emerged. The American col-onies attracted few European-trained practitioners, so European distinctions between physicians trained in schools, surgeons trained by apprenticeship, and apothecaries who prepared and dispensed medicines were often ignored. With few barriers to entering medical practice, physicians competed with midwives, bonesetters, botanic practitioners, and other lay healers.

Many types of practitioners compounded and sold medicines and treated patients. Physician entrepreneurs competed with businesses that sold med-ical cures, referred to as *patent medicines* or *secret nostrums* because sellers did not disclose their contents. These medicines were not patented: that would have required disclosing their contents. They were proprietary drugs, with copyrighted trademarks and trade names.

Physicians sold medication that they compounded and sometimes repackaged patent medicine with Latin labels to hide the source. They often earned most of their income from selling medications. Because they sold drugs, physicians had incentives to prescribe them. Later, when individuals specialized as apothecaries or physicians, they often formed partnerships "with resultant division of labor, but without sacrifice of drug profits on the physician's part."[5]

John Morgan, who founded the Medical School of the College of Philadelphia in 1765, was an early proponent of separating pharmacy from medicine. He argued that each required different skills and that it was more efficient to divide the work. Moreover, he wrote, "it is as desirable, as just in itself, that patients should allow fees for attendance, whatever it may be thought to deserve. They ought to know what it is they really pay for medicine and what for physician advice and attendance."[6]

Three important developments reshaped medicine during this period: the creation of medical schools; the rise of public and charitable medical facilities; and the emergence of professional organizations.

Initially, either an apprenticeship or a medical school degree sufficed to enter practice. By 1800, all fifteen states had enacted licensing laws, but they did not require independent examination of individuals who completed apprenticeships or received medical degrees. Between 1817 and 1850, nine

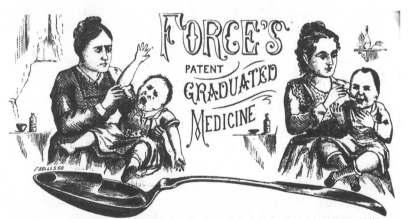

Advertisement for Force's Patent Medical Spoon.

U.S. National Library of Medicine, History of Medicine Collection.

of the thirty states repealed licensing laws because of public concern that they conferred a monopoly on privileged practitioners.[7] Even as conventional medicine grew, alternative schools of healing thrived, schools that allopathic physicians condemned as irregular.

Medical schools proliferated in the early nineteenth century; by the 1850s, there were forty-two.[8] Most operated for profit and divided tuition among physicians on the faculty. Many were degree mills. The financial interests of faculty members lay in turning out as many students as possible rather than promoting standards, developing curricula, or undertaking research.[9] Admission requirements, standard curricula, and accreditation were virtually nonexistent before 1870. Medical education typically spanned two years, included little if any clinical training, and offered no laboratory science.

Hospitals emerged from public and charitable institutions during the same period. The first great historian of medicine, Henry Sigerist, observed that American hospitals followed similar developmental stages as European hospitals, only more rapidly. They originated in seventeenth-century almshouses, which were established to care for the poor and provided medical care along with lodging. In the nineteenth century, reforms separated almshouse functions into different institutions. As a result, some almshouses became publicly owned and publicly funded hospitals. Charities also established hospitals to serve more respectable groups. Around 1870, urban charities created public dispensaries that supplied medicine and outpatient services to those without means.[10]

Public and charitable hospitals and dispensaries challenged the medical profession's market orientation. Dispensaries posed the greater threat: they crossed the boundary between outpatient care, which was supplied by private practitioners in people's homes, and inpatient medicine, which was provided for the poor in public institutions. Physicians' concern for the sick was tempered by their need to earn their livelihood. In medical journal articles they argued that dispensaries treated many people who could afford to pay physicians and sought their abolition.[11]

The medical profession tamed the challenge of public medical facilities by integrating them into medical education. Using medical students allowed charities and public authorities to provide services at low cost. Dispensaries and hospitals remained the province of the poor, allowing physicians to continue selling their services to individuals with means unencumbered by oversight from institutions or the state.

State and local medical societies formed during the early nineteenth century but had few members and exercised little influence because membership conferred few benefits. In 1847, leaders of medical societies, medical schools, and hospitals founded the AMA. Its policy-making body, the House of Delegates, represented state medical societies and specialty societies.

The AMA's organizers sought to restrict entry into medical practice, competition between physicians and other health care practitioners, and competition among physicians; in short, they sought a protected medical market. They wanted to distinguish medicine from other trades and commerce and to govern it by different rules. To this end, the AMA adopted a code of ethics at its first meeting and periodically revised it thereafter. In 1855, the AMA decided that state medical societies had to adopt and enforce the code.[12] They could expel physicians for violating the code, but physicians could practice without medical society membership.

The original AMA ethics code declared that physicians could not "hold a patent for any surgical instrument or medicine" and that advertising was a "derogation of professional character." It deemed it unethical for physicians to sell any drug with a secret formula or to attest to its value.[13] Nevertheless, medical society journals advertised patent medicines, and some physicians

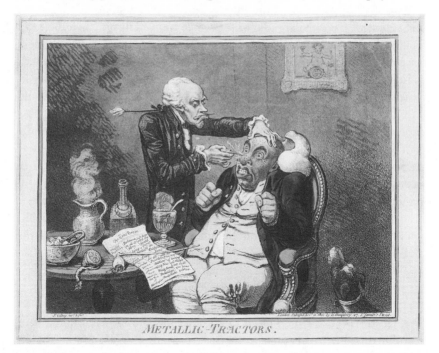

METALLIC-TRACTORS.

Metallic Tractors. In 1796 Elisha Perkins, a physician from Connecticut, patented the metallic tractors shown in this print. He claimed the tractors could cure disease through electric force. Artist Gillray's skepticism of this treatment is clear in this satire.

Boston Medical Library, Gift of C. J. White, 1921. Artist: James Gillray (1757–1815), Metallic tractors, London: H. Humphrey, 27 St. James's Street. 11 November 1801. This image is a reproduction from an example in the Harvard Medical Library in the Francis A. Countway Library of Medicine.

prescribed them. The AMA's 1849 plan to evaluate medicines faltered due to lack of funds.

OVERSIGHT OF PHYSICIANS, MEDICAL SCHOOLS, DRUGS, AND MEDICAL COMMERCE, 1870–1930

Licensing and Medical Education

Physicians who owned or taught in medical schools had conflicts of interest. Although claiming to train qualified physicians, their interest in tuition revenue encouraged them to accept lax admission and graduation requirements and to minimize their investment in medical education. They opposed laws that required doctors to pass a state exam, which would mean that medical degrees had value only if they prepared students adequately.[14] At the same time, the lack of licensing standards increased the supply of physicians, reduced their income, and diminished their reputation. An unregulated market hurt the interests of all practitioners, except physicians who earned income from medical school fees and individuals who might be barred from practice.

In the 1870s, the AMA started to lobby for state licensing, which would, in effect, limit the physician supply and competition. The United States then lagged behind France and Japan on licensing and education standards. At this time the Japanese government began to require that individuals receive training in Western medicine in state medical schools in order to be licensed to practice. The French government had required individuals to graduate from state medical schools and pass exams since 1803. In spite of its slow start, by 1898, every American state licensed physicians. Initially, states licensed any medical school graduate despite the lack of standards. But by 1905, all but three states required both graduating from a state-approved school and passing a state exam. Typically, licensing boards were comprised of physicians nominated by medical societies.

Individuals who were barred from practice challenged licensing laws. During this period, courts often interpreted the U.S. Constitution's Fourteenth Amendment due process clause as guaranteeing economic freedom and precluding many state economic regulations. However, in 1898, the Supreme Court held that licensing to protect the public was constitutional if standards were reasonably related to the occupation and applied uniformly.[15] Licensing boards were able to raise standards, in part, because Johns Hopkins and Harvard had started to reform medical education.

In 1904, the AMA formed a Council on Medical Education to establish standards. Rather than take the lead and risk criticism, the AMA invited the Carnegie Foundation to evaluate medical schools. Abraham Flexner's 1910 report criticized for-profit medical schools as being in the business of selling diplomas rather than training. He found admission standards minimal, training poor, and degrees conferred with little regard for ability or knowledge.[16] Flexner advocated reducing the number of schools, raising standards, and instituting state regulation.

In an article titled "Medical Colleges: The Duty of the State to Suppress Bad Ones and to Support Good Ones," Flexner argued that no group was capable of regulating itself in the public interest and that "the Government . . . represents the . . . interest of the people, and is alone in a position to make that point of view effective and controlling."[17] The idea that government should protect and advance the public interest and that experts should define policy was central to the American Progressive movement and propelled many of its social reforms. As standards were raised, medical schools consolidated; their numbers fell from 162 in 1906 to 95 in 1915. Most commercial schools could not upgrade training and either merged with university medical schools or failed.[18]

The Transformation of Hospitals

Once charities for the poor, hospitals became centers of medical treatment for all classes, precipitating conflicts over who should own hospitals and what relationship they should have to physicians. There were three likely options. One was for the state to own hospitals and employ physicians, as in France, other European countries, and Japan. Another was for physicians to become the main owners of hospitals, as occurred in Japan following World War II. Alternatively, lay-owned for-profit firms could own hospitals.

Instead, economic conflict produced a new alternative. Not-for-profit hospitals, subsidized by the state but under professional control, became the American norm. Physicians controlled patient referrals to hospitals and thus their revenue. Physicians used their intermediary role to promote their private practice. So physicians remained independent practitioners, billed patients, and used hospitals as their workshop—but without the burden of financing hospitals.

Formerly, hospitals had provided charitable medical care, typically in large wards. Most physicians had little or no hospital contact. Those who treated hospital patients did so without payment to gain experience. Between 1870 and 1930, however, the development of anesthesia, aseptic and antiseptic surgery, and X-rays created valuable services that solo practitioners could not offer and improved the effectiveness of hospitals, propelling them from the periphery to the center of medicine. Between 1873 and 1900, the number of hospitals in the United States rose from 178 to over 4,000. By 1930, there were nearly 7,000 hospitals with 922,000 beds.[19]

Hospitals began to serve paying patients, competing with physicians who previously treated them outside of hospitals.[20] By 1920, about half of hospital patients paid fees, which supplied nearly two-thirds of hospital revenue.[21] This change precipitated a crisis for physicians, who could not bill hospital patients and accused hospitals of stealing their patients. Some physicians started private hospitals, retaining their patients and earning hospital fees as well. By 1925, 32 percent of all hospitals and 7.5 percent of hospital beds were physician-owned.[22] When physicians started their own hospitals, not-for-profit hospitals lost paying patients who had subsidized their charitable care. In order to encourage physicians to refer paying patients to them, not-for-profit hospitals allowed physicians to bill patients in private rooms and, later, to bill all patients with means. In this way, charitable hospitals accommodated private practice.

Some physician-owned hospitals that did not distribute dividends were tax exempt. In 1928, the Internal Revenue Service (IRS) suggested that these hospitals were means for physicians to profit through professional fees and considered ending their tax exemption. In response, some physicians converted their hospitals into not-for-profit organizations but retained control through the governing board and restricted the right to use the hospital resources to a small group of physicians, an arrangement called a closed medical staff.[23] Reports of the AMA note that in 1933 there were 1,165 hospitals with closed medical staffs, and many physicians believed these functioned like physician-owned clinics.[24]

Initially, hospitals restricted which physicians could practice on their premises based on their status and social networks. They frequently excluded Catholic, Jewish, Italian American, and African American physicians. In response, racial-ethnic and religious groups and their mutual aid associations formed their own hospitals. Physicians in smaller communities also formed hospitals to avoid losing patients to urban hospitals. Hospitals with restricted medical staffs risked losing paying patients. Over time, most hospitals accommodated physicians by creating open medical staff bylaws that allowed all qualified physicians to obtain privileges to admit or treat patients.

Even not-for-profit hospitals with open medical staffs subsidized private practitioners. Physicians benefited from the services of nurses, residents, and interns and from access to medical equipment. Tax-exempt charities assumed the cost of construction and operation and serving the poor, leaving private practitioners to cater to paying patients. In the 1930s, not-for-profit hospitals lobbied for laws that exempted them from having to pay minimum wages, permit employee unionization, contribute to their employees' social security, or bear the risk of tort liability.[25] The law treated them as if they were charitable institutions in partnership with government, rather than firms that supported private practice.

Refinancing the AMA and Regulating Drug Markets

Organized medicine criticized secret nostrums, yet its livelihood depended on advertising them. The editor of the *Cleveland Journal of Medicine* lamented in 1900, "The greed for advertising patronage leads the editor . . . to prostitute his pen or his pages to the advertiser. . . . Our journals are filled with articles and editorials containing covert advertisements."[26] In 1900, the AMA pledged its journal would stop advertising patent medicine, but failed to do so. The problem, noted an AMA journal editorial, was that "a literal interpretation of professional ethics applied to patronage and advertising . . . would exclude the vast majority of them."[27]

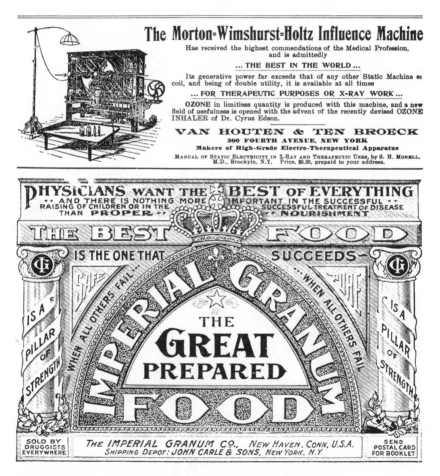

Advertisements in *Journal of the American Medical Association* **in 1900.**

Morris Fishbein, *A History of the American Medical Association 1847–1947* (Philadelphia: W B. Saunders, 1947), 982–85. *Permission granted by Elsevier Ltd.*

New sources of funding were needed to wean the AMA from advertising patent drugs. In 1901, the AMA reorganized and required its members to pay dues to local medical societies, which boosted income sufficiently to allow the AMA to stop advertising patent medicine. It also strengthened state medical societies that influenced physician licensing and hospital regulation. Membership in the AMA, only 8,000 in 1900, surged to 70,000 in 1910. Half of all physicians were AMA members by 1910, and 60 percent belonged by 1920.[28] Freed from dependence on advertising secret nostrums, the AMA then began to regulate drugs in a manner that required drug companies to advertise in the AMA journal. As a result, drug firms depended on the AMA for approval and the AMA depended on drug advertising revenue to fund its activities.

In 1905, the AMA created a Council on Pharmacy and Chemistry that approved drugs and became a private drug regulator.[29] At the time, most physicians dispensed medication, pharmacies dispensed drugs without prescription, and patients could refill and transfer prescriptions. There were two categories of drugs. Drugs listed in the United States pharmacopoeia and national formulary were called *ethical drugs*. Their manufacturers did not market under brand names and sold to physicians. Patent medicine manufactures marketed to the public and to physicians under brand names.

For drugs to be approved by the AMA Council, drug companies could not market to the public or indicate drug uses or dosage information on the label (a requirement intended to discourage self-medication). They had to disclose drug contents, which the AMA tested, to ensure accurate labeling. The AMA did not list drugs marketed to the public in its publication, *New and Non-Official Remedies*, or advertise them in its journals.[30]

AMA regulation forced most drug firms to market through physicians and patients to consult physicians for medication. The AMA and physicians became intermediaries between patients and drug firms, and this boosted their income. Physicians did not yet control all drug sales; however; they dispensed less than 5 percent of drugs in 1929. Only one-quarter of drugs sold in drugstores were narcotics and required prescriptions. Half of medicines in drugstores were proprietary nostrums.[31]

Yet the AMA journal's advertising of ethical drugs became the organization's main source of income. In 1912, the AMA began to channel advertisements to state medical journals, which increased its influence over state medical societies. By 1913, state medical journals advertised only AMA-approved drugs. From 1919 through the 1930s, the AMA journal's advertising income exceeded its subscription revenue.

The AMA joined muckraking journalists in urging Congress to enact the Pure Food and Drug Act of 1906, which required disclosure of all contents for narcotics and prohibited false labeling of ingredients.[32] The AMA also asked newspapers to cease advertising drugs and to expose fraudulent patent medicines. However, patent medicine advertising was a major source of newspaper revenue, and advertising contracts often stipulated that the newspaper could not disparage their products.[33] Newspapers' dependence on drug advertising compromised their reporting, just as medical journals' dependence on drug advertising had compromised their stance. The federal government did not regulate drug advertising for nonnarcotics or oversee claims regarding effectiveness until 1912.[34] Even then, proving intent to defraud was difficult, and drug marketing did not change much.

When Congress authorized the Federal Trade Commission (FTC) to prohibit false, misleading, and deceptive advertisements in 1914, it exempted those directed to physicians. People often say that the FTC assumed that physicians could evaluate medical claims.[35] However, the esteemed Dr. William Osler noted in 1902 that the most respectable drug firms generated a "bastard literature" with "advertisement of nostrums, foisted on the profession by men who trade on the innocent credulity of the regular physician, quite as much as any quack preys on the gullible public."[36] Marketing exclusively to physicians was not necessarily disadvantageous to drug firms, many of which were physician founded, including Abbot Laboratories, Upjohn, and E. R. Squibb. Even before the AMA's regulation, drug firms had marketed to physicians profitably. Moreover, firms selling infant formula often marketed exclusively through physicians, finding it preferable to marketing to consumers.[37]

Marketing drugs to physicians allowed drug companies to promote sales through financial ties to physicians and medical journals. In 1908, AMA president George H. Simmons accused the Abbott Alkaloidal Company (later Abbott Laboratories) of flooding medical journals with promotional material in the guise of articles. "The fact that the Abbot Alkaloidal Company spends thousands of dollars in advertising its products in the various journals that carry these 'original articles' and 'testimonials' might explain why they were published."[38] He contended that Abbott's publication, the *American Journal of Clinical Medicine*, was merely a means of promotion.

Adding financial interest to persuasion, Abbott sold physicians "guaranteed participation cooperative bonds" that gave physician-investors an interest in prescribing their drugs. As the firm explained, "We pay your 6 percent, we take 6 percent, and then divide the remainder evenly with you, dollar for dollar. . . . Doctor, this is as sure as the sun, as safe or safer than a bank and a money-maker according to the work we all put in." Simmons said this practice "induced physicians to become financially interested in its business and thus users and promoters of its products." He warned that no physician should "place himself in a position in which his own financial

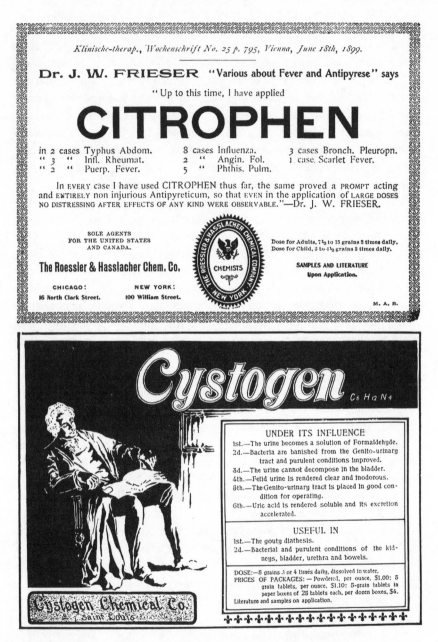

Advertisements for Citrophen and Cystrogen in *Journal of the American Medical Association* **in 1900**.

Morris Fishbein in *A History of the American Medical Association 1847–1947* (Philadelphia: W B. Saunders, 1947), 982–85. *Permission granted by Elsevier Ltd.*

interest might warp his judgment as to what is best for those who place themselves in his hands."[39]

Drug firms employed representatives known as detailers to meet with physicians and pitch their products. In 1929, speakers at an AMA symposium proclaimed "the need to replace the detail man as the main source of instruction in the use of medicines by professional, noncommercial sources of information." They decried the lack of an independent "guide in judging the claims of clever advertising and the detail men," the financial links between pharmaceutical firms and physicians writing articles on the drug's effectiveness, and the compromised ability of medical journals to assess drugs as a result of "receiving slices of the [advertising] appropriation."[40]

Starting in 1929, the AMA issued seals of approval for drugs that met stricter advertising standards.[41] In 1934, the powers of the Council on Pharmacy expanded. It could inspect production facilities and require drug companies to submit data to support advertising claims. It could withhold approval of a drug based on the firm's general marketing practices, precluding firms from marketing any unapproved drugs if it wanted to sell an AMA-approved drug. Firms with worthwhile drugs grudgingly accepted the rules. In 1932, the prestigious Committee on the Costs of Medical Care (CCMC) reported that "the opinion of physicians is taken as a criterion for the truthfulness of a manufacturer's statement. . . . Society has allowed the medical profession to be the judge of its economic competition, the 'patent medicine' industry."[42]

Following enactment of the 1938 Food, Drug, and Cosmetic Act, Food and Drug Administration regulations held that certain drugs are misbranded

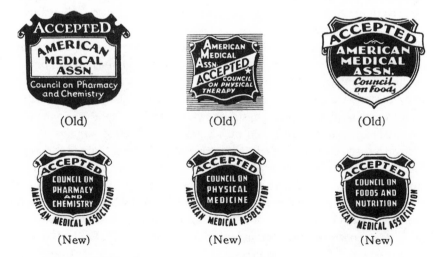

AMA Seals of Acceptance.

Source: American Medical Association, copyright 1947.

unless prescribed by a physician. Patients had to consult physicians to obtain prescriptions for them, which facilitated physician dispensing. By 1940, 25 percent of physicians dispensed drugs.[43]

Commerce, Kickbacks, and Codes of Ethics

As physicians became intermediaries between patients and others, they affected the fortunes of third parties. Many physicians exploited this role and boosted their income by charging for referrals or for prescribing drugs or services. These payments represent a conflict of interest because physicians can use their position to act in their own interest rather than for the good of their patients.

The AMA regarded commissions as the heart of a cluster of ethically dubious practices that emerged in the 1890s.[44] It defined commissions as "'rake offs,' or pro rata moneys sent for referring patients or for favors received, and not for medical and surgical services rendered by the receiver." Fee splitting was a special form of a commission, "the sharing by two or more men in a fee which has been given by the patient supposedly as the reimbursement for the services of one man alone."[45] Medical journals started to refer to fee splitting and commissions as kickbacks during the 1950s.

To investigate fee splitting in 1899, G. Frank Lydston, a prominent Chicago physician, corresponded with Chicago surgeons, posing as a rural general practitioner who offered to refer patients in return for a 50 percent commission. Lydston reported in the *Philadelphia Medical Journal* that over 60 percent of physicians solicited accepted the practice and some bargained over the percentage.[46]

Reports by the AMA and American College of Surgeons (ACS) attested to the persistence of fee splitting and commissions through the first half of the twentieth century. An AMA survey in 1912 found that commissions existed in every state. Surgeons paid physicians for referring patients. Medical suppliers and pharmacists paid physicians who ordered supplies for patients. Hospitals and sanatoriums paid physicians who admitted patients; some even advertised commissions. In 1914, the AMA's Judicial Council surveyed medical suppliers who reported that many physicians demanded commissions in secret while publicly denouncing the practice.[47] In 1914, Wisconsin made fee splitting a misdemeanor punishable by forfeiture of the medical diploma. By 1953, twenty-one other states prohibited fee splitting. Nevertheless, AMA reports documented fee splitting through World War II.[48]

Defenders of fee splitting claimed it did not affect their recommendations. They asserted that general practitioners could not receive fair fees because patients did not understand the value of their work; in their view, general practitioners used surgeons merely to collect services rendered before or following surgery. Some critics argued that fee splitting led to referring physicians to shop for the highest payer, compromising the patient's interest because they ignored the surgeon's qualifications or skill. Others charged that fee splitting led to unnecessary surgery.[49]

The AMA wavered over whether fee splitting and commissions were objectionable in themselves, or whether the problem lay merely in nondisclosure. In 1902, the House of Delegates resolved that members who split fees without patients' knowledge were guilty of misconduct. The AMA's 1903 code declared it unprofessional to pay, receive, offer, or solicit commissions in return for recommending patients.[50] In 1912, the AMA threatened to expel members who kept their fee splitting a secret, but not if they disclosed it. In 1914, the AMA's Judicial Council stated, "Physicians cannot . . . ethically partake of the profits of the manufacture and sale of their goods" when dealing with their own patients.[51]

The ACS, founded in 1913 to raise clinical and ethical standards, took a stronger stand. Members signed an oath to shun "unwarranted publicity, dishonest money-seeking and commercialism" and to "refuse utterly all secret money trades with consultants and practitioners." From 1918 to 1952, the ACS operated a hospital accreditation program and required hospital medical staff to pledge not to engage in fee splitting. However, the ACS lacked an institutional means to identify fee splitters, and evidence sufficient to expel members proved hard to acquire.[52] One journalist called the ACS's efforts to deal with fee splitting by pledges, codes, and laws as ineffective as Prohibition was in stopping drinking.[53]

PROFESSIONAL CONTROL OF MEDICAL PRACTICE
AND INSURANCE, 1920–1950

In the early twentieth century, alternatives to solo practice emerged, including physician employment by nonphysicians and group practice. Lay employment challenged the model of medical practice based on physician entrepreneurship. Conversely, group practice offered private practitioners a new business model and expanded revenue by allowing sharing of income from referrals with the group and supplying more ancillary services. Organized medicine resisted lay employment and embraced group practice. It maintained that only physicians had the expertise necessary to oversee medical practice. Through this argument, the AMA defended the position of physician entrepreneurs in a medical economy that restricted competition.

At the beginning of the Great Depression, France had state-sponsored mutual insurance for industrial workers, while Japan had mandated that industrial employers provide health insurance for their employees and had begun community-based insurance. The United States had neither public nor private medical insurance but, like many Western European countries, it considered proposals to extend medical access. The AMA mobilized to control the forms of insurance offered.

Several types of not-for-profit organizations began to supply medical benefits in the early twentieth century. Prepaid group practices supplied medical care through a limited network of physicians for a monthly premium. Some began as employer-sponsored programs, some as consumers' cooperatives, and others as physician-controlled group practices, but all tended to employ physicians. However, organized medicine blocked their growth. It favored hospital benefit plans called Blue Cross and, later, physician service plans called Blue Shield. Both subsidized private practice without insurer control over prices charged or services supplied and allowed physicians to control the medical economy.

Physician Employment and Group Practice

In the late nineteenth century, federal, state, and local public hospitals were the leading employers of physicians. At the turn of the twentieth century, fraternal lodges, consumer cooperatives, industrial firms, and PPGPs began to employ physicians. Mutual aid associations and medical cooperatives known as lodge practices served immigrants and urban laborers; they paid physicians poorly. Railroads, mining, lumber, and shipping firms employed physicians to treat their employees for occupational injuries and sometimes to provide primary care. Some employed physicians both to treat employees and to testify in court when employees were injured at work or the families of those who were killed in workplace accidents sued the company. By 1930, 14 percent of physicians were employees.[54]

Organized medicine initially opposed nearly every form of physician employment by nonphysicians, which it called *contract practice*. Horace Alleman articulated a key reason: "the physician is being exploited for the benefit of the middleman; his services are purchased at wholesale and sold at retail."[55] Another reason was that employed physicians would lose control over medical practice. Local medical societies first criticized contract practice in the 1890s and increased their opposition as it grew after 1905. The AMA first spoke out in 1907.

In 1911, the AMA established criteria to distinguish inappropriate from appropriate contracts, and in 1912 it directed local medical societies to reject contract work based on per capita fees, which made it "impossible [for a physician] to render adequate service to his patient."[56] In 1927, the AMA Judicial Council announced that physician employment contracts were unethical if: they restricted the patient's choice of physician; the contracts were secured by underbidding; patients were solicited; compensation was inadequate to ensure good medical service; or employment conditions made it impossible to provide adequate service. It declared that it was unethical for organizations to employ physicians and sell their services to the public, which it called the *corporate practice of medicine*. With this doctrine, it combated the growth of PPGPs.

Group medical practices emerged in close association with hospitals. Out of 237 groups surveyed by the AMA in 1932, 76 reported that the group or a group member owned or controlled a hospital or that a hospital owned the group practice; in other instances, all group physicians were on one hospital's staff.[57] Group practices bolstered private practice by owning or directing the hospital, their workshop. They thrived in part because they tapped revenue from ancillary services and also because reformers believed they improved medical care. Some groups focused on a single specialty; others included multiple specialists.

In a 1932 survey the AMA noted that of 227 physician group practices, 140 were organized as partnerships, 45 as corporations, and 42 were individually owned.[58] There were two business models. In the first, physicians shared expenses, but not fees. In the second, physicians shared income and expenses, which created collective financial incentives. Sometimes physicians received a salary supplemented by half of any surplus after expenses were paid. Other groups shared practice income equally. Still others gave physicians different ownership shares and divided income accordingly.

A few early group practices started when prominent practitioners employed physicians as assistants. Over time, they brought in the other physicians as co-owners to avoid losing patients as employed physicians left to set up competing practices. One of the most famous group practices, the Mayo Clinic, illustrates their evolution. It began in 1890 as the surgical practice of William and Charles Mayo and their father. At first, the Mayos employed physicians to support their work and retained ownership and management control, but shared income. Later, they shared management control with physician partners. In 1923, the Mayo Clinic was converted to a not-for-profit organization. All physicians became employees and received a salary, but the Mayo brothers controlled management. By 1929, the Mayo Clinic employed 386 physicians and dentists and a large support staff.[59]

Organized Medicine and Prepaid Group Practice

One of the first PPGPs began in 1929 when 2,000 employees of the Los Angeles Department of Water and Power contracted with Dr. Donald Ross and Dr. Clifford Loos to receive hospital and ambulatory care in return for a fixed monthly payment. By 1935, the Ross-Loos Clinic provided medical care to over 12,000 workers and their dependents. Prepayment plans also grew in Dallas, Fort Worth, and Houston, Texas, and covered employees of streetcar firms. Physicians created a PPGP in the Mesabi Iron Range mining community in Minnesota around 1900.

In 1933, Dr. Garfield contracted with a workers' compensation firm to provide medical care for 5,000 workers building the Los Angeles aqueduct. Employees paid a monthly fee to cover medical services unrelated to work injuries. Dr. Sidney Garfield extended this arrangement in 1938 for workers employed by Henry J. Kaiser in constructing the Grand Coulee Dam. This was the genesis of the Kaiser Permanente, which is the largest HMO on the West Coast today. The Health Insurance Plan of New York (HIP), founded in 1947, initially provided ambulatory care services to municipal employees through twenty-two physician group practices; later HIP became a full ser- vice PPGP.

Some PPGPs were cooperatives, which were considered radical. During Franklin Roosevelt's presidency, the Farm Security Administration spon- sored rural health cooperatives that enrolled 600,000 low-income mem- bers.[60] In 1947, four hundred families in Seattle, Washington, formed a cooperative, purchased a physician-owned hospital, and employed a group practice. That was the origin of the Group Health Cooperative of Puget Sound, which today is a large health care network.

Between 1927 and 1932, several philanthropies sponsored a prestigious commission, called the Committee on the Costs of Medical Care (CCMC), to assess the nation's medical needs and insurance options. The CCMC recommended the expansion of PPGPs. However, nine physician mem- bers, including AMA officials, wrote a dissenting report that quoted exten- sively from the AMA Principles of Medical Ethics and its 1927 statement on contract practice. They maintained that PPGPs "directly profited from the services of physicians by charging fees greatly in excess of what they paid the physicians."[61] The AMA House of Delegates endorsed the dissent.

In response to the CCMC regulations, in 1934 the AMA condemned lay physician employment in its ethical code. It also proclaimed principles that should govern all medical insurance.[62] These were remarkably similar to the French physician unions' 1927 Medical Charter, promulgated in response to similar challenges posed by mutual insurance, and to the 1934 principles of the International Association of Physicians. The AMA had published arti- cles on insurance developments in Europe, so the Medical Charter may have had a direct influence.[63]

The AMA 1934 insurance principles required physician control over prac- tice with these requirements:

- Physicians should control all phases of medical practice without interference.
- No third party should come between patient and physician.
- Patients should not be restricted from choosing any physician willing to provide services.
- Physicians should control all aspects of medical services, including those in institutions.
- Patients should pay when served. Public funding of medicine should be limited to those with incomes below the "comfort level."
- Any program should include all qualified physicians willing to participate.
- There should be no restrictions on physicians' choice of treatment or prescriptions except for those devised and enforced by the medical profession.
- The relationship between patient and physician is confidential.[64]

The AMA's 1934 insurance principles constituted a robust response to challenges from employers, workers, consumers, and the democratic state. Emphasizing the benefits to patients, they helped secure a protected medical market for physicians by preventing insurer oversight of medical practice. Armed with these principles, medical societies vigorously fought PPGPs. They expelled the founders of the Ross-Loos Clinic and leaders of prepaid plans in Milwaukee and Chicago. The local medical society condemned a medical cooperative in Elk City, Oklahoma, founded by Dr. Michael Shahid as unethical. It dissolved and reconstituted itself without Dr. Shahid and he was ostracized. The cooperative had to recruit physicians from outside the area, but the medical society tried to stop them from working for the cooperative.

Courts typically supported medical societies that expelled members who violated their policies against the corporate practice of medicine. Commenting on these cases in a 1939 *Yale Law Review* article, Joseph Laufer argued that the AMA's ethical code "constitute[s] the special law of a group, made, interpreted, and enforced by the group." Laufer found that courts deferred to AMA policies so long as they did not violate public policy and were applied fairly.[65] Laufer also noted that ethics codes influenced judicial decisions that later prohibited the corporate practice of medicine. Other writers missed the link between organized medicine's policies and court doctrine.

After the AMA developed its corporate-practice-of-medicine doctrine, courts interpreted medical licensing laws to implicitly preclude corporations from employing physicians. Courts held that corporations could not employ physicians because physicians would be their agents and so corporations would be practicing medicine, which they could not do because

corporations cannot pass licensing exams. This tangled reasoning overlooked the fact that corporations could employ licensed physicians and
let them practice medicine.[66] Later, organized medicine drew on these judicial decisions to sue firms that employed physicians, including PPGPs
and hospitals.[67] Even though many states allow physician employment, judicial decisions against the corporate practice of medicine remain in some
jurisdictions.[68]

When the Group Health Association formed in Washington, D.C., the
AMA tried to close it, arguing that it was unlicensed medical insurance. The
government disagreed, so the AMA and local medical societies convinced
local hospitals to deny its physicians practice privileges, consultations, and
referrals. In 1938, the Justice Department indicted the AMA for conspiracy
in restraint of trade that violated the Sherman Antitrust Act, and the AMA
was convicted in federal court.[69] Nevertheless, local medical societies continued to boycott physicians participating in PPGPs. In Washington state, the
King County Medical Society boycott of physicians in the Group Health
Cooperative ended only after a court order in 1951.[70]

After the AMA's antitrust conviction, Morris Fishbein, its medical journal editor, declared that the AMA would undertake a concerted effort to
"establish the . . . right of organized medicine to use its discipline to oppose
contract practices."[71] Starting in 1939, the AMA lobbied for legislation to
prohibit lay-controlled PPGPs. By 1949, twenty-six states had statutes that
required prepaid plans to be physician incorporated or specify that physicians constitute a majority of the board of directors, and to obtain approval
from the local medical society.[72] Seventeen states required that they allow
patients free choice of physicians, which prevented limited physician
panels.

The Birth of the Blues

Although the AMA vigorously opposed PPGPs, it accepted Blue Cross and
then Blue Shield because they subsidized physicians without controlling
their fees or overseeing their practice. By the mid-twentieth century, writes
sociologist Paul Starr in his influential social history of American medicine,
medical insurance emerged "under the control of hospitals and physicians
that sought to buttress the existing forms of organization . . . [and this] was
the basis for the accommodation of private insurance."[73]

The Great Depression left many patients unable to pay hospital bills.
In 1929, Baylor Hospital in Texas devised a prepaid service benefit plan
which it sold through employers. In return for a small weekly payment,
employees could use a fixed amount of services from Baylor Hospital if they
became ill. The Baylor plan inspired the creation of multi-hospital service

plans administered by private not-for-profit organizations under which individuals could be treated at any hospital in their service area. Blue Cross, as these service plans were called, was easily funded. Rather than reimburse expenses with cash, hospitals guaranteed that they would provide services, so they did not need large financial reserves.

In 1936, the American Hospital Association sponsored a model law eventually adopted in every state that authorized tax-exempt charitable associations to offer Blue Cross plans.[74] These plans had to extend benefits through at least 75 percent of hospitals in the service area and a majority of their trustees had to represent hospitals. They had to allow all individuals to enroll, a policy called *open enrollment,* and charge all enrollees the same premiums, a practice termed *community rating.* By 1939, thirty-eight states had Blue Cross plans. By 1946, Blue Cross plans enrolled 20 percent of Americans.[75]

Blue Cross plans accommodated the interests of physicians and hospitals while in part addressing the demands of organized workers, employers, and citizens for greater access to affordable medicine. They stabilized hospital funding and reduced the risk that patients would be unable to pay physicians. They allowed physicians to remain self-employed and set their own fees. Some Blue Cross proponents argued that private voluntary insurance made NHI unnecessary. The model Blue Cross established dominated subsequent health insurance and enshrined the authority of organized medicine over medical practice.

Commercial Insurers Enter the Market

When Blue Cross grew, commercial insurers sought a piece of the market by selling indemnity insurance, which reimbursed medical expenses. Commercial insurers excluded high-risk individuals. They also set individual premiums based on predicted risk, called *risk rating,* and set group premiums based on its claims experience, termed *experience rating.* Individuals with low risks were charged less than for Blue Cross, where everyone paid the same premiums. As low-risk groups switched to commercial insurers, Blue Cross costs rose and plans had to raise premiums, accelerating the exodus.

In 1946, the Blues had twice the enrollment of commercial insurers, but commercial insurer enrollment quickly surpassed the Blues.[76] By 1953, commercial plans insured 29 percent of Americans, Blue Cross 27 percent, and independent plans 7 percent.[77] In response, Blue Cross plans adopted practices similar to those of commercial insurers. They switched from providing service benefits to indemnity payments. Some ended open enrollment. They began to set premiums for individuals using community rating by class of risk—for example, age and sex—and for groups based on their claims experience.

After the start of Blue Cross, physicians formed Blue Shield plans for physician services, but, unlike Blue Cross, these plans lacked community boards. State laws that prohibited PPGPs generally allowed physicians to sponsor service-benefit plans. In 1942, the AMA House of Delegates bowed to the rising demands from its members to permit insurance that covered ambulatory services, and reluctantly revised its insurance principles to allow plans "sponsored by the constituent state medical society."[78]

Employer-sponsored insurance had started in the late 1930s and took off during World War II. Wartime wage and price controls prevented salary increases. However, firms could provide medical insurance as a fringe benefit. Employers provided medical benefits to attract employees. In 1943, the IRS ruled that employer contributions to group medical insurance were not taxable income for employees. As a result, medical benefits became more valuable to employees than an equivalent amount in salary.[79] In 1947, the Supreme Court held that fringe benefit plans were "conditions of employment," which the National Labor Relations Act requires that employers negotiate with unions.[80] Thereafter, labor unions made medical benefits a key item in contract negotiations. Less than a quarter of Americans had medical insurance in 1946, but half were insured by 1951.[81] These developments represented a decisive turn away from adopting a governmental NHI program. Much of the public then viewed state-funded medical care as welfare for those unable to obtain benefits through employment.

CONCLUSION

Between 1890 and 1950, organized medicine fostered a market that sheltered physicians from competition. The value of medical services increased, the medical market expanded, and physician entrepreneurship became profitable. By the mid-twentieth century, the key roles and relationships that defined the main physicians' conflicts of interest in the United States were firmly in place. Physicians acted as intermediaries between patients and hospitals, pharmaceutical firms, and other providers. While the physician-entrepreneur and private insurance were legitimate within American political culture, the conflicts of interest that they generated remained shielded from scrutiny.

Conflicts of interest arising from physicians' intermediary roles generated income. Pharmaceutical firms and other parties developed financial ties with physicians. Not-for-profit hospitals subsidized private entrepreneurial medical practice. Private insurance financed medical care but allowed physicians to control their fees and decide what services to supply and how to organize medical practice. Physicians were almost entirely exempt from insurer or state oversight.

5

The Commercial Transformation

The United States, 1950–1980

Between 1950 and 1980, changes in organized medicine, the market, and state policy commercialized the American medical economy. The American Medical Association (AMA) relaxed its ethical code to allow more physician entrepreneurship. In a particularly important shift, it also stopped regulating drug marketing and forged closer ties with the pharmaceutical industry. As economist Peter Temin notes, the pharmaceutical market "increased symbiosis between doctors and drug companies."[1]

State-subsidized private insurance boosted physician entrepreneurship, while the enactment of Medicare and Medicaid reinforced the trend. However, insurance also fueled spending and lured investor-owned firms. In response, the government tried to control spending, initially through rate regulation and control over hospital expansion, then by sponsoring prepaid group practices (PPGPs). Later, public policy promoted markets and courts prevented organized medicine from restraining competition. These changes upset the status quo. Physician entrepreneurship and its conflicts of interest expanded, but physician control over the medical economy eroded.

REVISING ETHICS FOR COMMERCE

In 1952, the AMA Judicial Council noted a rising number of requests "for interpretations of principles of medical ethics . . . which . . . increase income through devious means," including physician ownership of pharmacies and ophthalmologists employing opticians. Paul Hawley, director of the American College of Surgeons (ACS), declared that some physicians wanted to "re-code medical ethics . . . [to] legitimize practices which have . . . been regarded as inimical to the interests of patients."[2] The AMA initially resisted the pressure, but then dropped numerous prohibitions and expanded physicians' entrepreneurial opportunities just when insurance made them profitable.

In 1949, the AMA ethical code prohibited physician dispensing. Nevertheless, in a 1950 survey, 16 percent of physicians acknowledged dispensing drugs. As late as 1954, AMA Principles deemed it unethical to "engage in barter or trade in appliances or devices or remedies prescribed for patients." Then, bowing to member pressure, the AMA revised its code in 1955 and 1957 to allow physicians to dispense drugs and devices when it was "in the best interests of the patient." In 1959 and 1961, the AMA permitted physicians to own pharmacies if "there is no exploitation of the patient."[3]

American drug dispensing practice lay between that of Japan, where physician dispensing remains accepted, and that of France, where the Old Régime began to separate prescribing from dispensing, the Revolution reinforced the trend, and the Vichy régime fully implemented the policy. Without prohibition by the federal government and most states, the AMA's voluntary ethical code had served as a tepid restraint.

In 1964, the U.S. Senate investigated physician ownership of pharmacies and drug firms to ascertain whether "unfair practices and restraints . . . arise from the possible conflict of interest doctor-owners face."[4] The hearings revealed that one firm, Carrotone Laboratories in Metairie, Louisiana, had 2,700 physicians among its 3,040 shareholders in 1961.[5] Testifying for the AMA, Dr. George Woodhouse framed the issue as whether a physician "uses his position as a doctor in combination with his position as the owner of the pharmacy to the detriment of his patients."[6] When questioned, he admitted that in 1962 the Council on Ethical and Judicial Affairs (CEJA) recommended endorsing the principle that physician dispensing and, by extension, pharmacy ownership are unethical, but the Association of Medical Clinics and AMA House of Delegates did not support it.

In 1967, the Senate considered amending antitrust legislation to prohibit physician ownership of pharmacies and optometry practices and physician dispensing of eyeglasses. Senator Philip Hart (D-MI) noted that "the AMA . . . has softened its prohibition against the doctor-merchants. . . . So if there is a problem . . . Congress alone has the last clear chance" to address it.[7] Congress did not create new restrictions then, or when it reconsidered the matter in 1970. By 1972, 6 percent of pharmacies were physician owned. One study concluded that physician-owners of pharmacies overprescribed and incorrectly prescribed.[8] Repackaging firms sold individual doses, facilitating work for the 5 percent of physicians who dispensed drugs.[9] By 1974, nine states had restricted physician pharmacy ownership and five states prohibited physician dispensing.[10]

The AMA retained its prohibition on fee splitting—its symbol of opposition to conflicts of interest and medical commerce—but avoided taking action against the practice or other inducements for referrals. The AMA had supported legislation banning fee splitting in 1948. However, in 1953, when the ACS proposed that the AMA support state anti-fee-splitting legislation, it declined.[11] Interviewed by *U.S. News and World Report*, ACS director Paul Hawley said fee splitting was prevalent and led to unnecessary surgery. Members of the AMA condemned Dr. Hawley and called for his censure. The Chicago Medical Society initiated disciplinary proceedings against Dr. Loyal Davis, a prominent ACS and AMA member, for speaking out against fee splitting without its permission.[12] The AMA still deemed unethical "any inducements [for referral] other than the quality of professional services." Nevertheless, the AMA Judicial Council recommended "a moratorium from the constant discussion of 'principles' about fees."[13] From then until the 1980s, it neglected fee splitting and complained that the ACS's publicity harmed the profession.[14]

Some physicians got around the prohibition on fee splitting by engaging in practices that compensated them for referrals without technically violating the ban. The AMA accepted subterfuges it had previously condemned. Although in 1899 Dr. G. Frank Lydston had said that having referring physicians assist in surgery was a cover for fee splitting, in 1952 Dr. W. L. Downing argued that it was a means to eliminate fee splitting. He contended that surgeons should "utilize the general practitioner in caring for surgical patients . . . and charge a joint fee and divide it equitably with [the patients'] full knowledge."[15]

Massachusetts Blue Shield followed Dr. Downing's advice in the late 1950s. It developed schedules to pay 15 percent of surgical fees to compensate physicians who assist in surgery and 15 percent for physicians who perform follow-up care. Surgeons were to use the "deduction and allocation" arrangement only when they could not perform post-surgical care, but there was no means to confine the practice to such cases. The ACS opposed the reform, saying it "greatly restricts the . . . traditional definition of fee splitting." The AMA declared it acceptable in 1960.[16]

In the 1940s, some surgeons subsidized beginning general practitioners in order to create feeders for their practices. They initially paid physicians 110 percent of their fee for each patient referred, and progressively reduced the rate until it reached the standard 50 percent split.[17] Starting in the mid-1950s, hospitals subsidized physicians to promote referrals. They subsidized office rent, loaned money at below-market rates, and covered administrative expenses. Over time, hospital inducements increased in value and became more prevalent.

Hospitals and other health care providers formed joint ventures with physicians, giving physicians a share in medical facility profits. These arrangements resembled fee splitting since they gave physician-investors an incentive to refer patients. Granted, physician self-referral is not the same as fee splitting, but it allows physicians to boost their income by recommending services. Unlike France, which does not allow physicians to earn income from ancillary services directly or as co-owners of firms, the United States generally allows physicians to supply ancillary services.

In 1965, the AMA Judicial Council declared it acceptable for physicians to invest in nursing homes if patients could choose their own physicians. In 1969, it held that physician stock ownership in hospitals was acceptable. In 1976, the AMA allowed physician ownership of expensive diagnostic equipment if it did not "involve abuse or exploitation of the physician-patient relationship."[18] But it failed to establish a processes to determine whether these conflicts of interest led to exploitation.

SYMBIOSIS BETWEEN THE PHARMACEUTICAL INDUSTRY AND THE MEDICAL PROFESSION

After World War II, drug firms shifted from selling supplies in bulk to producing drugs for wholesalers and drugstores. They replaced unrestricted production licenses with limited sales arrangements. Although the pharmaceutical industry was twice as profitable as the manufacturing sector in the postwar years, earning profits of between 17 and 21 percent after taxes, patents did not confer an effective monopoly because multiple companies developed drugs in the same therapeutic class. So firms competed through promotion.

Spending on marketing rose rapidly, amounting to almost one-fourth of drug company revenue in 1958 and one-third by 1960.[19] The share of drug sales by prescription grew from 12 percent in 1940 to 40 percent in 1965. Since physicians controlled prescriptions, firms redirected advertising to physicians, reducing consumer-oriented publicity from 90 percent in 1930 to 20 percent by 1972.[20]

Drug firms studied what influenced physician prescribing and identified the effects of social networks and marketing.[21] They learned that physicians choose drugs using what economist Peter Temin calls *customary behavior*— habits, norms, and other influences—rather than on evidence of their effectiveness. The firms employed *detailers* to meet physicians, offer gifts, cultivate personal ties, supply promotional information, and influence norms. Temin explains that the relationship works through reciprocity: "The detail man gives freely to the doctors, and the doctor feels obligated to reciprocate . . . [by] prescrib[ing] the company's drugs."[22] In 1961, the twenty-two largest drug companies devoted nearly 60 percent of the marketing budget to detailing. Pharmaceutical representatives were physicians' main source of information on new drugs.[23]

Rather than resist this trend, the AMA was an integral part of its development and profited from it. It helped pharma market drugs. The AMA sold drug firms its physician registry, now called the *Physician Masterfile*, which identifies physicians by their license numbers, practice locations, and practice specialty. Pharmaceutical firms combined AMA data with prescription data purchased from pharmacies. They tracked individual physician prescribing and drug sales and evaluated the effectiveness of their marketing.[24] The AMA physician data became not only a crucial element in pharmaceutical marketing but also an important source of the organization's revenue. In the 1950s the AMA earned only modest income from selling physician data, but by 2004 it earned $44.5 million, about 16 percent of its revenue.[25]

As the AMA physicians and private practitioners increased ties to pharma, the AMA relinquished its drug regulation, which it had overseen since 1906. In 1946, it reduced requirements for drugs to receive its seal of approval.[26] In 1954, AMA journals ended their policy of advertising only drugs it approved and made the approval of advertising entirely separate from its evaluation of drugs. In 1955, the AMA stopped granting seals of approval, publishing lists of acceptable drugs, and testing drugs and monitoring drug manufacturing. It slashed the budget of the Council on Pharmacy from nearly $1 million in 1954 to $75,000 in 1958.[27]

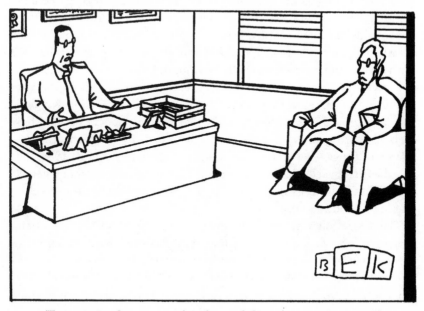

"I recommend an aggressive form of throwing money at me."

Bruce Eric Kaplan/The New Yorker Collection; Source: © www.cartoonbank.com.

What explains the AMA's reversal? It was not convinced that the Food and Drug Administration (FDA) was a better regulator. Indeed, in 1959 the AMA ended support for government regulation and aligned itself with the pharmaceutical industry. In Senate hearings, the AMA testified that only treating physicians can determine drug effectiveness and opposed legislation that required companies to demonstrate to the FDA that drugs are effective before receiving approval.[28]

Despite opposition from the Pharmaceutical Manufacturers Association (PMA) and AMA, Congress passed the 1962 Food, Drug and Cosmetic Act (FDCA) amendments, which strengthened drug regulation. Firms were required to demonstrate to the FDA that new drugs were safe and effective. In 1970, the FDA required drug companies to demonstrate drug safety and effectiveness through clinical trials that compared the new drug to a placebo or an approved drug.[29] The FDCA also prohibited marketing drugs for unapproved uses. However, the FDA does not regulate physicians, who can prescribe drugs for off-label uses that are not FDA approved.

The evidence suggests that the AMA's interest in advertising revenue and other financial support from pharma conflicted with its regulatory role, leading it to reverse its policy and to oppose stronger regulation of drug safety, advertising claims, and pharmaceutical marketing practices.

From the start of the AMA's drug approval program until the late 1930s, drug advertising in the organization's journals had increased as manufacturers sought AMA approval to promote sales. After the 1938 act establishing the FDA, however, AMA approval was less important, new advertising sources emerged, and AMA advertising revenue fell. In 1949, AMA advertising revenue was half the amount brought in by membership dues and subscription fees. From 1948 to 1952, advertising space decreased 3 percent in AMA journals but increased 40 percent in *Medical Economics* and *Modern Medicine*.[30] Following the AMA's 1955 policy changes, however, its journal advertising revenue rebounded. By 1959, advertising— mainly of drugs—generated over half the AMA's revenue. In 1968, journal advertising yielded about 43 percent of revenue, and another 8 percent came from selling exhibit space at professional meetings and selling mailing lists to advertisers.[31]

The AMA policy reversals followed systematic study and marketing advice. To increase journal advertising, the AMA employed Ben Gaffin and Associates (Gaffin), a market research firm, which wrote twenty reports for it from 1950 through 1956. Gaffin explained to the AMA that it had lost its monopoly on physician publications and needed to make changes to attract advertising. It recommended that the AMA speed up its drug evaluations, promote use of its approved drugs, drop restrictions on advertising trade names and products that mixed different drugs, reduce restrictions on advertising copy, create an advertiser index, and end cigarette advertisements, which tarnished its image.[32]

Following these recommendations, the AMA shifted advertising responsibility to a department that did not scrutinize advertisements closely. Edward Pinckney, associate editor of the *Journal of the American Medical Association*, later testified in Senate hearings that the committee was a sham, operated by a person without medical training who "glanced at the ads, and seemingly did nothing more than admire them for overall appearance."[33]

Surprisingly, one Gaffin report warned that financial ties between the AMA journal and pharmaceutical firms created conflicts of interest. "It is obvious that there necessarily exists a basic conflict of interest between the business office, whose primary interest is increasing advertising revenue, and the editorial office, whose primary interest is in turning out . . . [a] professional . . . publication. Often, what will increase advertising revenue will decrease professional standing."[34] Gaffin's comment anticipated tensions that emerged between commercial ventures to boost AMA income and its effort to speak with professional authority on public issues as well as conflict between physicians who championed rational therapeutics and those who promoted stronger ties to the pharmaceutical industry that resulted in "internal schisms within the AMA."[35]

One Gaffin report recommended that the AMA conduct a study on the effect of promotion on prescribing: such a study would "perform a service for the industry of such magnitude that [it will be] mindful of AMA publications when setting up advertising media allocations." The AMA discussed this proposal with industry representatives, who supported it.[36] In 1956, the AMA paid Gaffin to conduct the *Fond du Lac* marketing study, named after the Wisconsin community chosen because it reflected national demographics. This sophisticated study examined "all relevant facts which have bearing on the sale of a particular brand of the selected new and established products over competitive products, in this specific market."[37] It showed that the majority of physicians who prescribed a drug received samples and recalled meeting with a detailer and that most physicians who did not prescribe the drug did not.[38] It assessed the relative value of journal advertising, detailing, samples, and other promotions based on physician specialty, practice, and work setting. The AMA gave the report to the pharmaceutical trade associations.

The AMA also developed closer relations with pharmaceutical firms through cooperative boards, as Gaffin had suggested. In 1956, representatives of the AMA and the two pharmaceutical trade associations discussed "subjects of mutual interest and the creation of committees to meet and discuss matters . . . thereafter." These meetings led to joint efforts, such as surveys of medical students regarding pharmaceutical firms offering "non-educational entertainment, awards and prizes, lectures, visits to pharmaceutical laboratories, printed literature, and drug specimens."[39]

Pharmaceutical Funding for Medical Journals, Education and Associations

Gaffin proposed blurring the lines between advertising and continuing medical education (CME), articulating a strategy that became widely practiced. One report said, "The AMA can . . . make advertising a . . . force for helping the practicing MD keep current on developments which have occurred after he has completed his formal medical training."[40] Soon drug firms began to promote advertising as education and mix promotion with education. In 1959, Tobias Warner, marketing director for Smith Kline and French, wrote that "pharmaceutical promotion differs from consumer promotion to the laity [because it] . . . is dedicated almost as much to educating and imparting essential information as it is to selling." Dr. Austin Smith, president of the PMA, argued the same in Senate hearings chaired by C. Estes Kefauver (D-TN) that led to the 1962 amendments to the FDCA.[41] In other contexts, the presidents of leading drug firms defended their advertising in a more nuanced manner, claiming advertisements were merely "informative."[42]

Dr. Charles May, who served on the AMA Council on Drugs and was editor of *Pediatrics*, an AMA journal, criticized this view in his 1961 article titled "Selling Drugs by Educating Physicians." He warned that the "independence of physicians is . . . threatened by . . . drug manufacturers . . . [that] promote their products by assuming an aggressive role in the education of doctors." In Senate testimony he charged that advertising was "the masquerading of promotion as education" and that "pharmaceutical promotion cannot be accepted as [a] trustworthy means of bringing accurate information . . . to physicians as judged by the [AMA] code or the present statement of principles of the PMA."[43] He chronicled advertisements published in the *Journal of the American Medical Association* (*JAMA*) and elsewhere that made false or misleading statements or unsubstantiated claims, including one that claimed a drug was safe after an article in the same journal had warned of its health risks.

Dr. May exposed drug company gifts, which he said were no different from payola or graft. He charged that "medical organizations are given moneys to support a large part of their activities and then are in a poor position to criticize practices that infringe on the prerogatives of the medical educator." He described the "design" of a "network of promotion and education" that included: wining and dining and other entertainment and gifts including medical supplies and equipment; subsidies of medical journals;

grants for applied research and tests of products; sponsorship of conferences; invitations to contribute to paramedical publications for pay; the manufacture of numerous brands for similar products that complicated evaluation of drugs; clamorous competing claims for drugs; charges of censorship and socialism to silence critics; and contributions to the national fund for medical education.[44]

The hearings revealed the close links between medical publications and marketing. Dr. William Bean, chair of the Department of Internal Medicine, University of Iowa Medical School, testified that some medical journals "refused to publish articles criticizing particular drugs and methods of therapy, lest advertising suffer."[45] Some medical journals, such as *Current Therapeutic Research*, were mainly avenues for marketing. Pharmaceutical firms paid fees to place their articles in the journal, which published them promptly without peer review, and then sold expensive reprints to pharmaceutical firms, which distributed them to physician under the guise of informing and educating them about new developments, a practice that continues today.[46]

The AMA maintained that pharmaceutical advertisements were educational and as late as 1969 argued that therefore the revenue they yielded in medical journals should be tax exempt.[47] Nevertheless, some advertising executives touted ads' persuasive power: "Advertising is a selling force, not a postgraduate course in medical education." "If experience did not show beyond doubt that the great majority of doctors are splendidly responsive to . . . advertising, new techniques would be devised in short order."[48] AMA medical journals published at least sixteen advertisements that the FDA asserted were false and misleading between 1962 and 1969. In response to prosecution of Pree MT for misleading advertisements, the AMA said that responsibility for false advertising was "a matter for manufacturers."[49] The AMA acknowledged that it did not ensure the accuracy of advertisements it claimed were educational.

During this period, medical schools, too, began to look to pharmaceutical firms for financial support. In 1953, the director of clinical research for the drug firm Hoffmann-LaRoche, Dr. Elmer Sevringhaus, published an article in *JAMA* titled "Interdependence of the Medical Profession and the Pharmaceutical Industry." He reported requests that the industry make "larger contributions to medical education" and that "universities and larger hospitals are asking . . . for undesignated grants [for use] at the discretion of the staff" and requesting that pharmaceutical trade associations endow chairs in clinical pharmacology.[50]

Drug firms increased their financial support for medical journals, professional societies, and educational activities to help promote sales. By 1967, the Department of Health and Human Services (DHHS) reported that "many of the functions of the AMA and other national, state and local medical groups are financed to a very large degree by PMA member companies."[51] Some physicians were alarmed. In 1969, Dr. James Faulkner testified, "No organization which purports to represent the medical profession should allow itself to get in a position of being largely dependent on income from drug advertising." Dr. Robert Seidenber endorsed that view in 1971 Senate testimony. He noted that in opposing proposals for national health insurance (NHI) the AMA said third-party payers should be kept out of the picture, but "we were not told that another third party was waiting in the wings; [or that] the drug industry was deemed a more acceptable (or more generous) bedfellow."[52] All the while, drug firms continued extensive marketing, spending about half their $900 million total on detailing. On average, firms devoted 20 percent of sales revenue to promotion and only 9 percent to research.[53]

The idea that advertising might be educational had credence at the time, in part because physicians received little formal training following internships and residencies. Until the 1940s, medical schools offered few courses for practicing physicians and few physicians participated. At the time of the Kefauver hearing, there was no organized continuing medical education.[54] Physician opposition prevented the AMA from requiring physicians to receive CME. In 1968, the AMA promoted CME by granting participating physicians recognition awards. In 1971, state medical societies began to require that members receive CME, but in 1978, only six states required CME for physicians to keep their licenses.[55]

Although accredited CME was supposed to help physicians maintain competence, there was no attempt to specify a curriculum, make CME rigorous, evaluate its effectiveness, or establish accreditation. Academic medical centers and state medical societies offered most CME to supplement their revenue. Some drew physicians by holding meetings at resorts, on cruise ships, or in foreign countries. Many physicians chose courses that doubled as vacation, although tax-deductible as a business expenses.

Some for-profit firms, called medical education and communication companies or medical education service suppliers, offered CME. So did publishers, insurers, a managed care trade group, and Eli Lilly. Many CME providers simultaneously did marketing or public relations for pharmaceutical firms; others hired employees who had worked for drug companies and marketing firms. Initially, most commercial CME providers organized programs under the aegis of not-for-profit medical schools or state medical societies, but a few organized programs independently.

By 1975, medical societies and journals debated how to pay for continuing medical education.[56] Senator Gaylord Nelson's (D-WI) hearings on the pharmaceutical industry from 1967 to 1977 linked the debate about advertising and education to drug firm–financed CME. In opening the hearings Nelson said "The courses which doctors take for their postgraduate education, the books, journals, and other printed material they receive, . . . the closed circuit TV and radio programs they see and hear, are virtually all sponsored by the drug industry. . . .. [T]he almost complete takeover by the industry of postgraduate medical 'education,' is cause for alarm."[57] Richard Crout, the FDA's Bureau of Drugs director, testified that CME was becoming a form of drug marketing unregulated by the FDA or the Federal Trade Commission (FTC) and that it also undercut the medical profession's integrity.[58]

The pharmaceutical industry became "a silent partner" in CME.[59] By 1980, pharmaceutical companies could shift from selling drugs by educating physicians through advertising to selling drugs by funding CME. Drug and medical device firms soon became the main funders of even *accredited* CME and shaped curricula to promote sales.

MARKET CONTROLS AND MARKET PROMOTION

Medicare and Medicaid

In 1965, only 60 percent of senior citizens had hospital insurance, compared to 85 percent of those under 65, and even fewer had physician insurance.[60] Retired persons could not purchase insurance through an employer, and relatively few labor unions had contracts covering retirees' health benefits. Insurers that sold policies to individuals considered the elderly high risks and shunned them or charged exorbitant premiums. The poor lacked funds to buy insurance.

Some proponents of private insurance acknowledged these market failures and joined NHI advocates to support government insurance for the elderly and the poor.[61] In 1964, President Lyndon Johnson, known as *the master of the Senate* for his legislative savvy, brokered the enactment of Medicare and Medicaid.[62] It created three programs supported by different constituencies: an obligatory national hospital insurance program for the elderly (Medicare, part A); a voluntary national physician insurance program for the elderly (Medicare, part B); and a federal-state program for the poor in which the federal government subsidized state government spending (Medicaid).

Medicare served the interests of physicians and hospitals, along with the insured. It financed medical services, but the statute's preamble said it would not exercise "supervision or control over the practice of medicine and the manner in which medical services are provided." It paid physicians their usual, customary, and reasonable fees. Medicare let physicians decide what medical treatment patients needed. Its open-ended commitment to pay for medical care created new entrepreneurial opportunities without checks on physicians' conflicts of interest. Private insurers earned money by processing claims and payment but had no incentive to control spending.

Ample funding lured investor-owned firms, creating what the business press and liberal left critics dubbed a medical-industrial complex. The first investor-owned hospital chain, Hospital Corporation of America, started in 1968. It was joined later by Humana, American Medical International, National Medical Enterprises, Charter Medical Corporation, and Republic Health Corporation. In the 1970s, these corporations grew mainly by purchasing hospitals, but about 20 percent of their facilities required new construction. Later, several hospital corporations merged.[63]

Academic medical centers had shied away from practice plans in which faculty generated money for the institution since the reforms that followed the Flexner report, but some revived them in the mid-1950s. Faculty practice plans proliferated after Medicare and Medicaid guaranteed funds, increasing from only 6 in 1960 to 118 in 1985. Medical schools created faculty tracks with reduced teaching loads and time for research. Clinical scholars practiced half-time, and patient fees supplied half their salary. Other faculty practiced 95 percent of their time and generated 75 percent of their salary.[64] In 1965, less than 6 percent of medical school revenue came from physicians' fees; by 1980, clinical revenue surpassed research funding and became the main revenue source.

Cost Containment and Health Planning

Although political leaders continued to propose the expansion of government insurance, by the early 1970s, researchers had documented overuse of medical services, and growing spending shifted federal attention to cost control.[65] Controlling expenditures confronted stubborn obstacles. Cutting provider payments or restricting coverage would generate opposition. It was easier to attack pilfering of public funds, which congressional investigations had publicized. Congress passed the Medicare and Medicaid Anti-Kickback Act in 1972. When it proved insufficient, amendments expanded the definition of kickback several times.[66]

Fraud was not the main cost driver, however, so public officials searched for other solutions. One approach was *utilization review*: insurers reviewed medical bills and records and denied payment for unnecessary services. Medicare required hospitals to have utilization review committees, but they lacked authority to deny payment and hospitals had no incentive to control costs. By the 1970s, twenty states employed utilization review for

Medicaid, and in 1972 federal legislation created physician standard review organizations (PSROs) to perform utilization review. However, the law did not establish norms for medical necessity or require approval prior to elective surgery. Later, reviewers determined in advanced whether surgery was appropriate, or monitored ongoing treatment to set the hospital length of stay. By 1979, studies revealed that Medicare utilization review cost more than it saved. In an effort to achieve better results, Congress replaced PSROs with peer review organizations (PROs) in 1982. In 1990, Medicare gave the AMA a major role in evaluating PROs; volunteer physicians evaluated the PRO (and their colleagues and hospital) while working as the PRO's reviewers and consultants.[67] This clear conflict of interest undermined evaluation.

Meanwhile, states regulated hospital reimbursement and expansion. Starting with New York in the late 1960s, states authorized insurance departments to set hospital per diem charges and fees. Congressional legislation in 1972 promoted the trend, and by 1980 thirty states regulated hospital rates.[68] New Jersey developed a method to pay hospitals a set amount based on each patient's primary diagnosis that served as the model for Medicare's 1983 prospective payment system.

Inspired by Professor Milton Roemer, who coined the aphorism "a built bed is a used bed," states initiated health facility planning.[69] Roemer advocated using licensing laws to limit the number of hospital beds based on need. In 1964, New York required organizations to obtain a state-issued certificate of need before constructing a new hospital or nursing home, expanding existing facilities, or purchasing capital-intensive imaging equipment. The state did not allow insurers to reimburse facilities lacking certificates of need.

In 1965, Congress passed the Comprehensive Health Planning Act, funding state and local health planning agencies to coordinate growth of hospitals and capital-intensive equipment. By the end of 1972, twenty states had similar programs, and Medicare could deny reimbursement for capital costs not approved by planning agencies. Planning agencies lacked control over construction or reimbursement, however, which undercut their effectiveness. In 1974, Congress passed the National Health Planning and Resources Development Act, creating a health planning system overseen by federal health agencies that included consumer representatives in addition to providers.[70] The results varied. Often, hospitals lobbied state legislatures to overturn denials of certificates of need. Moreover, the law did not authorize agencies to control purchase of magnetic resonance imaging (MRIs) and other expensive equipment outside of hospitals, so they could not limit the entrepreneurial activities of private practitioners and independent firms. Both developed these revenue-generating opportunities.

The HMO Act of 1973: From Pre-Paid Group Practice
to Managed Care

In 1969, President Richard Nixon declared there was a health cost crisis, imposed temporary price controls in Medicare, and searched for ways to control spending that avoided regulation, which Republicans opposed as intrusive government intervention in the market. He was familiar with Kaiser Permanente from his years in California, and Republican governors Ronald Reagan of California and Nelson Rockefeller of New York supported prepaid group practices. Studies showed they reduced hospitalization by 20 percent without sacrificing quality.[71] Nixon embraced PPGPs that the political right had previously criticized as socialistic and set in motion a remarkable transformation.

The Nixon administration renamed PPGPs health maintenance organizations (HMOs) and promoted them to control medical spending. In 1971, it sponsored HMOs with grants and made them available to Medicare and Medicaid recipients. Then it backed the HMO Act of 1973, which authorized grants for HMOs that offered comprehensive benefits, charged everyone the same premiums, and allowed everyone to enroll.[72] Many PPGP advocates wanted HMOs to include only not-for-profit organizations and only entities that employed physicians. However, the legislation included for-profit firms and independent practice associations (IPAs) that contracted with self-employed physicians. These were modeled on foundation medical plans that physicians had started earlier in the century to compete with PPGPs that employed physicians.

Three types of HMOs emerged. Staff-model HMOs employ physicians, pay them a salary, and own hospitals and other medical facilities. Network-model HMOs resemble the staff model, but contract with two or more physician groups and hospitals. Another variation, the IPA-HMOs contract with one or more IPAs that contract with self-employed physicians. Their physicians are typically paid fee-for-service and can treat patients outside the HMO. By 1980, there were 217 HMOs with eight million enrollees; but they covered only 4 percent of the nation's population.[73] All HMOs countered incentives to increase services. But for-profit and IPA-HMOs maintained entrepreneurial incentives for physicians and created incentives to reduce services.

Many people did not join staff- or network-model HMOs because they did not want restrictions on their choice of physician or hospital. In response, in the 1980s, insurers created preferred provider organizations (PPOs), a hybrid between HMOs and indemnity insurance. These organizations offer medical care through a network of preferred providers with whom they contract, just as IPA-HMOs do, and patients are responsible for small copayments. The PPOs also reimburse services from other providers, but then patients pay a copayment as in indemnity insurance, usually 20 percent. HMOs and PPOs—collectively called managed care organizations (MCOs)—differ from indemnity insurers in that they can influence practice through rules and incentives. They contract with a network of physicians and hospitals to obtain lower prices, monitor medical practice, limit services through utilization review and other controls, and offer physicians financial incentives to control spending.

Managed care organizations changed physician payment, first by paying salary instead of fee-for-service and later by using financial incentives and risk sharing to induce physicians to control spending.[74] For example, primary care physicians often receive a capitation payment to cover their own services and also the cost of laboratory tests or referrals to specialists as well as their own services. Alternatively, physicians receive fees for services that are adjusted for patient resource use.

Typically, IPA-HMOs and PPOs contract with an IPA, group practice, or other intermediary organization that contracts with individual physicians.[75] The MCO can spread financial risk across the physician group rather than having each physician shoulder the burden individually. Policy makers anticipated that risk sharing would lead providers to reduce only unnecessary services. They overlooked the fact that risk sharing substituted new conflicts of interest for the fee-for-service conflicts it replaced.[76]

Initially, most MCOs were staff- or network-model HMOs, and typically not-for-profit. However, IPA-HMOs and PPOs, which were usually for-profit firms, offered a wider choice of physicians and hospitals. They grew quickly because they were not saddled with fixed costs, and in the 1980s they came to dominate the market. They often avoided federal qualification so they could set premiums based on the insured group's claims experience and exclude high-risk patients for individual policies.

The Demise of Professional Control over Medical Commerce

The HMO Act of 1973 allowed HMOs to employ a limited physician network and advertise, overriding state laws and the AMA's ethical code. Antitrust law weakened the AMA's control further.

In 1952, the Supreme Court had created an exemption from antitrust law prohibitions for learned professions, particularly law and medicine, by holding that they were not engaged in commerce. However, in 1975, the Supreme Court ended the learned profession exemption under the Sherman Antitrust Act and struck down bar association ethical code restrictions on advertising.[77] Then courts chipped away at the authority of state and professional medical societies to sanction physicians for their economic behavior, even if the declared purpose was to promote professional ethics or quality of health care.[78]

In 1975, the FTC sued the AMA, charging that its ethical code violated antitrust laws. In 1979, an appeals court ruled in favor of the FTC and ordered the AMA to cease enforcing restrictions on physician contracting with organizations that offer services to the public, physician employment by organizations owned or managed by laypersons, and restrictions on physician payment. The FTC also ordered the AMA to rewrite its constitution, its Principles of Ethics, and all its ethical opinions, reports, and bylaws to conform to the ruling.[79] However, some states still have judicial decisions and statutes that restrict organizations from employing physicians.

Subsequent FTC cases struck down other market restrictions by organized medicine, including restraints on optometrists selling eyeglasses and contact lenses; ceilings on the number of offices that optometrists can have; controls on physicians affiliating with physical therapists; collective refusal of dentists to provide X-rays to insurers that sought to determine whether treatment is appropriate; and prohibitions on physicians cooperating with chiropractors.[80]

Antitrust laws also stymied physicians' attempts to bargain collectively with insurers. In 1979, a federal court declared illegal provider boycotts of Medicaid aimed at raising fees. In 1982, the Supreme Court held that medical society fee schedules constitute illegal price fixing. As MCOs increased their market share, they obtained fee discounts. Many physicians proposed forming unions to bargain with MCOs, along the lines of what physicians had done in France. However, the National Labor Relations Act exempts collective bargaining from antitrust prohibitions only for employees, not for self-employed practitioners.[81] Unions do represent some employed physicians, such as residents, interns, and physicians working in the public sector. In 1997, there were between 14,000 to 20,000 physician union members: 6,000 to 9,000 were interns or residents; approximately 3,000 were physicians employed in independent practices; and the rest were public employees. But unionized physicians made up only 5.5 percent of practicing physicians in 1999.[82]

CONCLUSION

Between 1950 and 1980, the American medical economy underwent a commercial transformation that increased physicians' conflicts of interest. Organized medicine spurred the process by dropping ethical restrictions on physician entrepreneurship and aligning itself with the pharmaceutical industry on policy issues just as it turned to drug companies to fund medical journals, associations, and educational activities. The AMA helped the pharmaceutical industry develop new forms of marketing, and together they blended drug marketing with physician education.

The expansion of insurance removed financial restraints on what services physicians could sell, and investor-owned firms entered the medical market. When medical costs soared, the federal government attempted to control spending through regulation, by promoting HMOs and, paradoxically, by promoting market competition. Antitrust law ended restraints of trade that had allowed physicians greater profit than a competitive market would yield. At the same time, it ended any remaining professional restraints on entrepreneurship. However, physicians no longer worked in a market that organized medicine controlled. The stage was set for a reconfiguration of the medical economy in the 1980s, based on market logic, that generated new and more numerous physicians' conflicts of interest.

6

The Logic of Medical Markets

The United States, 1980–Present

Ronald Reagan's election in 1980 signaled a policy shift that reduced government regulation and promoted markets. This set the stage for the fourth phase of the American medical economy, which is characterized by the logic of markets. The federal government ended health planning and states ended hospital rate setting. These changes did not result in the *perfect competition* of economic theory, however. The medical economy was characterized by medical uncertainty and imperfect information, the regulation of professionals and institutions, the powerful presence of insurance, and the government's dominance as payer. Nevertheless, policy changes allowed market forces greater sway in medical care and shaped contemporary physicians' conflicts of interest.[1]

Market logic encouraged physician entrepreneurship. Physicians invested in medical facilities when they could profit by referring patients to the facility. Dr. Arnold Relman, editor of the *New England Journal of Medicine* (*NEJM*), warned in celebrated articles of dangers from physician investment, conflicts of interest, and investor-owned firms.[2] Concern that physician entrepreneurship created conflicts of interest led Congress to restrict physician self-referral in Medicare. But physicians retained similar entrepreneurial conflicts of interest within group practices, where they began to supply profitable services previously available only in hospitals. At the same time, for-profit firms increased their market share of hospital and ancillary services, concentrating on profitable niches. Their competition reduced the income of not-for-profit hospitals, which then deepened financial ties with private practitioners to encourage them to refer patients.

In response, public policy granted insurers authority and financial incentives to reduce expenditures. They enlisted physicians as cost-control agents by shifting financial risk to self-employed physicians. Financially squeezed, hospitals needed to cut their costs. They offered physicians financial incentives to use resources frugally. Some employers began to adjust physicians' salaries based on their financial performance. These changes blurred difference among incentives of private practitioners, physician employees, and insurers. As insurers developed greater influence over medical practice, they created new physicians' conflicts of interest. However, they also became a source of countervailing power that helped cope with some physicians' conflicts of interest.

Markets led not-for-profit hospitals and insurers to compete with their for-profit counterparts by using similar strategies. As they adopted entrepreneurial behaviors, so did their affiliated physicians. These changes reduced the differences in the behavior of not-for-profit and for-profit medical facilities.

Meanwhile, market logic exacerbated conflicts of interest arising from physician ties to drug firms. Drug companies influenced choices at multiple strategic junctures, including the initial research, evaluation of drugs, continuing medical education (CME), and physician prescribing.

Let us now explore in detail how market logic influenced physicians, hospitals, insurers, and drug firms.

PHYSICIANS

Kickbacks and Self-Referral

Medicare had earlier prohibited kickbacks and cast a cloud over many related practices. Nevertheless, in the 1980s, businesses and physicians formed joint ventures in which profits rewarded physicians for referrals. Critics argued that they created the same problem.

Physicians often invested as *limited partners*, an arrangement in which a *general partner* owns a majority share and bears full management, financial, and legal responsibility. The other investors, designated *limited partners*, earn profits in proportion to their ownership share; they lack management authority, legal liability, or financial risk beyond their investment. The business decision to create limited partnerships requires a strategic choice. Limited partners contribute capital, but firms can acquire funds in other ways, usually at lower cost. Publicly traded firms have access to capital through the stock market, and not-for-profit organizations can acquire money by issuing tax-exempt bonds. Medical facilities can also borrow funds from banks.[3] Businesses often create limited partnerships, not to obtain investment capital but other contributions from limited partners.

My review of prospectuses that solicited physicians as limited partners in the 1980s reveals that these documents often specify the number of patients each limited partner needed to refer for the venture to be profitable.[4] Moreover, these firms obtained most investment capital through their own funds or bank loans. In short, firms offered physicians limited partnerships for their patient referrals.

Critics coined the term *physician self-referral* for physicians who refer patients to medical facilities in which they invest, to highlight its similarity to *self-dealing*. Self-dealing refers to individuals who are on both sides of a financial transaction and can use their position to promote their personal interests rather than those of others whom they are supposed to serve. For example, a corporate officer or manager may direct the corporation to contract with a business that she owns. Although expected to serve the corporation, the manager can promote her personal interests.

There are similarities between kickbacks and self-referral. Individuals who pay kickbacks for patient referrals can often convert their arrangement into a limited partnership investment. Consider the example of Walter Ford, a physical therapist, who paid Dr. Anthony Cabot 45 percent of his fees as a kickback for patients referred. After four years, fearing legal sanctions, the men decided to "formalize" their agreement by creating a limited partnership. Ford was the general partner; Cabot, his colleague Sylvia Urratia, and their spouses each invested $3,000 as limited partners. Ford performed the work and received 55 percent of the income; the limited partners who referred patients earned 45 percent. The partnership continued the financial and referral arrangement, but made it legal. However, in 1982, Georgia prohibited self-referral in physical therapy. Ford then told Cabot they could no longer continue the partnership. Cabot ceased referring patients; Ford's practice went bankrupt, and he sued Cabot.[5]

Over a dozen studies conducted between 1970 and 1992 reveal that 12 percent to 80 percent of medical facilities had physician investors, depending on the region and service, and that physician investors order more tests and services than physicians who have no share in the facility's profits.[6] A 1989 study found that 25 percent of clinical laboratories reimbursed by Medicare had physician investors who referred patients and that they ordered 45 percent more tests for their patients than comparable physicians who were not inventors. A series of studies in Florida in the 1990s found that physicians invested directly in more than 80 percent of Florida medical facilities and corporations owned in part by physicians invested in the remaining 20 percent. The studies found that physician-owned laboratories performed nearly twice as many tests per patients and charged over twice as much per patient as labs without physician investors. Other physician-owned facilities use many more medical services than the norm, even radiation therapy, which is harmful to patients if used inappropriately.[7]

In the 1980s, physicians invested in medical facilities that relied on their referrals, particularly clinical laboratories and centers for diagnostic imaging, radiation therapy, and ambulatory surgery. Physicians also formed joint ventures with investor-owned hospitals. The investor-owned firms owned multiple hospitals as general partners, while physicians and group practices invested as limited partners in their local hospital. Three hospital chains—Hospital Corporation of America (HCA), Tenet Health Care System (formerly National Medical Enterprise), and Quorum Health Resources— made physician investments central to their business plan. HCA owned more than 350 hospitals, 145 outpatient surgery centers, and 550 home care agencies in 1996, many of which had physician investors. Starting in 1997, HCA sold many physician-owned hospitals after prosecution for Medicare and Medicaid fraud. In 2004, Tenet Healthcare Corporation shared ownership in 650 subsidiaries; physicians invested in 4 percent of these subsidiaries.[8]

Physicians invested in ambulatory surgery centers (ASCs), which boomed after Medicare promoted their use to reduce hospital spending. By moving surgery from hospitals to ambulatory centers, physician-investors tapped profits from the facility. Because ASCs are smaller than hospitals, the link between individual physician referrals and profits are stronger. Only 239 ASCs existed in 1983, but there were over 1,800 in 1993 and nearly 5,900 by 2008. By 2002, 61 percent of independent ASCs were entirely physician owned; physicians and other investors jointly owned over 90 percent.[9]

More recently, physicians invested in specialty hospitals, which focus on a single practice area such as cardiac, orthopedic, surgical, or women's services. Proponents claim they organize medical services efficiently and improve quality. Perhaps—but they focus on profitable services. Studies reveal that after physicians become part owners of specialty hospitals, their referrals for surgery, tests, and treatments increase.[10]

The number of specialty hospitals grew from twenty-nine to ninety-two between 1990 and 2003. Nearly 70 percent were partly owned by referring physicians. Typically, physicians owned about 50 percent of each hospital. In 10 percent of these hospitals, a single group practice owned more than 80 percent. From 2003 to 2005, Congress placed a moratorium on Medicare payments to new specialty hospitals. Between then and 2008, the number of physician-owned specialty hospitals has risen to 177 and an additional 85 were being developed. In 2010, health reform legislation stopped the creation or expansion of physician-owned hospitals.

The AMA did not oppose this trend. Instead, in 1986, the AMA's Council on Ethical and Judicial Affairs (CEJA) issued conflict of interest guidelines that allowed physicians to self-refer if they disclosed their ownership to patients. Despite the guideline, in a 1989 AMA member survey, nearly one-third of physicians reported that they did not disclose their ownership to patients.[11]

Representative Pete Stark (D-CA) thought that medical facilities with physician investors produced the same harm as kickbacks. He urged the Department of Health and Human Services (DHHS) Office of Inspector General (OIG) to prosecute self-referral under the Medicare Anti-Kickback Act (Anti-Kickback Act) and in 1989 sponsored legislation to restrict certain self-referral. Dr. James Todd, senior deputy vice president of the AMA, testified that legislation was unnecessary because "history has repeatedly shown that the inherent conflict of interest in the doctor-patient relationship has been decided in favor of the patient." Failing to find this assertion persuasive, Congress passed the Stark law, prohibiting physician self-referral in Medicare for clinical laboratories and required reporting of other self-referral to the OIG.[12]

The AMA's Council on Ethical and Judicial Affairs (CEJA) revised its self-referral guidelines in December 1991, just before long-scheduled Senate

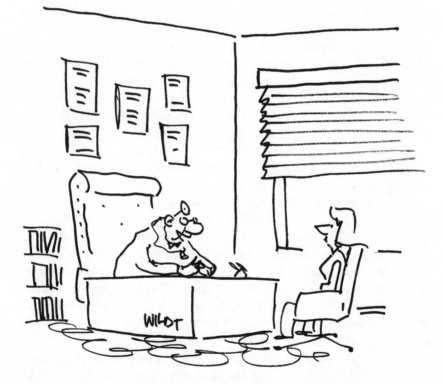

"We'd like to run some tests to help pay for our expensive new testing machine."

Artist: Chris Wildt. Acknowledgment: www.CartoonStock.com.

hearings. Its new guidelines declared that self-referral was "presumptively inconsistent" with the physician's obligation to patients but acceptable if existing facilities were "not adequate" in number, quality, or location.[13] How should physicians decide if existing facilities were adequate and what travel distance rendered another facility unsuitable? The guidelines were silent. Yet, the AMA testified that its guidelines made broader legal restrictions unnecessary.

Moreover, many AMA members believed the CEJA guidelines were too restrictive and some state medical societies opposed them. In June 1992, the AMA House of Delegates resolved—contrary to the guidelines—that self-referral was appropriate if physicians disclosed their ownership and informed patients of alternative facilities. The standoff between the House of Delegates and the CEJA continued for six months. Then, a House of Delegates committee offered a resolution that supported the guidelines, arguing that they helped counter "overly restrictive legislation" and noting that the guidelines allowed exceptions. The House of Delegates passed the resolution to stop enactment of stricter self-referral laws, not to restrict physician conduct.[14]

Testifying in 1993 hearings for the AMA, Dr. Nancy Dicey opposed expanding self-referral prohibition and cited its new guidelines. Nevertheless, Congress broadened the Stark law, barring self-referral for eleven additional service categories in Medicare and extending the ban to Medicaid. However, the law included over twenty exceptions. Most important, doctors can refer patients within group practices, to hospitals, and to ASCs.[15] These loopholes encouraged physicians to form group practices and invest in hospitals and ASCs.

Drugs, Tests, and Ancillary Services

Physicians combined prescribing and selling by dispensing drugs that they prescribed and through investing in pharmacies. Taking notice in 1987, Representative Henry Waxman (D-CA) investigated and considered amending the Food, Drug and Cosmetic Act to prohibit physician dispensing. He opened hearings by quoting a *New York Times* editorial: "The physician/pharmacist has an obvious potential conflict of interest. Might he be tempted to write unnecessary prescriptions or prescribe a drug he sells when another he doesn't sell might be preferable, or to sell brand name drugs with high markups when cheaper generics are available?"[16]

Testifying for the AMA, Dr. Nancy Dicey opposed prohibiting physician dispensing, but acknowledged that AMA guidelines hold that "physicians should avoid regular dispensing . . . when the needs of patients can be met adequately by local ethical pharmacies or suppliers." The Federal Trade

Commission also opposed the bill as a restraint on competition and the bill died.[17]

The growth of pharmacy chains subsequently made it difficult for individual physicians to operate pharmacies profitably. Still, in the 1990s, investor-owned pharmacies sought physicians as limited partners, typically with thirty to thirty-five limited partners per pharmacy. Physicians also dispensed drugs, assisted by firms that sold them individual packaged prescriptions. However, insurers countered this trend with pharmaceutical benefit managers, who controlled drug formularies and required patients to obtain drugs through designated pharmacies or by mail. In 2002, only 7 percent of physicians dispensed drugs.[18]

Physician sale of injectable medications, in contrast, grew rapidly after 1990, when chemotherapy administration moved from hospitals to ambulatory facilities. Oncologists earned a significant part of their income by selling chemotherapy drugs. A 1999 Medicare coverage advisory meeting discussed the problems that result from incentives for oncologists to prescribe expensive therapies. Studies revealed that even after cancer did not respond to treatment oncologists often continued to prescribe chemotherapy. In 2007, the *New York Times* reported that oncologists and nephrologists earn high profits from injecting anemia medication and routinely overuse it.[19]

Shifting laboratory testing from hospitals to physicians' offices, which was designed to limit costs, had the opposite effect because it gave physicians incentives to order more tests. From 1984 to 1988, Medicare spending on laboratory services grew from $936 million to $1.9 billion, while they shifted from hospitals to ambulatory settings, particularly physicians' offices.[20] Press reports and congressional hearings revealed quality problems, erroneous billing, false billing, and kickbacks in ambulatory laboratories, nearly half of which were in physician offices, which Congress had exempted when it set laboratory quality standards in 1967. The Clinical Laboratory Improvements Amendments of 1988 (CLIA'88) required physicians' offices to meet the same standards as independent laboratories, raising their costs. Some physicians stopped all testing, and others only performed simple tests.[21] Physicians' market share of laboratory tests decreased from 28 percent in 1986 to 11 percent in 1996, after CLIA'88 and managed care restrictions.[22]

Group Practice and Physician Employment

Group practices facilitate supplying tests and ancillary services. The proportion of physicians practicing in groups rose from 25 percent in 1980 to 32.6 percent in 1991. The Stark law spurred their growth; by 2001, 62 percent of self-employed physicians were in group practice. Some groups are loose affiliations of physicians in multiple locations with little coordination or sharing of income and expenses except for ancillary services. A few subcontract with others for ancillary services. Through contracts, physicians can reallocate income derived from collective services.[23] This arrangement dissolves the line that separate services provided within a medical practice from those outside it.

A few group practices offer a full range of services. As they grow, the distinction between a group practice and an integrated health care system becomes moot. Large physician groups even purchase hospitals. In 2004, Physicians of Midway, Inc., purchased the 225-bed Midway Hospital Medical Center in Los Angeles from Tenet HealthCare Corporation.[24] The Mayo Clinic and other early twentieth-century multi-specialty group practices developed organizational cultures that promoted excellence and efficiency. However, the large physician groups that consolidated disparate physicians into networks in the 1990s did not. Physician managers were subject to the same incentives and market pressures as lay managers. Some large group practices sold their practice to investor-owned firms called physician practice managers (PPMs), and others became managed by PPMs.

During this period, physician employment grew apace. By 2001, 35 percent of all physicians were employees.[25] Private hospitals employed physicians as hospitalists and for anesthesiology, radiology, and pathology. Medical schools employed physicians in faculty practice plans and to staff freestanding ambulatory care practices. Some health maintenance organizations (HMOs), independent practice associations (IPAs), and physician-owned group practices also employed physicians.

Physicians' employment conflicts of interest are a function of the employer's ownership status and mission, control over physicians, and how the employer pays physicians. In public hospitals, physicians generally have secure employment, professional discretion, and a fixed salary, all of which minimize the risk that they will practice in ways that promote their employer's financial interest. In contrast, physicians employed by private entities have less secure employment; their employers seek profit and use financial incentives to manage the care they provide.

Traditionally, salary did not encourage physicians to change medical decisions. It occupied a middle ground between incentives to increase services, such as fee-for-service payment, and incentives to decrease services, such risk sharing. Now, however, many private employers adjust salary to reward revenue generation and expense reduction. Medical school faculty practice plans often adjust physicians' salaries to reflect the fees they generate.[26]

The surgeon Atul Gawande captured the effect of market logic on physicians in his 2009 *New Yorker* article on McAllen, Texas, the most expensive medical market in the country. Investigating why medical spending was higher there than in other communities that had similar demographics, he asked doctors what was different. The usual explanations for ordering more tests and procedures—physicians practicing defensive medicine, or sicker patients—could not explain the difference. But interviews revealed that an "entrepreneurial spirit" took hold of the medical community. Many doctors viewed practice "primarily as a revenue stream" and "profit growth to be a legitimate ethic in the practice of medicine." The most expensive medical equipment was not high-tech machines but the doctor's pen used to write prescriptions. Doctors "rack up charges with extra tests, services and procedures."[27]

Private practice organized on an entrepreneurial model is the core problem. Market logic, however, applied to insurance, hospitals, and drug firms amplifies rather than tames the problem. It undermines values associated with professionalism, such as public service, fidelity to patients, and practice based on knowledge.

HOSPITALS

Revenue and Referrals

Market logic made hospitals more profit oriented and reduced differences between not-for-profit and for-profit hospitals. Lured by new opportunities offered by the start of Medicare and Medicaid, investor-owned firms supplied hospital services. By 1980, they owned nearly 9 percent of community hospital beds and owned or managed 12.4 percent of all hospital beds. By 2008, for-profit firms owned 19.6 percent of hospital beds.[28] Focused on lucrative niches, they located in middle-class and affluent communities, offered only profitable services, and shunned uninsured patients. This business strategy undermined not-for-profit community hospitals that supplied the full range of medical services and offset losses from uncompensated care with income from profitable services. When for-profit hospitals siphoned off profitable patients and services, that strategy no longer worked. The growth of specialty hospitals, ASCs, and physician-owned facilities also cut community hospital revenue.

Market logic led even not-for-profit hospitals to compete for patients. In the 1980s, hospitals offered physicians incentives to refer patients. Some hospitals, particularly in rural areas, offered physicians practice privileges and induced them to relocate in the vicinity with financial support. To assure physicians that they would have a financially viable practice, hospitals guaranteed their income for the first three years; if the physician earned less than the guaranteed amount, the hospital paid the difference. Hospital contracts with these physicians typically stated that in return for these income guarantees, physicians would refer all their patients to the hospital.[29] Today, hospitals offer subsidies but cannot legally require physicians to refer patients in return. In the 1990s, some hospitals prohibited physicians with practice privileges from referring patients to competitors.[30]

Some hospitals created *physician-bonding* programs, which subsidized physicians' payment for office space on their campus and supplied staff assistance, dictation and billing services, and other support. Hospitals attempted to become "indispensable" in order to strengthen their hold on physicians.[31] The Anti-Kickback Act prohibits many subsidies. But in 2006, regulations exempted from Anti-Kickback prosecution hospitals that donate technology to physicians for electronic medical record, prescribing, scheduling, and billing.[32]

Hospitals formed joint ventures with physicians to provide ancillary services or ambulatory surgery in order to dissuade them from offering these services independently. Consultants recommended these ventures to hospitals as a way to "harmonize" the incentives of physicians with the interests of the hospital. The Stark law and stricter enforcement of the Anti-Kickback Act reduced the use of joint ventures in the 1990s.

Employing physicians in ambulatory facilities allowed hospitals to receive patient referrals without risk of legal liability. The employers forbade their physician employees from competing with them by supplying ancillary services or forming joint ventures with other hospitals. Most hospital-owned physician practices were unsuccessful. Many hospitals had purchased primary care practices, but they yielded fewer referrals than specialists. Physician employees were less productive than when self-employed. Later, many hospitals sold primary care practices because they were unprofitable.

Cost-Containment, Cost Shifting, and Collection

In 1983, Medicare started to pay hospitals based on each patient's diagnosis, rather than the length of hospital stay or volume of services supplied, in order to create an incentive for hospitals to reduce expenses. However, self-employed physicians, who are paid separately and lack incentives to reduce hospital costs, make clinical decisions that affect hospitals. So hospitals created financial incentives and administrative rules to change physicians' behavior.

In 1985, the Paracelsus Health Care Corporation, a for-profit hospital chain, paid physicians between 10 percent and 20 percent of any surplus it earned from each of their Medicare patients, comparing the cost of treating each patient with what Medicare paid. When Congress learned about this practice, it prohibited such payments. However, industry lobbying ensured that the legislation did not prohibit sharing profit or loss across a physician group or physicians sharing profit or loss across a patient group.

Hospitals changed physician practice in other ways as well. Some instituted *economic credentialing;* they revised medical staff bylaws to allow them to deny or revoke privileges of physicians who generated high hospital costs.[33] Hospitals that employed physicians varied compensation to reward cost control. Many hospitals created profiles for each physician that revealed the costs of treating their patients. Profiles documented patients' length of hospital stay, tests, and other expenditures. Managers sent physicians a chart that compared their patients' costs with those for other physicians' patients. Some managers publicized each physician's profile to all medical staff, hoping to enlist peer pressure to change practice.

Incentives to cut expenses translated into harsher policies for patients without means. Previously, insurers reimbursed hospitals full costs, and overhead included charity care and unpaid bills. In effect, insured patients subsidized uncompensated care. However, when insurers sought to pay only for their patients, hospitals could not shift costs. Medicare also reduced cost shifting by paying a standard fee for each patient, and many state Medicaid programs cut payment rates. As hospitals' surpluses declined, so did their ability to fund uncompensated care.

When states stopped regulating hospital charges in the 1980s, hospitals could charge rates as high as they wished. In practice, they negotiated payment with insurers individually. Managed care organizations with a large market share obtained discounts. When insurers did not increase reimbursement and hospitals raised rates, patients paid larger copayments. No one negotiated discounts for uninsured patients.

Unable to shift costs, some hospitals transferred uninsured patients to public hospitals. Humana, Inc., made this policy official.[34] Even charitable hospitals dumped patients. Hospitals' denial of emergency services created scandals that led Congress to enact the Emergency Medical Treatment and Labor Act in 1986.[35] It required hospitals that receive Medicare or Medicaid funds to screen and stabilize all patients who come to the emergency room. However, Congress allocated no funds to pay hospitals, so they still have incentives to dump uninsured patients despite the liability risk.

Furthermore, hospitals can collect payment from emergency room patients after they are treated. Sometimes hospitals used harsh tactics to collect unpaid bills. They attached wages, repossessed cars, placed liens on property, foreclosed mortgages; they charged very high interest rates on unpaid bills. Some hospitals sought court orders called "body attachments," or "writs of capias," for the arrest of debtors who missed court hearings. These individuals remained in prison until they posted bail and paid a fine. When the *Wall Street Journal* exposed these practices in 2003, hospitals said

that Medicare policies required them to attempt to collect in full. In the wake
of publicity, Congress held hearings, lawyers filed class action lawsuits, and
Medicare revised its policy. The problem persists, however, and medical bills
are a prime cause of bankruptcy for individuals in the United States.[36]

While incentives encouraged supplying fewer services in hospitals, other
incentives promoted the growth of spending and services outside of hospitals, undermining the goal of controlling total spending.

Conversions and Consolidation

Although not-for-profit hospitals differ from for-profit hospitals, market competition created pressure for them to adopt similar strategies to generate revenue and cut expenses, including creating physician incentives that engender conflicts of interest. For-profit hospitals contended that not-for-profit
hospitals competed unfairly because the monetary value of their charity care
was less valuable than their tax subsidy. Some states revoked the tax exemption of a few not-for-profit hospitals, adding to their financial problems.[37]

When a charitable hospital's survival is jeopardized, state regulators can
allow it to convert into a for-profit firm. The hospital's assets must remain
for charitable use, so typically a for-profit entity purchases the assets and its
payment funds a charitable foundation. Between 1980 and 1993, 137 not-for
profit hospitals converted into for-profit facilities. Seeking to reduce their
expenses, some local governments divested their public hospitals, converting 241 into not-for-profit organizations and 89 into for-profit firms.[38]

Fiscal constraints led hospitals to form multi-hospital systems. For-profit
hospitals did so first. Not-for-profit hospitals followed, in order to purchase
supplies at bulk prices and obtain other benefits available to larger enterprises; they soon owned the majority of beds in multi-hospital systems.
These changes reduced local control and promoted more businesslike practices. In 1980, nearly one-third of community hospitals were part of a multi-
hospital system and nearly 80 percent shared services with other hospitals.
By 2002, there were 321 hospitals or integrated health care subsystems: 265
not-for-profit (56 religious, 209 secular); 51 investor owned; and 5 owned by
the federal government.[39]

INSURANCE

Conversion

The Blues were a cornerstone of the protected market that benefited physicians. They did little to control hospital and physician fees and did not stem

their subscribers' rising premiums and copayments. When commercial insurers competed with the Blues by risk selection, the Blues moved away from community rating and adopted other business practices of commercial insurers. Sylvia Law raised questions about the transformation of the Blues in her 1976 book, *Blue Cross: What Went Wrong?* By the 1980s, commercial insurers argued that tax exemption gave the Blues an unfair competitive advantage. Some scholars questioned whether the tax exemption was the best way to fund medical insurance, and others asked whether the Blues still deserved it. Congress repealed federal tax exemption for the Blues in 1986, but taxed them at lower rates than for-profit insurers if they had low financial reserves.[40]

Once the Blues paid taxes, there was no need for them to remain not-for-profit, and by 1997 two Blue Cross plans (WellPoint in California, and WellChoice in New York) had converted into for-profit firms. Blue Cross directors that sought to become for-profit argued that it was necessary to obtain capital to compete with commercial firms. Critics noted that not-for-profit organizations could raise funds by issuing tax-exempt bonds and charged that directors favored converting because they would earn enormous profits from stock options in the new firm.[41]

Consumer advocates often intervened to stop conversions or ensure that for-profit firms did not underpay for assets. When Blue Cross of California converted, it appraised its assets at $100 million. Consumers Union assessed the assets independently and found they were worth much more. Eventually, they were sold to WellPoint for $3.2 billion, creating two of America's largest charitable foundations, the California Endowment and the California HealthCare Foundation. By 2004, four plans that cover over a quarter of all Blue enrollees were for-profit.[42] Some not-for-profit Blues created for-profit subsidiaries. A 2004 state audit of Pennsylvania's Blue Cross revealed that it had amassed over $6 billion in reserves, more than $2 billion in for-profit subsidiaries.[43] Such arrangements blurred the distinction between not-for-profits and for-profits.

Health maintenance organizations (HMOs), initially mostly not-for-profit, became largely for-profit. For-profit HMOs grew rapidly because most offered an open provider network that consumers wanted and cut fixed costs by not owning facilities or employing physicians. Some not-for-profit HMOs also converted to for-profit enterprises. For-profit firms enrolled 12 percent of HMO members in1981 and over 63 percent by 2000.[44]

Managing Risk and Resource Use

By 1990, 38 percent of insured employees were enrolled in managed care organizations (MCOs), which were designed to reduce the use of medical resources. These organizations earned profits by reducing provider pay-ment, cutting unnecessary services and, perversely, by reducing beneficial services. Economist Uwe Reinhardt called them *bounty hunters*.[45] The MCOs managed resource use by having primary care physicians serve as gate-keepers, developing practice guidelines, and conducting utilization review. Some MCOs deemed their guidelines proprietary and did not disclose them. By 1997, 75 major organizations had over 1,800 practice guidelines.[46] Indem-nity insurers also adopted utilization review.

Managed care organizations gave physicians incentives to limit services through *risk sharing*, which varied their compensation based on the cost of their patient care. Sometimes MCOs reserved part of physician payment to cover shortfalls if the cost of designated services exceeded a specified level. Alternatively, MCOs paid physicians a bonus if treatment costs were lower than specified. Risk sharing made physicians financially responsible for their medical management. But it also made them assume insurance risk, because their income declined when their patients had higher rates of illness than the population average.

A 1987 study found that 85 percent of HMOs used risk sharing, typically placing as much as 20 to 30 percent of physician compensation at risk.

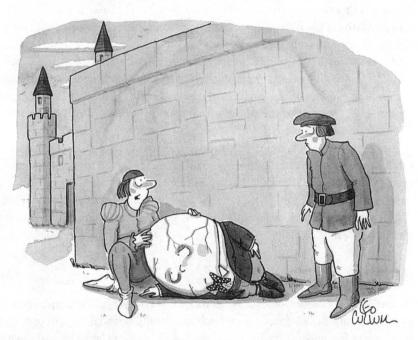

"He's in an H.M.O. Get some of the King's horses and a few of the King's men."

Leo Cullum/The New Yorker Collection; source: © www.cartoonbank.com.

Some group practices entered into *full-risk* capitation contracts with MCOs. They received all premium revenue earmarked for medical services and assumed full responsibility for organizing and paying for medical care; the MCO retained a portion of premiums for marketing and administration. Other physician groups created their own MCOs, called provider-sponsored networks, or captive insurance companies. They hoped to earn income that otherwise flowed to third parties and gain clinical autonomy.[47]

Most MCOs shared financial risk with group practices that spread responsibility across many physicians. However, some MCOs shared financial risk with small physician groups or individual physicians, strengthening links between individual physicians' treatment choices and their compensation. Critics warned that patient care would suffer. In 1996, Medicare regulations required that MCOs have stop-loss protection.[48] Since then, MCOs can place no more than 25 percent of a physician's income at risk without the MCO limiting the physician's loss for treatment of any individual patient.

Surveying the research literature in 1996, Fred Hellinger found that "in virtually every study, measures of utilization . . . were lower when physicians faced incentives to control their use of resources." Incentives to reduce costs may be a useful antidote to fee-for-service payment and indemnity insurance. However, Dr. Lawrence Casalino, who conducts research on medical outcome and effectiveness, notes that MCOs "may provide health care at relatively low cost . . . because they ration services." Economist James Robinson, who usually celebrates health care markets, writes that "capitation . . . creates undesirable incentives for physicians to err on the side of withholding potentially beneficial care."[49] He favors blending payment methods to balance incentives to control costs with incentives to provide services. But blended payment can also create multiple conflicts of interest that operate simultaneously.[50]

Since the late 1990s, many payers have used some mix of fee-for-service, salary, capitation, and risk sharing. Still, combining insurance risk and medical management in physician compensation was fraught with difficulties. By the end of the 1990s, most physician groups opted for partial risk sharing rather than full-risk capitation.[51] The use of capitation payment has also decreased since 2000.

Managed Care Backlash

In the 1990s, exposés of MCOs' denial of services became staple news stories. Highly visible innovations, such as limiting hospital stays to twenty-four hours for normal births, galvanized a public backlash. In response, MCOs offered statistics showing that their members fared well, but data were no match for the visceral impact of images of MCOs booting new mothers out of hospitals to save a few bucks. The press also publicized MCO payment incentives for physicians to reduce services. Rather than rely on experts, the public judged quality for itself and supported regulation. The AMA believed that MCOs restricted physicians' income and clinical freedom, so it supported consumer groups.[52] Previously it had lobbied to restrict physician malpractice liability; now it championed bills to allow patients to sue MCOs for lost income, pain, and suffering.

Forty-seven states adopted legislation establishing a patient bill of rights.[53] These laws allow patients to appeal any denial of services that an MCO deems unnecessary or experimental. Independent physicians decide the appeals, and MCOs must supply the services that reviewers find necessary. The laws often allow patients to consult certain specialists without referrals and to see physicians outside the MCO network in certain circumstances. Managed care organizations must supply sufficient providers close to patients to ensure accessible medical care and disclose whatever physician incentives they use. Patients injured by poor medical care can often sue MCOs for damages; MCOs must allow birthing mothers and women receiving mastectomies to remain hospitalized for a designated period.

In 2001, both houses of Congress passed bills similar to state patients' rights laws. They were directed at the more than half of employees who receive health benefits through plans regulated by the federal Employment Retirement Income Security Act instead of state law. Differences between the bills were never reconciled and the legislation died. The backlash cooled, and political attention shifted after 9/11. However, the reforms in 2010 gave all patients the right to appeal denials of coverage when their insurer claimed medical care was unnecessary or experimental.

State legislation and markets led MCOs to reduce gatekeeping, utilization review, and risk sharing, and to broaden provider networks. In 2001, economist James Robinson heralded "the end of managed care." Yet, private insurers promoted managed care to oversee drug and behavioral health benefits. In addition, over 69 percent of Medicaid recipients were in MCOs at the beginning of 2009. Since 2005, Medicare has promoted managed care plans; in 2008 nearly a quarter of Medicare beneficiaries enrolled in managed care plans. And 40 percent added drug benefits through stand-alone managed care drug plans.[54]

PHARMACEUTICAL FIRM INFLUENCE

The symbiosis between the pharmaceutical industry and the medical profession, forged during the postwar period, has become stronger since 1980. Obtaining a prescription from a physician is the necessary for patients to obtain medication. However, the process of marketing medication spans drug development to dispensing. Drug firms systematically deepened their financial ties to physicians and influenced medication choices at eight critical junctures, including:

- research on drug safety and effectiveness;
- Food and Drug Administration (FDA) review of drug safety and effectiveness;
- publication in medical journals;
- development of practice guidelines;
- insurer and hospital drug formulary choices;
- continuing medical education;
- views of opinion leaders and medical societies;
- physician prescribing.[55]

Research

Legislation encouraged joint ventures between industry and universities to develop commercial applications of research. The 1980 Bayh-Dole Act allowed research institutions to retain patent rights on products of federally funded research if they shared royalties with the inventor. Industry-funded university research grew from $200 million in 1980 to over $2 billion in 2000, when commercial interests funded 62 percent of biomedical research. Patents from joint industry-university research multiplied from 250–400 per year before 1980 to 3,000–4,800 per year by the end of the 1990s.[56] Researchers estimated commercial firms funded $58.6 billion for all U.S. biomedical research in 2007, 58 percent of the total.[57]

Joint ventures between drug companies and medical schools to commercialize research findings created institutional conflicts of interest. Universities often had a stake in a product while overseeing researchers who evaluated it. By 1990, more than 100 universities funded firms to commercialize faculty research.[58] Most made only small investments in joint ventures, but there were significant exceptions.

In 1975, Boston University (BU) invested heavily in Seragen, created to commercialize the drug Interleukin 2, developed by one of its professors. By 1987, BU had invested a substantial portion of its endowment, and the president and members of the board of trustees also invested as individuals. The company, in turn, funded university research on drug development. The Massachusetts attorney general intervened to ensure that the trustees fulfilled their fiduciary obligations, diversified the university endowment portfolio, and took steps to ensure that conflicts of interest did not compromise university-company relations. The company was not successful, and in

1998 the *New York Times* reported that the value of the university's investment had plummeted.[59]

By 2000, drug firms funded 70 percent of clinical drug trials, allowing
them to influence the questions posed, research design, protocol, and
methods.[60] By funding research, drug companies control the evidence that
the FDA uses to decide whether to approve drugs for sale, creating the risk
that it will approve drugs that harm patients or be ineffective. They influence the formation of practice guidelines, insurer coverage decisions, and
the choice of drugs included in formularies.

Of the seventy-seven most frequently cited controlled trials from 1994 to
2003, sixty-five received industry funding; eighteen of the thirty-two most
cited studies in 1999 were entirely industry funded. Numerous studies
demonstrate that industry-funded research tends to reach conclusions
that favor the funder.[61] A study of publications from 1980 to 2000 revealed
that industry-sponsored research was 3.6 times more likely to produce
results favorable to the sponsor than other studies. Drug firms buried unfa-
vorable results, published favorable findings multiple times, and forbade
researchers from publishing results without permission.[62]

Food and Drug Administration Review

Drug companies have ties with physicians who serve on FDA advisory committees. The FDA does not police these conflicts well.[63] These ties are not as
dramatic as those brought to light in 1960, when Dr. Henry Welch, head of
the FDA antibiotics division, earned substantial income as editor of an antibiotics promotion journal. Nevertheless, they compromise the review of
applications to approve new drugs and review of safety of drugs on the market. Moreover, since 1992, drug companies have paid the FDA user fees to
permit it to hire additional personnel to expedite their drug review.[64] Drug
company payment to the FDA increased their influence and reduced the
FDA's ability to insist that firms meet a high standard of proof that drugs
are safe and effective.

Publication in Medical Journals

Medical journal articles are also compromised by conflicts of interest.[65]
Many authors of medical articles have financial conflicts of interest that they
are supposed to disclose, but studies show that they frequently conceal
them. Moreover, disclosure does not eliminate bias.[66] Neither does peer
review. Dr. John Abramson provides a careful analysis of two articles published in *NEJM* and the *Journal of the American Medical Association* that
claim statins significantly reduce stroke risk although their data and other

literature did not support that conclusion. Both journals published reviews that suggested Celebrex and Vioxx were safer than ibuprofen for treating pain when both drugs posed greater risk of cardiac death and the FDA had warned producers their safety claims were misleading.[67]

Dependent on drug companies for advertising revenue, medical journals are vulnerable to their influence. In 1992, after the *Annals of Internal Medicine* published a study exposing misleading drug advertisements, drug firms reduced advertising in the journal for several months. In 2004, the journal *Dialysis Transplantation* dropped an editorial that questioned a drug's efficacy because, the editor reports, he was "overruled" by the marketing department.[68]

Drug companies ghostwrite articles, drafting manuscripts favorable to their products and then paying physicians to submit them for publication. Dr. Troyen Brennan of Harvard University reported in a 1994 article that he was offered payment merely to sign his name. In 2005, the *Wall Street Journal* exposed medical ghostwriters who advertise their services and listed articles published under others' names. In 2008, a study of litigation documents revealed that individuals employed by Merck drafted dozens of articles about its drug Vioxx, which was found to have serious side effects these articles concealed. Court documents made public in 2009 revealed that Wyeth paid ghostwriters to produce twenty-six papers advocating post-menopausal hormone replacement therapy.[69]

Practice Guidelines

Drug companies create financial ties with physicians who serve on committees that develop guidelines. A 2002 study found that drug companies who produced relevant medications had financial ties to 59 percent of physicians who drafted forty-four clinical practice guidelines for ten diseases. The physicians received payment for speaking or consulting, were given grants, or owned shares in the firm. Another study revealed drug company ties with physicians who served on panels that developed the *Diagnostic and Statistical Manual of Mental Disorders*. Other research documents extensive drug company funding of specialty societies that develop practice guidelines. They supply the main funding for these societies through so-called education grants and fund "pamphlets, books, web sites, registries, and quality initiatives"; they also purchase advertising and exhibit space at these societies' professional meetings.[70]

Formulary Choices

Insurers and hospitals develop drug formularies that limit physician choices, in part to prevent inappropriate prescribing because of the influence of drug firms. In order to ensure that their drugs are preferred, drug companies try to influence physicians who serve on committees that make formulary decisions. They offer physicians grants, consulting contracts, gifts, or kickbacks. Tap Pharmaceuticals offered a physician on an HMO formulary committee a $50,000 unrestricted grant in return for his help in placing their drug on his HMO's formulary. More typically, drug firms make grants first and then ask the recipient for favors, and then cut support if the physician does not reciprocate. Studies reveal that physicians who receive drug firm support request that their funder's drug be added to a formulary more than other physicians.[71]

Continuing Medical Education

Drug firms have long disseminated misleading product information and blurred the distinction between advertising and education to influence prescribing. Symposia, lectures, and conferences are often called educational, but most of these activities are unaccredited. Even in 2006, less than 9 percent of the nearly 500,000 physician meetings and symposia in the country were accredited as continuing medical education. Pharmaceutical companies were closely associated with 89 percent of these meetings.[72]

Furthermore, in the 1980s, drug firms expanded their funding of accredited CME providers as part of their drug promotion. When the AMA and six other organizations formed the Accreditation Council for Continuing Medical Education (ACCME) in 1980, there were only a few commercial CME providers (called medical education and communication firms or medical education service suppliers). Since then, their numbers have soared: 10 commercial providers had been accredited by 1990, 68 by 2000, and 158 by 2006.[73] Medical schools and medical societies competed with for-profit firms for CME revenue.

By 1980, eight states required CME for physicians to maintain licenses, and forty-four states did by 2008.[74] Eager to avoid footing the bill, physicians accepted company-sponsored CME. States did not set curricular requirements, so drug firm funding determines the topics offered; these firms support seminars on medical conditions that their drugs are used to treat.[75] The ACCME standards place some constraints on CME providers, but in the early years these were minimal. Today, ACCME attempts to reduce industry bias in CME, but it is an uphill struggle.

Supplying CME is lucrative. In 2007, physician membership organizations earned profits of 32 percent and commercial CME providers earned profits of 26 percent. Industry spending on CME is substantial: $302 million in 1998, over $1.71 billion in 2004 (with another $197 million for CME advertising and exhibits), and over $2.5 billion in 2007. In 2008, pharmaceutical firms, medical device manufacturers, and other businesses supplied 71 percent of income for commercial CME providers, over 59 percent of CME income from medical schools, and over 47 percent of income for physician membership organizations.[76] Drug firms typically paid physicians' CME expenses for registration, travel, and lodging until AMA and the Pharmaceutical Research and Manufacturer's Association (PhRMA) declared the practice unacceptable in 1990. Despite the guidelines, in 2004, over a quarter of physicians reported that commercial firms paid their personal CME expenses.[77]

Senate hearings in 1990 documented the use of CME to market drugs. David Jones, former vice president of Abbot Laboratories and former CIBA-GEIBY executive director for government and public affairs, testified that "medical education today is now determined by what the marketing department wants." "Promotion disguised as education is sponsored by bogus organizations" on behalf of marketing departments and routinely promotes "unapproved and unproven" drug uses. Furthermore, "Doctors . . . are recruited to publish helpful articles which are produced by company medical writers who assure that the marketing messages are featured."[78]

In 1997, the FDA concluded that some drug companies used CME to promote drugs. They changed the text of presentations, over faculty objection, in order to market products, and linked educational grants to hospitals placing their drug on its formulary. They used CME programs to promote unapproved drug uses. Some programs recommended calcium channel blockers, approved to control arrhythmia, for use after heart attacks; this off-label use resulted in tens of thousands of deaths according to the FDA.[79] These practices continue. GlaxoSmithKlein sells Valtrex, the leading herpes drug. Although not approved for neonatal herpes, in 2006 GlaxoSmithKlein funded a CME program that advocated testing pregnant women for genital herpes to treat neonatal herpes, and a study found that 20 percent of its prescriptions are for unapproved uses.[80]

Drug companies publicly maintained that CME providers were independent, but one individual reports that these companies sometimes refer to CME providers as their "agency," the same term they use to refer to medical communication companies who develop promotional and advertising materials."[81] Moreover, CME providers traditionally sought funds from one firm per program, because, as a manager of a CME provider explained to me, drug firms believed a provider supported by two or more firms with competing drugs would have a conflict of interest.[82]

Studies demonstrate that CME funding creates bias in programs. Researchers who reviewed two courses on calcium channel blockers used to treat high blood pressure and angina in the mid-1980s, each funded by a firm that sold them, found that speakers in these courses made more positive statements about the CME funder's drug than about other drugs. Other research showed that physicians increased prescribing of the CME's funder's drugs after a course. Physicians who attended hospital grand rounds of a physician employed by a drug company later prescribed the firm's drugs more frequently for inappropriate as well as appropriate uses.[83]

In 2001, CME providers that solicited grants proclaimed they helped market drugs. One firm's Web page said it creates "educational programs . . . designed to gain a higher rate of acceptance at the launch of a new product and to increase return on investment."[84] Until the OIG promulgated Anti-Kickback Act compliance guidelines in 2003, drug firms often directed the CME programs they funded.[85] They chose CME faculty, with whom they had significant financial ties, and supplied them with slides and written materials.

Documents from a lawsuit settled in 2005 reveal Parke-Davis's use of CME to market Neurontin. Four years after its introduction, 90 percent of its prescriptions were for unapproved uses.[86] Parke-Davis funded studies on unapproved drug uses but only publicized favorable results. It hired medical education companies to produce articles, review papers, and write letters to medical journals that advocated unapproved uses and paid physicians to sign as the authors. It sponsored studies as a means to teach physicians drug doses for unapproved uses. Then it made grants to a firm for CME while employing it to market Neurontin. Parke-Davis employees met with the CME provider to develop the curriculum, and CME faculty advocated unapproved drug uses.

Opinion Leaders, Medical Societies and Physician Prescribing

Drug companies employ and support physicians who are opinion leaders among their peers.[87] They hire medical school department chairs and other prominent physicians to promote their products at conferences and to the press, even arranging their speaking engagements. Eventually, such blatant conflicts of interest attracted public criticism, but they persist.

In addition, drug firms spend large sums on official promotion: between $28 billion and 58.5 billion in 2004, according to various sources. They employ representatives to develop personal relations with physicians and lubricate these relations with gifts that facilitate access to physicians, generate goodwill, and beget physician reciprocity. Physicians who meet with detailers increase nonrational prescribing, prescribe new drugs more rapidly, and decrease generic drug prescriptions.[88]

Drug firms still pay physicians kickbacks. Senate hearings in 1990 revealed in-kind payments based on the number and cost of drugs prescribed. Roche Pharmaceuticals paid physicians $1,200 for each patient started on a

third-generation antibiotic, Rocephin. For physicians who used their vaccine, Connaught Laboratories awarded them points toward computers,
VCRs, or televisions. Wyeth Ayerst awarded 1,000 frequent flyer airline
miles for every patient started on its drug, Inderal LA. In the fall of 2010,
Genetech, owned by Roche pharmaceuticals, offered rebates to some ophthalmologists who prescribe and inject in patients their drug Lucentis,
approved to treat macular degeneration. According to the *New York Times*,
physicians can earn tens of thousands of dollars each quarter from the
rebates by their substituting Lucentis for alternative drugs that work just
as well, and this could raise Medicare costs hundreds of millions of
dollars a year. The rebates, which may be legal, also encourage doctors to
recommend more frequent doses and to use the Lucentis for unapproved
uses.[89]

Post-marketing clinical trials allow drug companies to pay physicians for
every patient who receives a drug in return for their filling out simple forms.
Often the aim is to get physicians to switch drug brands. Today, drug firms
also fund sophisticated randomized trials that pay physicians to prescribe
drugs.[90] These blatant conflicts of interest are widely known, but tolerated,
even though the harm that inappropriate prescribing does to patients is
sometimes the subject of scandal.

CONCLUSION

Physicians decide what services and therapies patients receive, who provides the services, and in what setting. As a result, physicians allocate
income through their clinical choices. Market logic heightened the effects of
arrangements that create physicians' conflicts of interest. Hospitals,
insurers, drug firms, and firms selling other medical services all understood
that physicians' decisions controlled their financial success. They sought
out physicians for joint ventures and created incentives to align physician
financial interests with their own.

Physicians' conflicts of interest grew because the state placed relatively
few legal restraints on physician entrepreneurial activities while the complex
medical economy generated an increasingly wide variety of opportunities.
Some were created by new ways of supplying services and organizing practice, finance, and insurance arrangements, or changes in public policy;
others emerged from the growth of medical knowledge and technology.
Physician entrepreneurship blossomed in group practices and in partnership with lay-owned or lay-directed not-for-profit and for-profit entities. Even
employers sometimes rewarded physician employees who boosted income
or cut expenses. Physicians and medical organizations tapped resources

from drug firms, which liberally funded medical activities in order to influence prescribing.

When managed care or governmental programs oversaw physicians or restricted certain entrepreneurial practices, they did so selectively. As public policy tried to control spending, it rewarded insurers for cutting resource use. In response, insurers oversaw medical practice, changed its organization, and restricted physician incentives and opportunities to supply services. Insurers also enlisted physicians as economic partners. Physicians profited by restricting services and resource use.

Policy makers had consciously created incentives to channel the entrepreneurial instincts of physicians and laymen. Ironically, some measures that helped cope with conflicts of interest from fee-for-service and private practice created new ones in their place. Although their aim was to create incentives to promote desirable goals, the incentives were never well enough honed to avoid unanticipated and undesirable effects.

7

Coping with Physicians' Conflicts of Interest in the United States

ALTERNATIVE APPROACHES

The United States copes with physicians' conflicts of interest through three approaches that interact: (1) professional and industry self-regulation, (2) managed care, and (3) law.

The American Medical Association (AMA) and state medical societies exercised significant de facto authority over medical practice for the first three-quarters of the twentieth century. They restricted some activities that create conflicts of interest but neglected many others and opposed controls that mitigate conflicts of interest. Moreover, the AMA allied itself financially with the pharmaceutical industry and increased conflicts of interest from physician ties to drug firms.

Prepaid group practices (PPGPs) emerged during the 1930s as an alternative to entrepreneurial practice and a means to expand access to medicine, although organized medicine stymied their growth. But in the 1970s, policy makers turned to PPGPs to control medical costs and promoted health maintenance organizations (HMOs). HMOs, however, included not only not-for-profit organizations that employed physicians but also for-profit firms that contracted with self-employed physicians and facilitated physician entrepreneurship. Health maintenance organizations and related entities, collectively called managed care organizations (MCOs), curbed fee-for-service conflicts of interest by changing physician incentives and by applying administrative controls. Yet many MCOs also created incentives to cut services, a new conflict of interest.

State policies are shaped by the contest for power among different economic and political groups seeking to protect and advance their interests. The bureaucratic state oversees relations among interest groups and sets rules within which the economy and politics function. Organized medicine and commercial interests sometimes promote legislation but other times oppose it, and always attempt to influence its implementation.

Since 1975, state action has dismantled many policies that protected physicians and organized medicine. Antitrust law ended organized medicine's control over markets and that allowed MCOs and other insurers to become countervailing powers. The state also regulated insurers and medical practice directly. Courts, legislatures and regulatory agencies then addressed physicians' conflicts of interest. Sometimes they complemented managed care; at other times they oversaw the conflicts of interest that MCOs created. As public oversight increased, organized medicine and trade associations for MCOs and pharma developed voluntary guidelines and proposed legal standards that tolerated many conflicts of interest. Sometimes the state adopted these ineffective standards.

Professional and Industry Self-Regulation

In the early twentieth century, organized medicine held that when employed by laypersons, physicians compromised their professional independence. Its ethical code condemned firms that employed physicians to care for their employees and lay-owned firms that employed physicians to provide medical services to the public. These policies curbed employment conflicts of interest but fostered physician entrepreneurship with its conflicts of interest.

The AMA maintained that insurers should not control physician payment or clinical choices and adopted insurance principles that precluded national health insurance (NHI), PPGPs, and private insurance that paid physicians directly rather than reimbursing patients' expenses.[1] These policies delayed the emergence of insurers as a countervailing power. Without oversight by third-party payers or the state, conflicts of interest neglected by organized medicine proliferated.

Until the mid-1950s, the AMA ethical code restricted many entrepreneurial activities. But it distinguished between acceptable and unacceptable entrepreneurship, which allowed many conflicts of interest to thrive. The AMA prohibited physicians from owning pharmacies but not hospitals or clinics that dispense drugs and ancillary services. It condemned fee splitting and inducements for referrals but not group practices that share income and profit from referrals within the group. It recognized that capitation payment discourages providing services but not that fee-for-service increases their provision. Most important, the AMA failed to acknowledge the entrepreneurship inherent in most private practice, which had become a cornerstone of American medicine and enjoyed social legitimacy.

The AMA always had difficulty enforcing its code because it represents physicians, a role that clashes with implanting policies that restrict their income. In the 1950s, however, members convinced the AMA to drop many restrictions.[2] The revised code allowed physicians to own pharmacies and drug companies and to dispense medicine. The AMA then opposed new drug regulation, ceased its oversight of drug marketing, and boosted its income through increased drug advertising. Since then, the AMA and pharma have developed professional and industry self-regulation in tandem, usually to resist oversight and limits on activities that generate income.

Following Medicare's enactment, the AMA lost its ability to control the medical economy.[3] Rising public spending gave the state a reason to regulate medical payment and practice, while oversight of Medicare and Medicaid supplied the means. The HMO Act of 1973 struck down the AMA's prohibition on PPGPs and positively promoted them. In 1979, the Federal Trade Commission required the AMA to end its ethical prohibition on physician advertising and employment.[4] Thereafter, the AMA lacked meaningful sanctions or the ability to control practice. In the 1980s, public policy promoted markets in medical services and insurance, which further reduced the AMA's power.

In response, the AMA used advocacy to influence policy. Starting with its 1986 report on conflicts of interest, the AMA developed guidelines on physician self-referral, drug firm gifts, and physician incentives.[5] It opposed regulation of physicians and pharma, arguing that professional codes adequately addressed conflicts of interest. Today, AMA ethical guidelines serve contradictory aims: they discourage certain practices, but they also stave off government regulation so physicians can engage in these very activities.

Managed Care

Managed care changed financing and organization in ways that countered conflicts of interest arising from fee-for-service payment and from activities that encouraged physicians to recommend services. Most PPGPs and staff-model HMOs employed physicians, so physicians could not boost their income by increasing services and tests or dispensing drugs. They lacked incentives to make clinical choices that cut costs and had few or no financial ties to third parties that could influence their prescriptions and referrals. These organizations minimized employment conflicts of interest because they were not-for-profit, had a public service mission, and gave physicians broad clinical discretion and relatively secure employment.[6]

In independent practice association (IPA) HMOs and preferred provider organizations (PPOs), by contrast, physicians remained self-employed, retained entrepreneurial incentives, and were usually paid fee-for-service or by capitation. To control costs, these MCOs varied physicians' compensation based on how well they managed medical resources. In effect, physicians partnered with insurers and profited by cutting costs; this created new conflicts of interest. Today, MCOs have policies to check underuse of services because laws, federal programs, and private accreditation organizations require them.

Managed care organizations also countered incentives to increase services by supervising medical practice. Primary care physicians oversaw each patient's medical care and acted as gatekeepers whose referral was needed for access to specialists or hospitals. MCOs developed guidelines for cost-effective treatment and promoted compliance by monitoring physicians. Utilization reviewers could deny authorization for medical care that falls outside their guidelines.

In principle, practice guidelines, gatekeeping, and utilization review can serve as alternatives to financial incentives that create conflicts of interest. Whether they do so depends on the aims and content of practice guidelines, which vary. In practice, administrative controls and financial incentives often work in tandem. For example, many MCO primary care physician-gatekeepers bear financial risk for the cost of treating their patients. Thus, MCO oversight reinforces financial conflicts of interest.

Organizations seldom develop guidelines through a process that ensures public accountability. They rarely disclose the basis for their standards and many say their guidelines are proprietary and confidential. Guidelines may reflect typical practice and hold individual physicians accountable to group norms. Alternatively, when based on expert opinion or evaluations of medical practice, guidelines can change norms. Some guidelines recommend treatment only when benefits exceed costs. Others limit expenses regardless of the clinical benefit. Rather than being neutral, guidelines reflect the value choices and conflicts of interest of those who create them.[7]

Managed care organizations turned to pharmaceutical benefit managers (PBMs) to control drug spending, and PBMs supervised over 60 percent of all retail drug prescriptions in 1998. The process illustrates how MCOs address physicians' conflicts of interest.

Pharmaceutical benefit managers establish a formulary, which limits drugs that patients can receive and may offer only one drug in a therapeutic class. Some PBMs substitute generic for brand-name drugs, or one brand for another; others require that physicians receive their permission before using a brand-name drug when a generic is available. Both methods curb drug company incentives that lead physicians to prescribe particular brands.[8] Pharmaceutical benefit managers distribute drugs through mail or designated pharmacies, and this precludes physicians from prescribing drugs to earn income from dispensing drugs or referring patients to financially related pharmacies. In addition, PBMs can counter drug firm misinformation by employing pharmacists to meet physicians face-to-face to discuss prescribing, a practice called *counter* or *academic detailing*. It is more effective than simply supplying physicians written material, improves prescribing, and saves money.[9]

However, PBMs often have their own conflicts of interest. Some, such as Merck's Medco, were subsidiaries of drug firms and promoted their drugs. Even when PBMs are independent, they are driven by cost control and marketing, not appropriate drug use. Drug firms negotiate rebates with PBMs, increasing their market share in return for discounts.[10] PBMs can fail to purge from formularies inexpensive drugs that present high risks or are known to be used inappropriately.

Law

Medicare and Medicaid account for about 35 percent of national medical spending and are the prime vehicles for regulation of the medical economy. The Medicare and Medicaid Anti-Kickback Act (Anti-Kickback Act), Stark Law, and Civil Monetary Penalties Law play key roles, complemented by the Food, Drug and Cosmetic Act (FDCA) and tax law. State laws oversee not-for-profit and for-profit corporations, health care institutions, professional licensure and accreditation, insurance, and managed care. Taken together, this patchwork of regulation controls physicians' conflicts of interest only in part, because it sets very modest goals and seldom changes incentives that create conflicts of interest, and because those individuals and organizations it regulates find ways to flout the law's objectives.

State regulation can be divided into three broad categories. The first two address incentives in medical practice: incentives to increase services, and incentives to decrease services. The first supports managed care while the second supplies remedies for problems created by managed care and cost-containment policies. The third category of regulation addresses financial ties between physicians and pharma, medical device firms, and other commercial interests. I examine each category in relation to professional and industry self-regulation and managed care oversight.

LEGAL CONTROLS ON INCENTIVES TO INCREASE SERVICES

Peer and Utilization Review

In 1972, Medicare required hospitals to create physician standard review organizations (PSROs) to assess whether medical services they provided were appropriate. These organizations had hospital medical staff audit admissions and length of stay and determine whether they were justified.

Hospitals had no incentive to cut costs, however, so PSROs produced dismal results, and Congress ended the program in 1982. In its place, Congress created peer review organizations (PROs), which reviewed hospital records to assess quality. Unlike PSROs, PROs could deny payment for unnecessary services and recommend that Medicare exclude doctors with poor quality records.[11] But PROs, like PSRO, did not eliminate overuse of services.

In 1986, Congress reorganized PROs to monitor quality rather than identify unnecessary services, shifting their goal to improving patient outcomes rather than inspection and regulation. In 1992, Medicare redefined PROs' role as providing technical assistance on quality. Later, PROs were renamed quality improvement organizations (QIOs). The Center for Medicare and Medicaid Services (CMS) says that QIOs focus on quality assurance but also assist in enforcement.[12]

State promotion of peer review and utilization review continues with only moderate effects on the overuse of services. Much greater reductions occurred after Medicare replaced cost-plus based hospital payment with prospective payment in 1983. Outside of Medicare, the federal government promoted the use of MCOs with their cost-control incentives. Utilization review was much more effective when MCOs oversaw it because they had an incentive to cut spending and often linked utilization review to physician incentives. Around 2004, the federal government promoted the growth of managed care in Medicare with subsidies. It paid private MCOs on average 14 percent more than it cost to supply services through traditional Medicare, so this increased federal spending.[13]

Ancillary Services, Kickbacks, and Self-Referral

Private practitioners typically can earn income by supplying ancillary services in their practice or by referring patients to facilities in which they share ownership. Physician prescribing of services that increase their income is a major conflict of interest. Here American medicine contrasts starkly with practice in France, where most physicians cannot legally earn income from ancillary services.

American law, however, prohibits some kickbacks and restrict other arrangements that encourage physicians to prescribe ancillary services or refer patients to third parties that supply them. In response to investigations revealing that kickbacks and fraud thrived in Medicare and Medicaid, Congress enacted the Anti-Kickback Act in 1972. Thereafter, regulation resembled a game of cops and robbers. Some providers disguised kickbacks by claiming that payments were for services rendered, or used in-kind payment rather than cash. Amendments in 1977, 1980, and 1987 prohibited covert, indirect, and in-kind payments to induce referrals.[14] As the statute became stricter, firms sought physician investors. Profits provided an incentive to refer patients, but without an explicit payment per referral.

In the 1985 case *U.S. v. Greber*, a federal appeals court held that even if there are legitimate grounds for remuneration, if one purpose is to induce the provision of services, the payer violates the Anti-Kickback Act. This interpretation precludes gifts, physician self-referral, and other practices not previously prosecuted. Providers complained that the amended Anti-Kickback Act jeopardized normal business practices, lobbied for limits on prosecution, and sought guidelines to specify safe business practices. In 1987, Congress directed the Office of Inspector General (OIG) to draft regulations that designate financial practices it would not prosecute.[15] The OIG proposed safe harbors for physician investment in 1989.

By then, Congress had passed legislation that restricted certain physician self-referral. Viewing physician self-referral as producing harm similar to kickbacks, in 1989 Congress passed the Stark Law, which prohibited self-referral for laboratory tests covered by Medicare. In 1993, it extended the Stark Law ban to Medicaid and added eleven service categories: radiology, radiation therapy, durable medical equipment, home health care, physical therapy, rehabilitation services, occupational therapy, speech pathology, parenteral nutrient equipment and supplies, prosthetics, and outpatient prescription drugs. However, the law created over twenty exceptions, the most important of which allowed referrals to group practices, hospitals, clinical labs in rural areas, and publicly traded firms.[16]

The OIG first prosecuted self-referral under the Anti-Kickback Act in a 1991 case, *Inspector General v. the Hanlester Network*. However, the Hanlester arrangement resembled traditional kickbacks more than typical self-referral, so the risks of prosecution for typical arrangements remained uncertain. The 1993 OIG final Anti-Kickback Act regulations specified *safe harbors* for physician investment and supplied further guidance. To be protected, referring physicians cannot collectively own more than 40 percent of the facility or generate more than 40 percent of its revenue in any twelve-month period. Thus the rule protects facilities that would be unprofitable without self-referral, but not those that receive most of their revenue from self-referral.[17]

Several developments gave the state powerful tools to deter conflicts of interest arising from kickbacks. Legislation in 1996 and 1997 allowed government agencies to use a portion of money recouped from Anti-Kickback Act prosecutions to enforce the law. Prosecutors began to combine Stark Law and Anti-Kickback Act lawsuits with charges under the False Claims Act, which triples the fines and funds agencies retain. The law rewards individuals who report evidence of fraud to prosecutors with 25 percent of any settlement when they initiate *Qui Tam* lawsuits.[18] Federal sentencing guidelines created incentives for firms to create compliance programs that promote fraud detection and reporting of misconduct by treating such firms more leniently if an employee violates the law without corporate authority.

LEGAL CONTROLS ON INCENTIVES TO DECREASE SERVICES

Four main strategies help cope with the incentives to reduce services that are built into insurance and physician payment systems. Medicare regulates physician risk sharing. State laws regulate MCOs in several ways; one important rule mandates that when MCOs deny medical treatment on certain grounds, patients can appeal this decision to an independent reviewer. Patients can sue MCOs. Finally, accreditation organizations and laws require MCOs and hospitals to have quality assurance programs. Yet each strategy allows practices that create conflicts of interest with minor changes.

Regulating Risk Sharing

In 1986, Congress prohibited hospitals and HMOs from using *individual* physician incentive payments to reduce services to *individual* Medicare patients. It did not preclude hospital or MCO incentives that reward physicians for reducing costs for a group of patients. Moreover, Congress delayed the law's implementation, during which time MCO lobbying led to amendments. The revised statute prohibited only physician incentives that restrict medically necessary services, which is harder to prove. It required HMOs that place physicians at "substantial financial risk" to provide stop-loss protection. The 1996 risk-sharing regulations required that Medicare HMOs with fewer than 25,000 patients in the risk pool obtain stop-loss insurance for physicians when more than 25 percent of their income is at risk. At that point, physicians cannot bear more than 10 percent of the additional cost of referral services.[19] The regulations also require stop-loss coverage for physician groups (IPAs and group practices) that assume financial risk.

In the 1990s, several hospitals adopted or proposed *gain-sharing* programs, under which the hospital gives physicians a share of hospital savings that come in part from physicians reducing the use of medical suppliers or services, using less expensive products, or changing the manner in which they practice. In 1999, the OIG declared that some gain sharing violates the Anti-Kickback Act and Civil Monetary Penalty law, but in 2000, it said it would not prosecute gain sharing under specified conditions. Institutions must identify and limit cost reduction, limit the amount and duration of the reward, and monitor patient care and quality. Physician earnings must be limited and equally distributed, and patients must be informed that a gain-sharing plan is in place. In 2005, the OIG issued five advisory opinions approving proposed gain-sharing plans.[20]

Independent Review and Other Managed Care Regulation

As public backlash against managed care grew, patient advocates and providers proposed legislation referred to as Patients' Bill of Rights or Patient Protection Laws to regulate MCOs. Forty-seven states enacted such laws and federal legislation in 2010 extended the right nationally to be governed by federal regulations.[21]

Independent review, or *external review*, was a key requirement of these laws. If insurers deny medical care or a specific procedure on the grounds that is not medically necessary or that it is experimental, patients can have an independent physician review the merits of their request. An independent review organization (IRO) chooses the physician to conduct the review. Insurers must pay for medical care if the reviewer judges it necessary. Patient protection laws, however, do not require independent review for disputes over whether insurance policies cover specific services, an area of equal concern. In Medicare, where a review organization examines all denials of service, 65 percent of disputes in 1999 concerned coverage.[22]

Most states require that reviewers have no significant financial ties with the insurer or patient. However, that does not preclude bias. In many states the MCO selects two or three IROs from which the patient chooses. These IROs are likely to favor MCOs over patients because MCOs decide which IRO to employ in the future. Moreover, IROs frequently depend on MCOs for other work: supervising internal appeals and peer review; overseeing quality assurance programs; and designing clinical protocols.

Patient protection laws use four additional strategies to counter underuse of services. They (1) set minimum covered benefits; (2) establish rules to ensure access to physicians; (3) regulate MCO finance, require transparency, allow patients to sue MCOs, and encourage competition; and (4) mandate quality assurance programs. These yield some benefits but treat symptoms rather than the problem's source.

Standard Benefits: Several states require insurers to pay for emergency room visits prompted by symptoms that would have led a prudent patient to seek urgent treatment, even if the examination reveals no emergency. Other states require insurers to pay out-of-network providers for urgent care or if no adequate provider is available within their network. Many states require MCOs to cover a minimum length of hospital stay for childbirths and mastectomies.

Access: Several states set standards for an adequate provider network. Others require that patients have direct access to specialists without gate-keeper approval, particularly for patients with chronic illness and women seeking gynecological or obstetrical care. Some states require that MCOs have an ombudsperson to help patients. States sometimes require that MCOs employ only accredited utilization reviewers.

Financial Regulation, Transparency, Legal Liability, and Competition: Some states establish financial reserve requirements or regulate physician risk sharing. Many require MCOs to disclose information, including measures of patient satisfaction and quality, the provider network, plan operations, performance measures, physician incentives, and utilization review standards. Other states make MCOs liable for negligent decisions regarding patient care coverage or make MCOs potentially liable for their physicians' negligence. Some states preclude MCOs from seeking indemnification from physicians for their liability.

Quality Assurance: Many states require MCOs to have quality assurance programs to check for underuse of services or set other quality standards. Others require that MCOs be accredited.

Court Remedies

Americans turn to courts to resolve vexing policy issues, yet court remedies have proved inadequate to cope with physicians' conflicts of interest. Courts have held that most managed care cost-containment policies are legal.[23] The Supreme Court has held that Congress expressly authorized risk sharing and utilization in the HMO Act of 1973 and acknowledged that HMOs ration medical services to control spending.[24]

Patients can sue MCOs for malpractice, alleging that their risk-sharing incentives caused physicians to deny appropriate treatment or that their utilization review programs denied appropriate medical services.[25] To succeed, plaintiffs must show that the particular incentives or utilization review program violated prevailing norms and so constitutes negligence and also were a proximate cause of their injury. However, the expense of litigation deters lawsuits. Plaintiffs' lawyers are paid only if they win the lawsuit, when they receive a percentage of the award, so they take on cases only when the chance of winning and amount they can recover are high. Only one of every 7.5 hospital patients injured because of negligence files a malpractice claim, and only one of every 15 negligently injured hospital patients is compensated.[26]

Some patients have alleged that utilization review or risk sharing violate the federal Racketeer Influence and Corrupt Organizations Act of 1970 (RICO), or state laws on consumer deception and fraud. Most such lawsuits have been unsuccessful. Other patients have alleged bad faith breach of contract when MCOs have not paid for medical care. This litigation has led MCOs to moderate incentives to reduce services and to balance them with incentives for quality of care.[27]

Would-be plaintiffs face one more barrier. Most lawsuits against insurers based on state laws (including malpractice, bad faith breach of contract, and consumer deception) are unavailable to the more than half of all employees who are covered by employer self-funded benefit plans governed by the Employee Retirement Income Security Act (ERISA). In 1987, the Supreme Court held that ERISA preempts suits for bad faith breach of contract, consumer protection, and other state law remedies. Subsequently, it held that ERISA precludes other tort claims related to denial of benefits.[28]

Some patients have sued MCOs for not disclosing physician risk-sharing incentives. The circuit courts of appeal are split regarding whether ERISA requires disclosure. Requiring MCOs to disclose physician incentives might lead some to end their use. More likely, however, MCOs will reveal the information in ways that discount the risk. Clear disclosure of incentives may enlighten patients, but it will not help individuals choose among MCOs.[29] Because of the complexity of risk sharing, laypeople can rarely determine which of two incentive plans places physicians at greater financial risk. Moreover, disclosure does not increase patient choice. Typically, employers select the health plans or the options among which their employees choose.

Quality Assurance

Monitoring quality of care can help address problems that arise from conflicts of interest. Starting in 1982, Medicare required hospitals to have PROs to monitor quality. However, PROs were designed to detect overuse of services. They can investigate overuse but cannot follow up on patient complaints of underuse. In addition, it is much harder to detect underuse of services than overuse. No record exists for services or tests that might have been, but were not, provided. Some PROs expressed concern about their ability to track underuse.[30] Later, PROs were renamed quality improvement organizations and their function shifted to promoting quality through means other than oversight. Managed care organizations also have quality assurance programs that provide a check on underuse by examining quality measures for the population of patients served and medical outcomes.

However, MCOs have financial incentives to reduce services, which under-cut their vigilance.

LEGAL CONTROLS ON TIES WITH PHARMACEUTICAL OR MEDICAL DEVICE FIRMS AND OTHER SUPPLIERS

Legal oversight of financial relations between physicians and commercial interests arise mainly from the Anti-Kickback Act and the FDCA. These focus on kickbacks, gifts, and industry funding for professional activities.

The Battle over Gifts

Current policy has been shaped by jockeying between organized medicine, pharma and other commercial interests, and the government. The AMA's ethics code prohibited gifts from the early twentieth century until 1960 and then neglected the problem until the late 1980s, when pressure from Congress, the Food and Drug Administration (FDA), and the OIG led the AMA to adopt guidelines.[31]

In 1974, Senator Edward Kennedy (D-MA) chaired hearings that investigated drug promotion abuses. Testimony showed that Pfizer and other firms rewarded physicians for prescribing drugs by awarding them points they could redeem for gifts. As the price and volume of prescriptions rose, the value of the gifts increased. Gifts included phonographs, cassette tape players, color televisions, clocks, watches, microwave ovens, freezers, lawn-mowers, luggage, bicycles, and golf clubs.[32] The record included photographs of the gifts from the catalogues sent to doctors.

The AMA's Dr. William Barclay testified that gift giving was "limited to a handful of manufacturers and recipients," but retracted that statement when confronted with the committee's survey of twenty companies that revealed nearly 13 million gifts.[33] Kennedy charged that the AMA and pharma had done nothing to stop these practices and said that Congress might prohibit gifts. The AMA and the Pharmaceutical Manufacturers Association (PMA) pleaded to be allowed to end abuses through self-regulation.[34]

A decade and a half later, when nothing effective had been done, Senator Kennedy announced he would renew hearings on drug promotion in 1990. To deter government regulation, the AMA and PMA jointly developed organizational policies that discouraged obvious kickbacks and the most offensive gifts but permitted pharma funding for most professional activities. The AMA wrote an ethical opinion, drafted guidelines on gifts, and solicited comments from the PMA.[35] The PMA endorsed the guidelines, the AMA published them, and the PMA adopted a similar code of conduct.[36]

Senator Kennedy promptly held hearings and asked PMA president Gerald Mossinghoff if it had means to enforce its new code. He replied "We do not . . . but I firmly believe that the voluntary code will work." He reported that the PMA received no complaints about companies violating its 1988 code. Kennedy angrily responded: "We heard in 1974 and 1975, let the industry police itself; we don't want to get the Federal Government into this . . . and for you . . . to suggest . . . that you haven't had a single instance that has come before the PMA with regard to either ethical issues or inappropriate conduct by any of the members . . . then one has to really wonder what in the world your organization has been doing."[37]

Kennedy also pressed the AMA to explain how it would enforce its guidelines. Dr. Daniel Johnson, vice speaker of the House of Delegates, said "the AMA has some difficulty with how best to enforce the code of ethics. . . . We are constrained . . . by the legal system." Antitrust law hampered it from disciplining physicians. Then he added a vague and grudging acknowledgment of the problem: "we have . . . [a] belief in the goodness of people in general and physicians in particular; . . . [yet] even good people need to have some guidance."[38]

The AMA and PMA guidelines differ from the Anti-Gift Law overseen by the Order of Physicians in France in that they do not approve of drug companies reimbursing physicians for travel, lodging, and fees to attend professional meetings. But like the French law, they distinguish between *normal* and *abnormal* corruption.[39] Normal corruption consists of financial relationships between commercial firms and physicians, which frequently engender reciprocity and compromise physicians' judgment and loyalty to patients. These conflicts of interest are inherent in, but often concealed by, many business practices. Abnormal corruption consists of overt kickbacks, which violate commonsense ethics, and often law. Most physicians and businesses support prohibiting overt corruption but accept normal corruption.

The 1990 AMA guidelines and its subsequent reiterations prohibited doctors from accepting "substantial gifts with strings attached," namely kickbacks.[40] It allowed gifts worth up to $100 per item that had educational value or primarily benefited patients. Under that rubric, the AMA allowed gifts that subsidize practice but do not reduce patients' costs, including textbooks, gram stain test kits, and stethoscopes. Drug firms could pay for meals, sponsor receptions, and for physician consulting or speaking on their behalf. They could also pay the expenses of medical interns, residents, and fellows to attend conferences when medical schools chose the recipients and conferences. The guidelines did not limit the total value of multiple gifts from a drug firm.

Neither the AMA nor the PMA monitored compliance or required any reporting of gifts or financial support. The guidelines were widely breached and business continued as usual. The *Journal of the American Medical Association* reported in 1991 that one-third of the gifts offered at one medical meeting violated guidelines. A1992 survey by the Department of Health and Human Services (DHHS) found over one-third of physicians who wrote more than fifty prescriptions a week were offered disallowed gifts. The AMA's *American Medical News* documented widespread violations.[41] Throughout the 1990s, drug firms invited physicians to conferences at resorts, paid physicians to attend promotional dinners, and offered them tickets to sporting events and theaters.

Around 2000, the OIG focused on pharmaceutical firm kickbacks. In response, the AMA and the Pharmaceutical Research and Manufacturers Association (PhRMA, the renamed PMA) mounted a million-dollar campaign to publicize the AMA guidelines. Nine drug firms pledged $675,000 and joined the working group to disseminate the guidelines.[42] The press expressed outrage that the AMA used drug firm funds to publicize guidelines that restricted drug firm gifts. But the news media failed to see that, rather than having conflicting interests, the AMA and PhRMA shared interests in reducing gifts because they wanted to deter more stringent legal restrictions on drug firm funding for continuing medical education (CME) and other activities.

In 2002, PhRMA and the AMA each issued slightly revised guidelines. Then the OIG proposed Anti-Kickback Act compliance guidelines which, "at a minimum," required drug firms to comply with the PhRMA code. PhRMA responded that the OIG should grant "the benefit of the doubt" to firms that followed its code. Nineteen drug firms urged the OIG not to make PhRMA guidelines a "minimum standard" since that would discourage future industry standards.[43] They requested that the government not prosecute firms for violating the Anti-Kickback Act if they followed their own guidelines and wanted the AMA and PhRMA guidelines to preclude stronger regulation. That would empower the AMA and PhRMA, rather than courts or government agencies, to define what the Anti-Kickback Act prohibited and preclude Congress from adopting stricter legal standards than voluntary professional and industry guidelines.

The AMA and PhRMA prevailed. The OIG adopted guidelines in 2003 which stated that following the PhRMA code "demonstrates good faith efforts to comply" with the Anti-Kickback Act, in effect calling it a proxy for compliance. However, the OIG added a criterion to determine whether remuneration was illegal: "Would . . . remuneration diminish, or appear to diminish, the objectivity of professional judgment?"[44] This provision homed in on the conflict of interest that drug firms' gifts to physicians and CME funding involved. It left open the option for stronger restrictions in the future.

Since the OIG did not require firms to report gifts, some states have done so. In 2002, Vermont require pharmaceutical firms to report any gifts to a physician worth over $25, and similar bills were proposed in fifteen states. By 2007, five states required reporting of gifts to physicians or regulated pharmaceutical firms' gifts in other ways. Disclosure, however, does not stop gifts from compromising medical practice. In 2009, Senator Chuck Grassley (R-Iowa) introduced a bill that would have prohibited physicians participating in Medicare or Medicaid from accepting more than $25 in gifts from pharmaceutical or biological product companies. He also asked that the AMA disclose the funds that the organization and its officers received from drug and medical device firms.[45]

Starting in 2013, the Patient Protection and Affordable Care Act of 2010 requires manufacturers of drugs, biologics, medical devices and medical supplies to report payment or transfer of in-kind benefits greater than ten dollars to physicians or teaching hospitals. Reports include the name and address of the recipient, the nature and amount of payment and the date paid. They will report the information in electronic searchable format bi-annually to the DHHS, which will make the information public.[46]

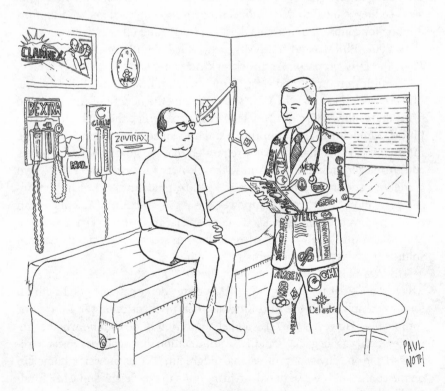

Paul Noth/The New Yorker Collection; source: © www.cartoonbank.com

Funding Continuing Medical Education

Senator Gaylord Nelson's (D-WI) 1976 hearings documented the dominance of pharmaceutical industry funding in CME;[47] and Senator Kennedy's
1990 hearings revealed that drug firms used CME to market drugs for uses
that the FDA has not found to be safe and effective. In 1991, the FDA
announced plans to curb that practice because drug firms are not allowed to
promote drugs for unapproved uses. The announcement worried the AMA,
since it might reduce funding for professional activities. Kirk Johnson,
senior vice president of the AMA, told *Medical Marketing and Media*, "our
position is that industry support of education is . . . critically important. . . .
we'll die for that position, and . . . vigorously defended it in our meetings
with [the FDA] Commissioner."[48]

The FDA's 1992 draft policy held that *drug firm–controlled* programs could
not suggest using drugs for unapproved uses, but that independent educational programs could, even if drug firms funded them. To qualify as being
independent, the FDA required CME providers to have a written agreement
specifying that the program is not promotional and granting them control
over its planning and content. Commercial supporters could not script the
program or specify its emphasis but could propose individuals as faculty, if
they disclosed this in the program. If presenters discussed off-label drug
uses, they had to note that they are not FDA approved. Continuing medical
education providers and faculty had to disclose their financial and other
relationships with commercial funders. The FDA said that it would rely on
accrediting organizations, such as the Accreditation Council for Continuing
Medical Education (ACCME) to monitor compliance.[49]

In 1992, the Washington Legal Foundation (WLF), a pro-business, free-
market advocacy group that generally opposes government regulation of
the pharmaceutical industry, asked the FDA to withdraw its draft guidelines, claiming they violated constitutionally protected speech. The FDA
response noted its authority over drug marketing and solicited additional
comments. Commercial firms contended that they should be allowed to
help design and implement CME. They objected to requiring faculty to disclose financial ties to commercial supporters and pharmaceutical firms
because it "unfairly raises the specter of bias as to that presenter."[50] Yet that
was precisely the point!

In its 1997 final guidelines, the FDA did not require written agreements
between commercial supporters and CME providers and said it would not
prosecute firms that only failed to meet one criterion for independence. The
WLF sued the FDA, arguing that its CME guidelines, and guidelines that
restricted drug firms from disseminating articles on off-label drug uses, suppressed free speech, thereby violating the First Amendment. In 2000, a trial

court sided with the WLF. In oral argument before the appeals court, the FDA said it no longer interpreted the law to prohibit the dissemination of articles that discussed off-label drug uses and would withdraw its guidelines on distributing articles and on CME funding.[51] The case focused on restrictions on distributing articles, not CME funding. The court decision implies, but does not state, that the CME guidelines also violated the First Amendment.

In response to the FDA's activities, in 1992 the ACCME created its Standards for Commercial Support. These held that CME providers must be responsible for the design and production of their activities and that CME cannot advance the proprietary interests of financial supporters. Providers had to disclose their own and their faculty's financial interests in the products discussed.[52]

The OIG's 2002 proposed Anti-Kickback Act compliance guidelines would have restricted commercial funding of CME. Organized medicine and PhRMA begged the OIG to remove all restrictions on industry funding of CME, research, and scholarships. Twenty-five professional organizations submitted similar comments, including the AMA, the American College of Physicians, the American College of Surgeons, and the Association of American Medical Colleges.[53] Several specialty societies pleaded for the OIG to protect all drug firm grants to medical societies.[54]

The OIG adopted these suggestions, giving commercial firms wide latitude. Its final guidelines declared that "support for educational activities sponsored and organized by medical professional organizations raise little risk of fraud or abuse." However, following the FDA, it said firms risk prosecution if commercial funders control CME and unduly influence the information given to physicians. It recommended that drug firms separate marketing and grant-making departments.[55] Previously, drug companies' marketing departments disbursed CME funds. Furthermore, some CME providers had also helped firms market drugs. Now, separate entities organize CME and marketing. Sometimes, however, one company owns both a CME provider and a drug marketing firm.

In response to the OIG anti-Kickback compliance guidelines, the ACCME substantially revised its standards for commercial support in 2004. The revised standards held that financial ties between commercial firms and CME faculty or program managers disqualify those persons from participating in the activity unless they resolve the conflict of interest. Its standards say that CME providers can resolve the conflict of interest by having independent peer review of the program materials to rule out bias.[56] Other measures might also resolve the conflict according to the standards, but mere disclosure is insufficient.

Still, the ACCME appeared to allow providers to show potential and current funders their draft program and receive suggestions. Its 2004 Standards say, "A provider *cannot be required* by a commercial interest to accept advice or services concerning teachers, authors, or participants or other education matters, including content, from a commercial interest *as conditions* of contributing funds or services" (emphasis added).[57] That language does not prohibit commercial supporters from offering advice, CME providers from soliciting suggestions from them, or CME providers voluntarily following suggestions of commercial supporters. My interviews with CME providers indicated that these were common practices.

In 2007, the Senate Committee on Finance investigated industry-funded CME. Its report noted that the "ACCME's accreditation process relies almost exclusively on information supplied by the CME providers . . . [yet] detects a significant number of incidences of noncompliance." It concluded that ACCME standards were inadequate because the "provider can technically maintain 'control' of content . . . while continuing to accommodate suggestions from the companies that control their funding." Providers can "accommodate the business interests of their commercial sponsors and afford drug companies the ability to target their grant funding at programs likely to support sales of their products."[58]

In reply to the Senate Committee, the ACCME wrote in part, "The ACCME recognizes that CME *can* receive financial support from industry without receiving any advice or guidance, either nuanced or direct, on the content of the activity or on who should deliver that content (emphasis added)."[59] Later, in answers to frequently asked questions, the ACCME interpreted its standards for commercial support to preclude providers soliciting suggestions or advice from commercial supporters or showing them a program draft.[60] The ACCME continues to oversee commercial support with the aim of precluding influence of funders. It maintains that there is no evidence that since its 2004 standards went into effect that commercial funders influenced the content of CME.[61]

In 2009, the AMA's Council on Ethical and Judicial Affairs issued a report saying it is ethically preferable for medical organizations to avoid accepting funds for CME from firms with an interest in physician prescribing, but that it is permissible if disclosed and the medical organization directs the program.[62] Even that position was criticized as too restrictive and was not approved by the AMA House of Delegates. Criticism grows and in the absence of effective control by organized medicine, the stage is set for increased legal regulation.[63]

Industry-Funded Research and Industry Ties with Universities

The federal government oversees research conflicts of interest through several agencies with different missions and jurisdictions. The Public Health Service has conflict-of-interest policies for researchers receiving funds from the National Institutes of Health (NIH). The FDA requires that when firms submit studies in support of new drug applications they must disclose the conflicts of interest of the researchers who conducted the studies. It also has guidelines for advisory committee members. The Office of Human Research Protections sets rules to protect research subjects; these are implemented by institutional review boards at universities and other organizations that receive federal research grants. Looking at federal policy as a whole, the General Accounting Office (GAO) concluded, "Unless federal agencies uniformly require that universities implement financial conflict of interest policies, the government cannot properly safeguard against conflicts of interest."[64]

Public policy currently delegates to universities the responsibility for overseeing their researchers' conflicts of interest. However, universities are not impartial; increasingly they labor under conflicts of interest that arise from their financial ties with firms that fund research and their investments in firms that develop research into marketable products. These ties grew after the Bayh-Dole Act promoted technology transfer through industry-university joint ventures.[65] Medical research conflicts of interest run very deep. They compromise the integrity of science, distort research priorities, and inhibit less profitable but beneficial treatments.[66]

To reduce the risk that their investment compromises their oversight of research, some universities manage their investment or technology transfer and licensing through independent institutions or foundations. Other universities limit their equity in a start-up company. Nevertheless, academic administrators are usually aware of university investments, and some universities have succumbed to industry pressure.[67]

Supervision of faculty and researcher conflicts is not a university priority and compliance is poor.[68] University policies typically say researchers must disclose financial conflicts of interest. But a GAO study in 2000 found they rely on self-reporting, lack a process to verify compliance, and rarely impose sanctions for failure to comply. Some universities have a committee monitor the research of individuals with significant conflicts of interest. A few can ask researchers to divest conflicting investments, but they rarely do. When the GAO examined four universities, it identified 111 investigators with significant conflicts of interest. No university required divestment, and only three researchers resolved their conflict by divestment.[69]

A 2009 OIG study of how universities oversee conflicts of interest of NIH-funded researchers found similar problems.[70] Ninety percent of institutions relied on researchers to determine what they should report. The grantee institutions did not routinely verify information submitted, lacked ocumentation to support their over oversight, and rarely required researchers to reduce or eliminate their conflicts of interest. The OIG recommended, among other changes, that DHHS develop regulations for institutional conflicts of interest. In 2010, the DHHS postponed any oversight of institutional conflicts of interest but proposed new regulations for public health service funded research. These would require that an institution review all researcher disclosures, and when it determined a conflict existed, that it develop a management plan and report it to DHHS and the public. DHHS allowed managing conflicts of interest by disclosure or other means. If a researcher did not comply with the plan and it appeared to the institution that this biased the design, conduct, or reporting of the research, it would have to notify DHHS of what corrective action it took.[71]

CONCLUSION

Professional and industry self-regulation, MCO oversight, and law each help cope with conflicts of interest, yet each sometimes undermines the efforts and authority of the others. The combination creates checks and counterchecks as each actor responds to the actions of others.

Professional self-regulation failed to cope with important and systematic conflicts of interest, which led the state and insurers to intervene. It took changes in public policy to enable insurers to become a countervailing power to organized medicine and physician entrepreneurs. The state granted insurers authority to oversee private practice because it lacked sufficient legitimacy to regulate medical practice on its own and because leaders were committed to strengthening markets rather than public authority. Market-oriented policies allowed insurers to assume functions that the state often performs in other countries. They changed the organization of medical practice and managed physicians.

The measures insurers took to control incentives to increase services often created a new conflict of interest: incentives to reduce services. Insurers were not suited to counter the conflicts of interest they had created to further their own interests, so the state intervened when political conditions permitted. The federal government regulated practice for Medicare- and Medicaid-funded services; it moderately regulated physician risk sharing and physician self-referral. It also set quality standards for tests performed in all physician office laboratories. State laws regulated insurance and physician drug dispensing. Yet this patchwork regulation does not cope effectively with many conflicts of interest that arise from physician entrepreneurship and payment.

Market-oriented policies fueled conflicts of interest from physicians' ties with pharma. Physicians can dispense medication, and in oncology and nephrology, earn substantial income from selling drugs. The absence of uniform drug price regulation creates numerous opportunities for physicians, drug firms, PBMs, and others to increase income through changing the choice of drugs or increasing the volume prescribed. Conflicts of interest from pharma funding of physician activities continue because organized medicine and pharma formed an alliance to keep the money flowing, and the state deferred to them. Several factors hobble governmental oversight, including the power of pharma and organized medicine and the legitimacy of the market in American culture. Critics who argue that regulated groups often co-opt the agencies designed to regulate them reinforce public skepticism about a strong state role.

One feature that distinguishes the United States' response from those of France and Japan is the federal government's limited role. The main vehicles for federal regulation of medical care today are Medicare and Medicaid; however, their rules only apply to practitioners for services they bill to these programs. The division of authority between federal and state governments precludes uniform rules and produces a wide variety of practice arrangements. Private insurance is regulated differently by each state. More than half of employees and their families receive health benefits that are exempt from most state regulation. Enacting legislation that extends federal regulation over all health insurance and medical care would allow uniform policy. States and some interest groups may resist such change, however, because the federal government would assume some traditional state responsibilities.

When the federal government has regulated physician entrepreneurship, it has done so only tepidly. Unlike France, which has cut nearly all reimbursement for drugs, tests, and ancillary services supplied by private practitioners and from facilities to which they have financial ties, Medicare restricts only a few, narrow types of physician entrepreneurship. Partial regulation encouraged physicians to redirect their entrepreneurial activities where it is permitted. In addition, the United States allows the private sector to control a much larger share of medical practice than do France and Japan. The American public hospital system remains underdeveloped.

Nevertheless, opportunities for change will arise because long-standing problems keep health system reform on the political agenda. As policy makers and the public evaluate reform proposals, they should examine how well they control physicians' conflicts of interest rather than consider this a separate issue to be addressed later. The sources of conflicts of interest are deeply embedded in the primacy the country gives to entrepreneurial private practice and markets and its reluctance to impose public oversight.

Part IV

JAPAN

8

The Evolution of Japanese Medicine

In 1961, Japan extended its existing patchwork of community and employer health insurance and began national health insurance (NHI). Today all employers and employees contribute funds. There are numerous insurance plans, most of which cover one large firm. Most individuals obtain insurance through their employer or the plan for the employees of small firms managed by the Ministry of Health, Labor and Welfare (MHLW). There are separate plans for civil servants, employees of mutual aid associations, seamen, and other groups. Most other individuals are covered by community-based insurance administered by cities, towns, and trade associations for the self-employed, farmers, and unemployed adults.[1]

In 1963, the Elderly Welfare Act established insurance for all those over seventy years of age. Legislation has changed its organization and financing over time.[2] Today, it covers individuals older than seventy-five, and national and local governments and employers finance it jointly. Covered benefits are the same as for other insurance, but premiums and copayments are lower. Japan began publicly funded long-term care insurance in 2000.

The state regulates insurance finance, coverage, and premiums. The MHLW regulates payment and providers cannot balance bill. Since NHI began, facilities with twenty or more beds are designated hospitals and those with fewer beds as clinics. Both can supply all ancillary and inpatient services. The fee schedule does not differentiate on the basis of provider training or experience, or between inpatient and ambulatory settings; but rates differ for hospitals, clinics, dialysis centers, and nursing homes. Unlike in France and the United States, insurers make a single payment to reimburse the services of both the facility and the physician and self-employed physicians cannot practice in facilities they do not own.

In 2008, physicians owned 55.6 percent of hospital beds, mostly through medical corporations. Public authorities, which include national medical centers and local hospitals, owned just under 29 percent of hospital beds. Private not-for-profit university hospitals, which were publicly funded and managed until 2004, but are now quasi-independent owned 3.4 percent of

beds. About 11 percent of hospital beds were owned by charities or foundations, and less than 1 percent were owned by lay investors. Physicians own
most of the 11,500 clinics with beds and the 87,583 clinics that supply only
ambulatory care. There are additional beds in long-term care facilities
owned by medical corporations, not-for-profit foundations, for-profit firms,
and public facilities.[3]

Most private practitioners have entrepreneurial conflicts of interest
from owning facilities and from selling medication and ancillary services.
Other conflicts of interest arise from payment incentives to increase or
decrease services. Many physicians are employees in physician-owned
facilities and paid a fixed salary. Other physicians are employees in private
not-for-profit facilities, such as university hospitals, that are increasingly
subject to market pressures. A fourth group works in government-owned
facilities. Physicians sometimes have financial ties with third parties, particularly drug and medical device firms, which give rise to other conflicts of
interest.

Contemporary conflicts of interest have roots in traditional Chinese
medicine. Practice was transformed when the state adopted Western medicine in the late nineteenth century, by struggles over social welfare at the
turn of the twentieth century, by state control over medicine and insurance
during World War II, and by reforms instituted during postwar reconstruction. As these changes occurred, organized medicine shaped the
medical political economy to protect entrepreneurial private practice.

TRADITIONAL MEDICINE

In the sixth century, Chinese medicine, referred to as *Kampō*, was introduced to Japan, where it supplemented healing arts based on Buddhist
and neo-Confucian practice and then became the core of practice. In
the *Ritsuryō-sei* period (from the mid-seventh to the mid-ninth centuries),
government-trained and -employed physicians provided services without
charge. When the central government lost power in the ninth century, public
medical care ended. The feudal order grouped physicians into the social
stratum below farmers, along with craftsmen and manufacturers.[4] Physicians were self-employed, without support from the state or from charities.
Between the twelfth and thirteenth centuries, lay peddlers began to sell
medicine to the public competing with physicians.[5] During the Tokugawa
(or *Edo*) period (1603–1867), medical practice was unrestricted by guilds or
licensing. Private practice became well established. Physicians provided
ambulatory care in their homes or in patients' homes when patients were
very ill. Some physicians advertised.

Writers referred to medicine as a humane art (*jinjutsu*) that was different from other work. They described the physician-patient relationship as moral, not contractual or commercial, and expected physicians to act altruistically. Rather than charge fees, physicians received gratuities, typically biannually, to reimburse the cost of the medicine they dispensed.[6] Individuals paid what they could afford. Most physicians lived modestly, though some were financially successful.

The extent to which the *jinjutsu* ethic affected physician behavior is uncertain. Dr. Naoki Ikegami cites some texts that suggest it removed barriers to medical services. One physician asked patients to put their contributions in a vase so how much any individual gave could not be known. The attending physician to the Shogun Tokugawa Ienari reportedly prohibited his apprentices from learning the price of medications out of concern that they might reduce the dosage of expensive drugs, which conflicted with the principle that all life was equally precious.[7] This example also suggests awareness that physician dispensing generates a conflict of interest. Dr. Ikegami, however, also notes evidence that inability to pay restricted access to medicine. A popular eighteenth-century story recounts how a daughter prostituted herself to earn money for drugs her father needed. At that time, clinics charged more for scarce drugs. Perhaps in response to this problem, edicts in Nanbu in 1711 and Nagaoka in 1714 set standard fees for different services. An 1802 edict in Nihonmatsu priced medication according to social class.

Although a few hospitals were established by political leaders or monks, Japan lacked a developed tradition of religious and secular charities that supplied medical care or operated hospitals.[8] Unlike in France and the United States, where charitable hospitals shaped medicine and offered an alternative model to entrepreneurial private practice, individual physicians or the state shouldered the burden of medical charity.

IMPORTING WESTERN MEDICINE

The Dutch and Christian missionaries introduced Western medicine to Japan during the late Tokugawa period (1600–1867).[9] In the 1850s, Japan reopened the country to the West and the government began to promote Western medicine.

The Meiji Restoration of 1868 overthrew the feudal order and created the institution of emperor. The ruling political-economic elite made a deliberate effort to transform Japan into a developed industrial economy and a powerful military state. The Meiji government adopted Western legal, political, and medical institutions. For law, it drew mainly on the German and French civil

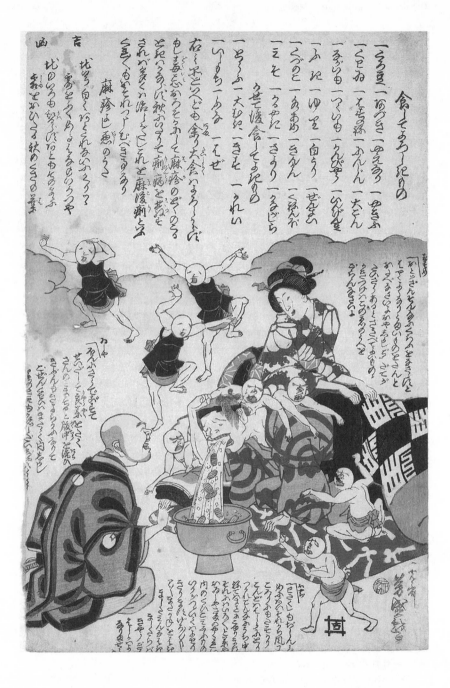

codes but adopted some American commercial law. It took specific features of its constitution and economic organization from Bismarck's Germany.

The Meiji government drew on the German model for medical education, hospitals, and insurance. At that time, there were five times as many traditional practitioners as Western-trained physicians, so the state created Western medical schools and hospitals and restricted Western practice to state-trained and -licensed individuals. In 1875 and 1883, it required new practitioners to have biomedical degrees. The government published a fee schedule in 1880 based on one used in Germany and encouraged patients to pay when served or within a month, rather than irregularly and voluntarily.[10]

The government regulated drug sales. It also tried to follow Western practice by separating prescribing from dispensing drugs, but it allowed exceptions for all practitioners of Chinese medicine and for Western practitioners who dispensed to their own patients, gutting the rule. Physician dispensing with its conflicts of interest, as well as efforts to end the practice, have continued ever since.

Two medical sectors emerged. Western medicine was practiced by physicians in elite public medical schools and affiliated hospitals and a few not-for-profit Western medical schools and hospitals, notably Keio University. Self-employed private practitioners, with lower status and less formal training, supplied ambulatory care, and over time shifted from traditional to Western medicine. This division set the stage for conflict between public and entrepreneurial private practice.

Public hospitals did not allow private practitioners to care for their patients on their premises. Since self-employed physicians risked losing patients when they entered public hospitals, they often created facilities to support their ambulatory practice. These facilities were not well equipped.

This print shows a man vomiting coins into a metal bowl, as his daughter and a doctor attend him. In a lengthy inscription, the man complains that his "purse is constantly drained for medicine and doctor's fees. I threw up money again. If I vomit nothing but money, can I recover from measles today?" The doctor agrees that if the medicine is taken faithfully he will recover, and that after all medicine's effect depends on money. As the man vomits, a crew of tiny figures the "good foods," their facial features rendered as characters for daionor yakifu (wheat gluten), clamber over the body and seem to remonstrate with the doctor. Measles personified as tiny figures wearing black aprons, their features made up of the characters ハ シ カ, or hashiku, gesture impotently above. At the top of the print are listed the good foods, as well as other helpful comments and diagnostic tips.

Artist: Utagawa, Yoshimori, 1830–1884. Source: UCSF Japanese Woodblock Print Collection. Archives and Special Collections, UCSF Library and CKM. University of California, San Francisco.

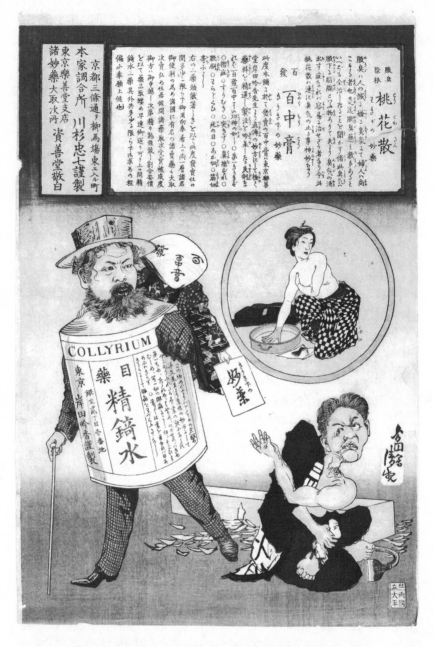

Lay Drug Peddler. Advertisements of drugs in late nineteenth century.

Source: The Naitō Museum of Pharmaceutical Science and Industry.

Nurses provided little patient care, and patients' families were responsible for food and bedding. The state designated those with ten or fewer beds as clinics, those with over ten beds as hospitals.

Anthropologist Susan Long writes that according to sociologists, professions require patrons to attain their position, and that the Meiji state served as the medical profession's patron.[11] It did so as part of a policy, established in the Japanese Civil Code, to control the formation of civil society groups. Article 33 requires all legal persons to conform to regulations. It creates a category for "public interest legal persons" which require government approval. Without this designation, not-for-profit entities lack state support, tax advantages, and legitimacy. When granting public interest status, Margarita Stevez-Abe explains, "bureaucrats . . . favor societal groups that represent specific sector interests."[12] Organized medicine received the government's blessing. However, lay-owned hospitals, mutual insurers, and charities did not, which strengthened both physician and state influence over medical institutions.

THE ORIGINS OF ORGANIZED MEDICINE AND INSURANCE

In 1891, responding to state promotion of Western medicine, traditional practitioners formed an association to defend their rights. Physicians trained in Western medicine then created their own associations. In 1906, the Medical Practitioners Law authorized the formation of local medical associations under state regulation. Associations elected leaders and could fine members or start proceedings to revoke a member's license through the prefecture. Prefectural governors could rescind association rules that they deemed detrimental to public welfare or contrary to law and, when permitted by the minister for Home Affairs, could dismiss its leaders, order new elections, or dissolve the association. In 1919 Japan's national legislature, the Diet, designated medical associations as *juristic persons*, organizations serving a public interest, and required physicians to join local and prefectural associations.[13] In 1923, the Diet reconstituted the Japan Medical Association (JMA), formed in 1916, to represent local associations.

Medical insurance emerged through mutual aid societies and employers. Local mutual aid started first, but national legislation, influenced by the German model, promoted employment-based insurance. As in France and the United States, citizen groups and communities seeking access to medical care developed social support arrangements. They pooled funds to contract with physicians. The JMA considered these efforts a threat to private practice and opposed them.

In the nineteenth century, rural communities started medical cooperatives called *Jyorei* societies that employed physicians.[14] In 1835, the Kami-
saigo village started a medical cooperative, or coop, and similar coops spread
to thirty-seven other villages in Fukuoka Prefecture by 1897. All members
contributed to compensate physicians with regular rice payments. When the
introduction of Western medicine increased costs, an annual household fee
supplemented rice payments. In the early twentieth century, when rural communities started agricultural cooperatives, Tadaatsu Ishiguro, a Ministry of
Agriculture official who later became the minister of Welfare, suggested that
they add medical services. The medical cooperative movement flourished,
and by 1931 there were more than 1,000 medical coops.[15]

From the 1880s on, medical societies opposed coops because they paid
physicians less than standard fees, undercutting private practitioners. The
two parties worked out a temporary compromise in 1909, but in 1915
medical societies asked medical coops to replace fixed payment with fee-for-
service. Medical coops phased out fixed payment by 1926. Tarō Kitajima,
JMA president, tried to stop medical cooperatives, without success.[16]

The industrial sector provided another insurance model. In 1905, the
Kanegafuchi Textile Company funded limited health benefits for its employees.[17] Other firms followed, in part to secure an ample and stable supply
of labor. Around 1911, some industrial firms started so-called cost-price
clinics that employed physicians and provided medical care for around a
third to half of the usual fees.[18] In the 1920s, medical societies opposed
employer-sponsored clinics that offered medical services below standard
rates. The Home Ministry reviewed these developments, studied German
policy and institutions, and proposed government-mandated employment-based insurance.

In 1922, the Diet enacted the Health Insurance Law, which required fac-
tories and mining firms to provide workers medical benefits. Implemented
in 1926–1927, the mandate was extended to all firms that employed five or
more manual workers by 1935. In 1939, the legislation extended coverage to
white-collar workers and their families. It used the JMA's fee schedule that
allocated points for each service, paid physicians a set fee per point, and
allowed payment for dispensing a drug during each visit, which encouraged
prescribing.

The 1922 Health Insurance Law was a part of a social welfare policy
intended to reduce labor strife and promote industrial development during
a time of social conflict. Between 1870 and 1930, agrarian and labor groups
and socialist, communist, and anarchist parties forged a social democratic
movement. Legislation to dampen social strife included the 1874 Relief Regulation and the 1911 Factory Law that limited working hours for women and
children. In 1918, rising rice prices and discontent with the social order

sparked riots. While the government passed social legislation as a carrot, it also wielded sticks. Among the most repressive measures was the 1925 Public Order Preservation Law, which allowed the government to disband leftist organizations and restrict speech and political activity.[19]

At this time, medical care remained beyond the means of many people. According to Dr. Tarō Takemi, who later became president of the JMA, the "practitioner . . . gave free medical care services to the poor while collecting large fees from the rich. In other words, the practitioner performed the function of income redistribution within a limited local area."[20] He notes, however, that physician clinic owners often had higher incomes than anyone else in their communities. Before World War II, physicians and employers owned about 46 percent of acute care hospital beds. In addition, assuming that on average clinics had five beds (half the maximum then allowed), physicians owned over 50,000 supplemental beds, or more than 41 percent of beds in the formal hospital sector.[21]

Physician fee adjustments based on patient means still left many uninsured patients with inadequate care. As Japan became a military state in the 1930s, the military became a leader in health and social policy in order to facilitate the war effort. The poor health of soldiers prompted the army medical bureau director, Lieutenant Chikahiko Koizumi, to start a campaign promoting public health and medical insurance.[22] In 1935, the Diet approved Citizen's Health Insurance and reorganized medical coops. The state sponsored twelve model Citizen's Health Insurance programs and built ten private hospitals to treat rural residents.[23] In 1936 cabinet meetings, the army minister reported on the high proportion of military recruits who failed physical exams, and in 1937 he proposed the creation of the Ministry of Welfare.

In 1938, the Diet passed the National Health Insurance Act, which established medical coops for farm workers, fishermen, and other self-employed workers. On the same day, it passed the National Mobilization Act authorizing the state (in the words of a Japanese history textbook) "to control national economics as well as people's lives without consent by the legislature."[24] The 1940 *Kokuho* convention set as a goal a coop in every municipality. When Koizumi became minster of Welfare in 1941, he planned to provide universal insurance through coops by 1944. By the war's end, 95 percent of communities had coops. But, because of the war's destructiveness, nearly half did not function and another one-fifth verged on insolvency.[25]

In 1942, the National Medical Care Law created a medical care corporation. This government-run organization administered insurance and directed the Japan Medical Care Corps, which assumed control of formerly private hospitals and employed physicians. The state appointed the JMA's director, required all physicians to be JMA members, and stipulated that they must treat insured patients for set fees. It allocated the JMA funds to pay physicians according to its fee schedule, but an insufficient budget forced the JMA to lower rates. Physician dissatisfaction led the state to revise the JMA contract in 1943 to pay the full fees set by the JMA schedule. When insurance funds were insufficient, it used general tax revenue. Physicians objected to treating all insured patients according to the fee schedule. A postwar report states that in one district with 400 physicians, only 40 accepted insurance.[26]

POSTWAR RECONSTRUCTION, 1945–1961

The American Plan

American forces occupied Japan from 1945 until 1952, overseeing the state's reconstitution as a parliamentary democracy. Until 1951, nearly all domestic policy decisions had to be approved by the Supreme Commander for the Allied Powers (SCAP), the American occupation authority. It restructured institutions to promote democracy, promulgated a new constitution, oversaw postwar legislation, and directed reconstruction. Ensuring the independence of organized medicine as a counter to state authority was an integral part of its efforts. After the war, the JMA militated against state control over medical practice, just as organized medicine did in France and the United States. However, only Japan had a legacy of all medicine being directly under state control.

Major Crawford Sams directed SCAP's public health section. His Social Security Mission, staffed with American Social Security Administration and Public Health Service employees, planned to extend health insurance and to end physician drug dispensing.[27] It sought to expand public hospitals and to complement them with physician-owned facilities overseen by prefectures. It transferred 497 military hospitals, with about 55,893 beds, to the Ministry of Health and Welfare (MHW), which made them national hospitals. It dissolved the Japan Medical Care Corporation and divided its 600 previously private hospitals with nearly 10,000 beds among national and local public authorities and three not-for-profit hospital leagues with a quasi-official status: the Japan Red Cross, the *Saiseikai*, and the *Koseiren*. It returned clinics to their previous physician owners. It introduced open medical staffs in national hospitals so that qualified private practitioners could use them. However, Japan ended open staffs after it regained control over policy.

The SCAP reconstituted the JMA as an independent, voluntary organization in 1947. Physicians elected local associations who were represented in the national organization. Its main constituents were private practitioners. The JMA wanted to administer payment under employment-based health insurance, but SCAP believed that would make it subject to state control and assigned that role to employment health insurance associations. The Social Security Mission thought that the JMA would assist in reorganization of insurance.

It did, but not as expected. The JMA organized demonstrations and participated in electoral politics through its affiliated Japan Doctors League, influencing the dominant Liberal Democratic Party (LDP). The JMA blocked many of the goals of SCAP and the Ministry of Welfare.[28] Physician-owned hospitals protected from competition by lay-directed not-for-profit, and investor-owned medical facilities became dominant, and the government subsidized them until the 1970s. Insurers were unable to conduct effective oversight. Physician dispensing continued. By 1961, the seeds were sown for the contemporary medical economy.

Securing Physician Hospital Ownership and Drug Dispensing

Legislation cemented physicians' control over private hospitals and clinics. The 1948 Medical Service Act (MSA) allowed physicians to own medical facilities as sole proprietors, and amendments in 1950 allowed physician-directed-and-owned medical corporations to own medical facilities. The MSA virtually banned firms that pay dividends (i.e., investor-owned firms) from owning hospitals and clinics.[29] It allowed prefectures to grant exceptions to the ban—but they have rarely done so. The MSA also restricted ownership by lay-directed charitable organizations. It grandfathered existing investor-owned and lay-directed charitable facilities.

Often misleadingly referred to as not-for-profit, medical corporations are for-profit firms that do not pay dividends. They distribute profits to physician owners through salaries, expense accounts, and fringe benefits. Their assets belong to shareholders who receive the proceeds upon the corporation's dissolution. They lack a charitable mission and do not provide uncompensated medical care or community benefits. They pay the same tax rate on surpluses as do other corporations, 37.5 percent.[30]

The events that led the Diet to enact the MSA remain obscure.[31] However, in light of the state's wartime control over physicians, the JMA probably wanted hospitals under physician control to ensure their independence. It certainly resisted proposals to expand public hospitals and opposed both insurer and state controls over private practice.

The history of alternatives to physician-owned hospitals is revealing. Before the war, some large firms operated hospitals for their employees, and some of these served the public as well. SCAP reported that just after the war, firms that operated hospitals for their employees treated a higher proportion of insured patients than physician-owned or public hospitals because they accepted insurance payment, which reimbursed less than two-thirds of what most physician-owned hospitals charged.[32] The JMA had grounds to believe that these hospitals were well positioned to compete with physician-owned practice. Investor-owned firms had easier access to capital, so they could expand more easily. They could withstand periods of low hospital profits, since medical care was not their main revenue source. Investor-owned firms might oppose increases in physician fees, since that would raise the amount they needed to pay their employed physicians who might otherwise form their own clinics.

SCAP's Social Security Mission criticized private hospitals' profit motive. Before the war, it reported that "over 80 percent of general hospital beds . . . were in proprietary and to some extent not-for-profit hospitals." With a tone of disapproval seeping through the bureaucratic prose, the report continued: "Hospitals and related facilities are frequently regarded as commercial undertakings which are expected to show an operating surplus." "There tends to be discrimination in the admission policy . . . against patients unable to pay full hospital charges." The report concluded: "The public service character of hospitals must be recognized." "Hospital care should be available to every one in accordance with his need, at a cost consistent with his ability to pay. To the extent that this principle cannot be implemented by private and charitable institutions and funds, it should be regarded as public responsibility."[33]

These opinions were shared by many American public health professionals, but they were regarded as radical by organized medicine and its friends in politics. Several members of the United States Congress attacked SCAP for advocating "state medicine" and "national health insurance." After all, why should the United States promote a policy in Japan that it did not accept at home? In response, in 1948 SCAP invited the American Medical Association (AMA) to review its work.[34]

The AMA mission advocated using the United States as a model, with not-for-profit hospitals supporting private practice. It argued, "The splendid hospital system . . . in the United States is the result of individual initiative on the part of physicians, lay personnel and voluntary groups."[35] Perhaps SCAP accepted the MSA as a compromise between existing private hospitals and public hospitals. The designation of medical corporations as not-for-profit may have convinced SCAP that these hospitals had a "public service character" and also drew on the "individual initiative of . . . physicians," which the AMA favored.

In 1951, the JMA published its first code of ethics with six principles. The sixth principle states, "The physician will not engage in medical activities for profit-making motives."[36] Since then, the JMA has championed the prohibition of investor-owned hospitals and portrayed physician-owned hospitals as the not-for-profit alternative. That allowed physicians free rein as medical entrepreneurs.

Then the JMA pledged to support the LDP if they subsidized physician-owned hospitals. The LDP first resisted, but in 1960, the Medical Loan Public Fund authorized $300 million for private hospital expansion. From 1957 to 1985, physicians developed medical facilities free from regulatory restrictions, while public hospitals needed prefectural approval. Usually, a local JMA representative directed the prefecture's hospital planning committee. Local medical societies lobbied prefectures to limit public hospital expansion.[37] In this way physician-owned medical facilities grew without competition from private facilities owned or directed by laymen and reduced competition from public hospitals.

In contrast, in France, no legislation favored physician ownership. Not-for-profit hospitals that employed physicians became an alternative to physician entrepreneurs. In the United States, lay-directed charities subsidized self-employed physicians by allowing them to practice in their hospitals. However, the hospital's mission and interests differed from those of physicians. Collusion was possible, but so were competition and oversight. France and the United States also allowed investor-owned hospitals. Japan precluded alternatives to physician ownership and its conflicts of interest more thoroughly than France or the United States did.

Major Sams of SCAP tried to end physician dispensing. He was supported by MHW, the *Kenpōren* (the National Federation of Health Insurance Societies), and the Japan Pharmacist Association. The JMA, the Japan Dental Association, and the Democratic Health Federation League (DHFL, the communist physician organization) opposed the change. The DHFL argued that national drugstores were capitalist and would monopolize the market if physicians could not dispense. The JMA claimed there were insufficient pharmacists to meet patients' needs. Nevertheless, in 1951, the MHW recommended separating prescribing and dispensing within two years.[38]

The Diet prohibited dispensing, except when medically necessary, a loophole that rendered the ban ineffective. In 1955, amendments allowed further exceptions.[39] The Kenpōren wanted to reimburse physicians who dispensed medicine only at cost, but the JMA obtained markup payments and delayed the law's implementation until 1956. A 1960 MHW survey found only 14 percent of pharmacies filled prescriptions more than once.[40] When NHI began in 1961, it rewarded physician dispensing more than it did providing medical services.

The JMA Struggle over Insurance

The American Social Security Mission and the Japanese Social Insurance Investigating Committee advocated universal health insurance. The Diet passed health insurance legislation in 1948 and a tax to support community health insurance in 1951. In 1955, the MHW proposed universal coverage within five years. Two years later, Prime Minister Nobusuke Kishi declared "Health Insurance for the Whole Nation" his top goal.[41] Despite the JMA's opposition, the Diet passed NHI in 1957 and it began in 1961. In the wake of this JMA defeat, the charismatic Tarō Takemi was elected president; he led the JMA's campaign to ensure that NHI would not control fees or practice until 1982.

The Social Security Mission had recommended paying physicians by salary or capitation. It sought to control doctors "who will claim reimbursement for more services than were actually rendered, or who will give the patient more treatments, or more expensive treatments than are warranted."[42] The MHW and Kenpōren wanted fee differences based on skills, training, and experience and the institutions in which physicians practiced. They advocated revising fees to promote training, research, and specialization and to discourage overmedication. (At that time, the injection of vitamin supplements, a profitable procedure, was notoriously overused.)[43] The MHW wanted to choose which facilities received payment and hold them responsible for fraudulent physician billing. Kenpōren wanted to limit the number of physicians, relocate them among regions based on need, and exert some control over practice through accreditation.

The JMA contended that these proposals would make physicians civil servants. It sought the right to strike, fee-for-service payment, and no insurer review of bills or limits on services.[44] The JMA secured its key goals in its famous Four Demands campaign of 1960–1961. It threatened mass physician resignations and noncooperation with NHI. It organized a work stoppage on several Sundays and held rallies while negotiating with leaders of the LDP and MHW.

Two JMA demands insisted on freedom to practice and prescribe; two pertained to fees. JMA physicians refused to supply insurers information except the patient's name, insurance number, illness or diagnosis, and the fee schedule points for their service. (This was more information than French physicians supplied, but insufficient for careful utilization review.) The JMA blocked restrictions on physician dispensing, covered services, or new technologies. It demanded recognition as the medical profession's representative on governmental policy committees. It challenged "the supervision and control of health insurance administrators" and asserted "claims to professional dominance."[45] It sought 30 percent fee increases, integration of separate schedules for clinics and hospitals, and leveling fee differences between regions and facilities.

Writing in 1982, Tarō Takemi recalled that through the JMA's efforts, "the inspection and examination of the doctor's bills practically ceased to exist, and we had an agreement that these measures could be taken only with the consent of the JMA." Yet he acknowledged that the JMA's success had distorted medical practice. "Doctors who had won professional freedom, want[ed] to make full use of it in augmenting their income. . . . This encouraged . . . [seeking] compensation . . . by finding a difference between the remunerations for the medicines they gave their patients and the prices they paid." The removal of oversight "was responsible for . . . physician[s] prescribing and dispensing a relatively large number of medicines."[46]

By 1961, insurers had little ability to oversee physicians by checking whether services were appropriate because physicians controlled information about diagnoses and treatment. The JMA had shaped insurance so that it subsidized physicians without overseeing their practice, just as organized medicine had done in France and the United States. But only in Japan did physicians own most private medical facilities and dispense drugs and the full range of ancillary services free from competitors other than the state.

CONTEMPORARY PRACTICE

Insurance and Fee Setting

In 1961, coverage and premiums differed widely under different NHI plans and favored well-off employees. Since then, Japan has reduced differences in premiums, copayments, and benefits so plans are roughly equivalent. Premiums are set as a percentage of income. In principle, patients have equal access to all hospitals and physicians. In 2009, copayments for most patients under age seventy were capped at ¥44,400 ($497) for multiple copayments, but varied between ¥24,400 and ¥83,400 ($273 to $934) based on income.[47]

National health insurance covers all services with a few exceptions which since 1984 the MHLW has designated as specified medical costs (SMC). Public and private facilities can supply these services for unregulated fees to patients who pay them. In 1984, the MHW designated private or semi-private rooms as SMC. Around 2002, hospitals charged around ¥3,000 ($34) a day for standard hospital rooms shared by four to eight patients. Patients paid supplemental fees to stay in semi-private, private, or luxury rooms.[48]

The Ministry of Health, Labor and Welfare (MHLW, renamed in 2001) renegotiates fees biannually through the Central Social Insurance Medical

Council (CSIMC, the *Chūikyō*), which until 2006 included eight providers (five physicians, a dentist, and a pharmacist), eight third-party payers, and four public interest representatives. The JMA chose the representatives to represent physician hospital owners and negotiate with the Health Insurance Bureau (HIB), the CSIMC secretariat. Publicly and privately employed physicians were not represented.

There are three stages of fee setting. First, the MHLW, Finance Ministry, and representatives of the political party in power (the LDP until September, 2009) negotiate overall increases or decreases. The government contribution to the MHLW-managed General Medical Health Insurance fund for small business employees is a fixed portion of total spending, so increases in total spending require the HIB to raise premiums for that fund. The Finance Ministry exerts significant influence through the HIB. The HIB supplies information on medical costs, changes in services used, hospitals' and physicians' finances, economic growth, and governmental budgets.

Since 1992, a second stage decreases drug expenditures and physicians' income from dispensing drugs. The HIB sets drug spending at a fixed percentage over the average wholesale market price. In stage three, fees are adjusted for more than 3,000 services. The points for each service are considered individually, taking all factors into account. When changes in population or other factors decrease one specialty's revenue, fee increases often compensate. For example, when falling birth rates reduced the number of children, the CSIMC raised pediatricians' fees. The CSIMC also reduces fees to compensate for unjustified increases in services by certain specialties.

Professors John Campbell and Ikegami characterize Japan's fee setting as "the art of balance." They contend that biannual revisions foster acceptance because those who are dissatisfied can press their claims in the next round. Incremental adjustments defuse conflict, because the process avoids sudden income shifts but allows change and accommodates the interests of different specialties. Differences between winners and losers are moderate, and multiple factors can justify particular changes. Adjustments balance competing interests and attempt a fair allocation.[49] However, power relations shape fee revisions. Moreover, it is unclear to whom the CSIMC public representatives are accountable or whether they represent patients' concerns.

For much of the postwar era, hospitals received separate fees for drugs, lab tests, radiology, and other services and a per diem for room, board, and physician and nursing services. Fee-for-service encouraged resource use. To address this problem, in the 1990s the MHLW began to use per diem rates to cover inpatient and most ancillary services for chronic and long-term care. However, the MHLW paid additional fees for rehabilitation care and increased per diem rates for facilities with higher nurse-patient ratios.[50] In 2004, the MHLW began to move to prospective hospital payment.

Private Practice

Since the start of NHI, hospital ownership has consolidated. Multi-hospital systems emerged during the late 1960s; by 1984, 250 hospital chains controlled about 30 percent of beds. A 1988 survey identified 259 integrated systems, 200 owned by medical corporations and 59 by public hospitals. Medical corporations owned 42 multi-hospital systems with over 1,000 beds each.[51] A few were large; a chain owned by Turao Tokuda included 50 hospitals and 170 clinics with 12,000 employees.

As hospitals consolidated, they developed a web of interlocking facilities that economist Ryu Niki dubbed "the medical-social industrial complex." Medical corporations owned hospitals, clinics, health or social service institutions for the elderly, and home care agencies. Integration of medical facilities created opportunities for the coordination of care, but it locked some patients into one chain, reduced their choice, and led to their being shuttled between different facilities within a system. It also created a class of physicians who resembled owners of other large corporations more than they did practitioners who owned small facilities.

Although physicians remain the dominant owners of both clinics and hospitals, the majority of physicians are employees. Dr. Aki Yoshikawa estimated in 1990 that 67.4 percent of physicians were employees in hospitals, clinics, or university hospitals and 3.8 percent were employees in health centers or other settings.[52]

Physicians who are employed in facilities owned by other physicians receive a salary and lack *direct* financial incentives to increase revenue or decrease costs. However, they have *indirect* incentives to advance their employer's economic interests. These hospitals can dismiss their physician employees, which makes physician employees attentive to the employer's financial goals. Management analysts write that most Japanese firms have organizational cultures that promote stronger employee loyalty to company goals than firms in other nations.[53] If private hospitals conformed to this pattern, they would have greater influence on physicians than do hospitals in other countries. However, I am aware of no studies that examine the behavior and loyalty of physicians in Japanese private hospitals.

Private hospitals typically adjust physicians' salaries yearly. Salaries can reward performance and reflect the hospital's financial health. An emerging trend is for physicians to negotiate salaries that rise with the revenue they generate.[54] The Kameda Medical Center has special contracts for department heads that set forth productivity expectations, and a small portion of salary may vary based on whether they meet productivity goals. Private hospitals typically inform physician employees about their productivity in relation to their peers. They note prescribing and utilization rates, expecting that physicians will want to perform well. Physician employees are sensitized to the financial interests of private hospital owners.

The process through which hospitals hire physicians affects their loyalties and may limit employers' influence. Since the Meiji era, medical school department chiefs have directed *Ikyoku*, a network that controls the employment of graduates. Some view the Ikyoku as a benign old-boy network; critics say it resembles a feudal order. It is very difficult for hospitals to recruit physicians outside Ikyoku or to replace a physician without the consent of the department chief who placed the physician there. Hospitals that act without the department chief's approval would have trouble recruiting physicians later. So physicians are less dependent on individual employers for job security.[55]

Public Hospitals

Physicians employed in public hospitals are tenured civil servants paid a salary based on seniority. Unlike public hospital physicians in France, they cannot earn income through private consultations. The law prohibits them, like all civil servants, from receiving kickbacks or gifts. Nevertheless, patients typically make cash gifts to publicly employed physicians, particularly obstetricians, surgeons, and medical specialists, especially at national medical centers and university hospitals in Tokyo and Osaka.[56] Public officials treat this practice with benign neglect.

A patient seeking treatment from a well-known surgeon obtains an introduction through someone who knows the physician and presents the physician with a gift, often a sweet, along with an envelope containing cash.[57] Gifts can be substantial. Writing in 1991, Naoki Ikegami reported patient gifts of $1,000 to $3,000 at University Medical School in Tokyo to have an attending physician perform surgery. More recently, one individual who sought information on the amount he should pay as a gift reported that colleagues informed him that patients typically pay a month's salary.[58]

Accepting gifts might lead physicians to give priority to patients who pay gifts, to favor patients who make large gifts, or allow patients making gifts to jump queues. The practice undermines the NHI ideal of equal access, treatment, and payment. Some writers view patient gifts as the equivalent of balance billing, which Japan prohibits. Since the mid-1990s, market proponents have advocated allowing balance billing. Both practices relieve pressure on payers to raise fees. Perhaps this consideration deters the government from prosecuting those who engage in the practice.

Private hospital rooms are typically separated from regular rooms, so nurses and physicians can easily give these patients priority. Private rooms may also be an informal means to balance bill. Hospitals can make it clear that patients must pay for private rooms if they want access to prestigious physicians, to whom they traditionally give gifts.[59] These practices create a problem similar to that in France, where public hospital physicians may favor patients who pay higher fees for private consultations.

Reforms, 2000 to the Present

Although at the start of the twenty-first century, Japan spent only 8 percent of its gross domestic product on medical care, compared to 10.4 percent for France and 15.2 percent for the United States, a decade-long recession made medical spending a public issue.[60] The government instituted major hospital and payment reforms. It also began trials for other reforms which, if developed further, would produce far-reaching changes.

The American Chamber of Commerce in Japan and other organizations that promoted market logic in the United States sought to promote medical markets in Japan. Japanese graduates of American law and business schools since 1980 returned with the Regan-era conventional wisdom that favored unregulated markets. As early as 1993, efforts to promote markets led to a new Administrative Procedure Act that made government agency decision making more transparent and reduced protectionist policies.[61] American medical device, pharmaceutical, and biomedical technology firms advocated related reforms. The United States supported their efforts through bilateral trade negotiations. Some Japanese interest groups also sought to promote markets. The development of international standards for medical institutions also encouraged markets.[62]

Junichirō Koizumi, elected prime minister in 2001, promoted markets in medicine through the Council for Regulatory Reform (CRR) succeeded by the Council for the Promotion of Regulatory Reform and the Committee on Decentralization. Several initiatives proposed shifting the financial burden for public programs, including medical care, from the national to the local governments. In 2002, the MHLW proposed reorganizing insurance in a single system administered by each prefecture.[63] This would vary the financial burden by region and reduce uniformity imposed by the national government.

The JMA's influence waned as the number of salaried physicians who did not own medical facilities rose and its electoral support diminished. The JMA opposed Koizumi's market reforms and lost supporters in the 2005 Diet election.[64] That set the stage for legislation in 2006 that reflected the JMA's diminished authority by reducing the JMA's representation on the

CSIMC, which negotiates fees. It now includes seven insurers, seven providers, and six public interest representatives.[65] The JMA chooses three physicians, and hospital associations choose two physicians. Government officials now hold a strong position in fee negotiations.

In 2004, the MHLW and the Ministry of Education initiated prospective hospital payment modeled on the U.S. Medicare program, using diagnostic procedure combinations (DPCs) set by each patient's principal diagnosis. DPCs assign payment points using primary and secondary diagnoses, procedures, complications, co-morbidity, severity, age, and gender.[66] Each hospital receives a per diem based on its historical average length of stay and the patient's DPC. Per diems decrease as the hospital stay lengthens. Introduced at eighty university hospitals and two national medical centers in 2004, physician-owned hospitals could opt for DPC payment if they billed electronically and submitted certain data, and met standards for nurse staffing and medical records. By June 2009, insurers used DPCs to pay just under 48 percent of hospital beds.

The government also made university hospitals—until then funded by the Ministry of Education—quasi-independent with fiscal and management autonomy. Previously, university hospitals incurred deficits. Their cost accounting was rudimentary; some did not even practice double-entry bookkeeping. The reform aims to make patient fees finance these hospitals. So far, the government still subsidizes them, but less than previously. Like other private hospitals, they seek new revenue and means to control costs. The new system places a premium on physicians bringing in revenue. Physicians have to see more patients, do more procedures, and have less time for research and teaching. Physician employees are public officials, but not civil servants.

Medical Liberalism

Polls indicated broad public support for Japan's egalitarian medical values, so market advocates promoted deregulation as a means to improve service, foster accountability, and limit public spending. They advocated (1) permitting investor ownership of hospitals; (2) allowing providers to offer services not reimbursed by NHI; and (3) letting providers balance bill—that is, charge more than MHLW fees with patients paying the difference.[67]

Starting in 2003, the government allowed limited *zones for deregulation* in which investor-owned firms can own hospitals devoted to high-tech medicine.[68] Patients treated in these hospitals pay the entire cost, which inhibits their growth. In 2004, the CRR renewed proposals made in 1995, which the JMA and MHLW had scuttled, to permit investor-owned hospitals across the country. The CRR argued it was unfair to preclude investor ownership because physician-owned medical corporations are really for-profit companies: their assets belong to shareholders and the proceeds revert to them upon the corporation's dissolution. Moreover, they typically rely on for-profit firms for capital.[69] Some Japanese businesses, the American Chamber of Commerce in Japan, and the United States trade representative agreed. They contended that since Japan allows investor-owned nursing homes and pharmacies, it should also allow investor-owned hospitals,[70]

As noted earlier, NHI covers all necessary medical services aside from the exceptions that the MHLW designates as SMC services, which patients must pay for themselves. No statute prohibits providers from offering uncovered services not on the SMC list. However, in 1989, the Tokyo District Court held that the SMC list of noncovered services that providers can bill to patients implies that they cannot bill patients for services not on the list as an integral part of medical treatment covered by NHI.[71] By 2000, the SMC list had expanded to include drugs and devices being tested in clinical trials; approved drugs not yet covered by NHI; high-tech services being tested; consultations with physicians by appointment, as opposed to walk-in clinic visits; certain consultations in hospitals with over 200 beds; and a 15 percent room and board surcharge starting after six months of hospitalization.

The second CRR proposal would allow patients to pay for all noncovered services as part of NHI-covered treatment. Providers could acquire revenue from new and high-tech services as rapidly as they emerged. Well-financed tertiary care medical centers, such as university hospitals, and investor-owned hospitals could develop this market niche. The JMA and MHLW opposed the proposal.

If in the future the MHLW limits coverage of new technology and services to control health care spending, and private insurers sell policies to cover them, the market for these services will grow. Since 1980 there is a limited market for supplemental insurance, mainly for cancer treatment and dementia. However, if NHI covered only basic services, that would undermine its egalitarian values, set up a two-tier system, and create an entrepreneurial medical sector with unregulated prices.[72]

In December 2004, the MHLW and the RCC reached a compromise. They replaced the SMC list with a list of services under investigation for coverage in 2006. They formed a committee to decide whether to allow off-label use of drugs, which other countries permitted but Japan did not. While the committee deliberated, these drugs became available as SMC list services. In addition, they permitted 2,000 hospitals to provide about 100 procedures and a list of designated high-tech services not covered by NHI. Hospitals were allowed to provide these services, certain preventive services, and translation services for non-Japanese speakers.[73]

In 2007, a Tokyo district court overruled the prohibition on providing noncovered services together with covered services, holding that it lacked a statutory basis. However, in the fall of 2009 the court of appeals reversed the decision.[74] Nevertheless, deregulation advocates still seek to allow physicians to provide any noncovered service.

The third RCC proposal would allow balance billing, which proponents claim would create incentives for quality, service, and accountability. If providers could supply uncovered services, Dr. Ikegami believes, it would be difficult to prohibit balance billing, which would generate much more revenue than the first two proposals.[75] If hospitals balance bill and offer noncovered services, they are more likely to grow. So would supplemental insurance for services not covered by NHI.

So far, these proposals have not been adopted. However, elite public hospitals, such as those at Tokyo and Kyoto universities, supported the RCC proposals. When they became self-funded in 2004, university hospitals searched for new sources of revenue. In 2005, Tokyo University Hospital announced a plan to join with a private firm and sell services on a members-only basis. In return for a ¥6 million ($67,195) membership fee, individuals would receive high-tech cancer screenings every eleven months as well as cardiac and cerebral nervous system testing.[76]

Public and university hospitals are so highly reputed that patients wait in long queues for ambulatory care in them. Patients typically make cash gifts to university hospital surgeons, so some patients would probably pay higher than regulated fees for services from prestigious physicians. Elite institutions could probably balance bill without reducing their number of patients. Physicians may prefer to receive undeclared and nontaxable cash gifts from patients than income from balance billing, but their views would change if the state began to prosecute physicians who accept gifts.

A related development is the growth of supplemental insurance. In 2000, the firm SECOM, which has invested in several hospitals, received approval to sell insurance that would pay hospitals 1.5 times the official reimbursement. This program was criticized for promoting two-tier health care and has not yet been developed. Market proponents, however, want supplemental insurance to create a market for services not covered by NHI, and for providers that charge more than the fee schedule. That would create entrepreneurial opportunities for investor-owned firms and elite physicians.

Japanese proposals to allow uncovered services and balance billing resemble proposed market reforms in France exemplified by the 2003 Chadelat report, which also proposed a new role for supplemental insurance. These market incentives would increase physicians' conflicts of interest from entrepreneurship and payment, similar to those that exist in the United States, but might also allow insurers to oversee physician practice to control costs. Health care liberalization and market reforms stalled when Prime Minister Koizumi left office in the fall of 2006. In August 2009, the Democratic Party of Japan (DPJ) swept the LDP from office, ending its domination of Japan and creating possibilities for significant change. The DPJ has opposed many market-oriented LDP policies, but some people think it might lift the ban on reimbursing mixed NHI covered and noncovered services.

9

Coping with Physicians' Conflicts of Interest in Japan

The Japanese state addresses physicians' conflicts of interest in two distinct ways: (1) it operates public hospitals with employed physicians, which avoids entrepreneurial and payment conflicts; and (2) it regulates the private sector: physicians, hospitals, and the pharmaceutical and medical device industries.[1]

The Ministry of Health, Labor and Welfare (MHLW) regulates medical practice mainly through controlling payment and primarily to constrain spending. However, reforms that reduce incentives to supply services have helped address conflicts of interest.[2] The Japan Medical Association (JMA) has blocked the state and insurers from using utilization review, practice guidelines, and other oversight. Unlike in France and the United States, organized medicine plays virtually no role in overseeing conflicts of interest or other aspects of practice through ethical codes, professional discipline, or practice guidelines.

Recent reforms target physician entrepreneurship. Legislation stopped the formation of new physician-owned medical corporations that can own hospitals and clinics. The MHLW offered incentives for physician-owners to convert their medical facilities into organizations that resemble American tax-exempt hospitals. It also promotes practice standards by requiring post-graduate medical school training, by offering incentives for physicians to receive specialty certification and continuing medical education (CME), and for hospitals to obtain accreditation.

The state bans kickbacks and gifts to publicly employed physicians. To promote open markets, the Japan Fair Trade Commission (JFTC) restricts individual drug firms from paying premiums to physicians and medical associations. Nevertheless, it permits pharma collectively to finance professional medical activities by supplying funds through foundations.

REFORMING PAYMENT

The MHLW recognized that fee-for-service and per diem payments created financial incentives for physicians to prescribe treatment, lengthen hospital stays, and overuse drugs, tests, and services. In response, it began to bundle payments for services. In 1981, the Ministry of Health and Welfare (MHW) revised the fee schedule to reduce the per-test fee as the number of different tests rose or when some tests are repeated frequently.[3] It also used the fee schedule to manage practice. To encourage low cost and effective treatment, it pays only for the preferred treatment for some diagnoses. For example, it reimburses stomach ulcer treatment by paying for antibiotics rather than more expensive alternative medications.

Reimbursement of treatment for end-stage renal disease illustrates the change. Initially, the MHLW paid dialysis fee-for-service and reimbursed dialysers much more than their cost, which increased spending and encouraged physicians to place patients on dialysis prematurely. A 1988 study by Michio Kodaka found that physicians started dialysis prematurely for at least 10 percent of patients. Dr. Seiji Yamagami suggests that physicians induce demand for dialysis.[4] Japan has 125 dialysis patients per 100,000 people, over twice the mean for Organization for Economic Cooperation and Development (OECD) nations; the United States has 100 dialysis patients per 100,000. The high number of dialysis patients is partly due to the relative lack of kidney donors, so alternatives are limited. However, financial incentives prompted physicians to invest in facilities; in 2006, physician-owned centers provided 80 percent of hemodialysis.[5] High fees also encouraged kickbacks for referrals.

Until 1981, providers received a fee for every bottle of infusion drip, leading to overuse. Subsequently, to discourage overuse, the MHLW reimbursed infusion drip only if more than one 500cc bottle was used daily and paid a fixed fee. Following a 1993 report by the Government Auditing Office that documented overbilling and kickbacks, the MHW bundled payment for drugs and medical management of dialysis patients, so hospitals had an incentive to conserve resources.[6]

Bundled payments, however, created incentives to cut appropriate services, a conflict of interest that can reduce quality. In a 1994 survey, 12.8 percent of dialysis patients reported that facilities substituted alcohol for iodine as a disinfectant and used 490 milliliters irrigation fluid per minute, while clinical guidelines called for 600. Facilities switched from Heparin to Flagmin, a less expensive anticoagulant, and personnel changed gloves infrequently. Five patients treated in a Tokyo dialysis clinic in the fall of 1994 contracted Hepatitis B, and four died; an investigation concluded that poor handling of syringes was the likely infection source.[7]

The MHLW made additional changes in 2002 and 2006. Instead of per unit drug fees, it paid a fixed fee per session. Today, outpatient dialysis centers receive prospective payment to cover management, dialysis fluid, anticoagulants, saline, routine lab tests, and technical fees. In addition, they receive individual fees for dialyzers, drugs, biologic tests, and special measurements.[8] Most inpatient dialysis is paid fee-for-service, but some receive prospective payment using diagnostic procedure combinations (DPCs). The effect of these changes on physician behavior and quality of care is not yet known.

Geriatric hospitals illustrate another payment reform. Geriatric hospitals had a history of overmedication, especially of lucrative injectable medicines. At the same time, they were understaffed. In changing payment for long-term care, the MHLW balanced incentives to reduce some services with incentives to increase others. In 1990, the MHW allowed geriatric and chronic care hospitals to adopt a per diem payment to cover most services, including nursing, laboratory tests, medicine, and injections. However, the per diem went up as the nurse to patient ratio increased; and geriatric hospitals received additional fees for services that were historically undersupplied, such as rehabilitation. Hospitals with patients who did not need intensive resources quickly chose the new payment system. Later, other hospitals also found it was more profitable if they reduced services. By 1997, the MHW paid for 89 percent of geriatric beds using modified per diems. When long-term care insurance began in 2000, it paid all facilities this way.

A 1991 MHW survey of eighty-six hospitals that chose the new payment system revealed decreased expenditure for items included in the per diem, while nursing and personal services, paid fee-for-service, increased. Hospital surpluses rose by over 62 percent. It is unclear whether facilities cut only unnecessary services or reduced the quality of care, however. A patient survey revealed increased satisfaction and improvements in activities of daily living.[9] Still, some observers worried that hospitals might not have admitted patients who required intensive services, since the MHW did not adjust payments for severity of illness.

Per-diem rates were more profitable for chronic than for acute care patients so providers increased their chronic care units. They often chose patients who did not need many services to increase their profits. In 2006, the Central Social Insurance Medical Council (CSIMC, the *Chūikyō*) replaced flat per diems with rates that reflected the acuity of care that patients required, their medical status, and clinical characteristics. The aim was to have payment accurately reflect the cost of patient care, discourage hospitalizing patients unless necessary, and encourage hospitals to admit patients needing high levels of care, which they had avoided.

The committee that developed the new categories used to determine patient needs expected payment rates would reflect the cost of each group. However, the prime minister made a political decision to lower overall medical spending and this required payment reductions. The brunt of payment reductions fell on chronic care beds, in part because they had higher rates of profits than other hospital beds. In addition, the JMA preferred to reduce payment for chronic care rather than other beds because their main constituents are physicians who own general clinics rather than chronic care beds. As a result, the new reimbursement for most chronic care patients was below the cost of supplying care. Only chronic care patients with the highest two levels of need were profitable to treat.

Providers protested and warned that they would have to discharge patients. In fact, the government intended for providers to close beds for patients with low levels of acuity. Instead, in the two years after the reform, providers reclassified their patients into categories that received higher payment. Thus, even though their revenue decreased, they still earned profits—less than previously—but more than the average for all hospital beds.

In addition, studies revealed an increase in patients with ulcers, urinary tract infections, and other indications of poor quality of care. This led the MHLW for the first time to issue quality directives based on outcomes and process and to require that hospitals document quality problems and their response for future inspections. As of yet, the MHLW cannot determine the true medical status of patients. In order to determine whether providers inappropriately classify patients into higher payment categories and whether they appropriately address quality problems, it needs to develop new patient data systems and conduct on-site inspections.[10]

Acute care hospitals also had incentives to increase services and prolong hospital stays. In 1993, Japan had the longest hospital stays of all OECD nations; the average was about three times longer than in the United States. Patients with acute myocardial infarction in teaching hospitals had an average stay of 25 days in Japan, 7.5 days in France, and 8.8 days the United States.[11] To discourage prolonged hospital stays, in 1997 the MHW reduced the per diem as stays lengthened beyond fourteen days. In 2007, hospital per diems varied between ¥9,000 and ¥15,000 ($76 to $127).[12]

Hospitals found ways to game the system. Some engaged in a practice called "playing catch with patients." When the daily per diem went down, the hospital discharged the patient and a cooperating hospital admitted the patient at the highest reimbursement rate. The cooperating hospital returned the favor by sending the referring hospital one of its patients. A Japanese television documentary on how a distressed hospital became profitable reported that the hospital manager negotiated swapping agreements with nearby hospitals. In 1998, the MHW disallowed resetting the fee scale when financially related hospitals transfer patients.[13]

In 2004, the MHLW initiated prospective payment based on the patient's diagnosis using DPCs in acute care hospitals. By March 2010, it used DPC codes to pay about half of hospital beds. Each hospital receives a per diem that declines with the length of stay. Rates vary, depending on the hospital's historical costs.

As incentives to reduce services become more prominent, they may cause more problems than they have in the United States because Japan's quality assurance is undeveloped and its consumer and patients' rights movements are weaker. Patients cannot appeal denial of treatment as they can in the United States, and the barriers to initiating medical malpractice lawsuits are higher.[14] So far, underuse of services does not appear to be a problem, perhaps because incentives to reduce services are relatively weak and countered by incentives to increase services. Still, medically inappropriate limits on services may not be detected because of ineffective quality monitoring.

NEGLECTED UTILIZATION REVIEW AND QUALITY ASSURANCE

When insurers and the state cannot preclude conflicts of interest, they can mitigate their effects through oversight. Controls over practice can address inappropriate provision of services in a way that price controls cannot. While low fees limit spending, they do not necessarily eliminate unnecessary services; they can even increase unnecessary services if physicians supply more to earn a target income as some economists argue they do.[15] Low prices without practice oversight help explain Japan's high drug use.

Because of the JMA's opposition, insurers lack many tools used in the United States to counter entrepreneurial and fee-for-service payment incentives. They cannot require individuals to receive authorization before receiving services. They lack primary care physician gatekeepers to coordinate patient care and reduce inappropriate referrals. They are also restricted in employing utilization review.

The JMA's four demands campaign in 1960–1961 precluded insurers from obtaining detailed information on patient care that would allow careful utilization review. Today, claims review includes two stages. Each prefecture reviews most claims employing physician reviewers nominated by the local JMA chapter; and a national board reviews the highest cost claims separately.[16] Then, insurance carriers perform a second level of review. Employment-based insurance societies contract with the *Kenpōren* (the National Federation of Health Insurance Societies) to perform this work. For local, citizen-based health insurance plans, reviews are delegated to the National Federation of Citizens' Health Insurance Associations.

When the MHW developed electronic claim filing and processing in 1985, the JMA opposed its use to monitor physicians. In 1990, it negotiated an agreement under which the MHW pledged that utilization reviewers would only examine paper claims even though insurers processed claims electronically.[17] That made the process very cumbersome, prevented analyses that would identify unusual patterns and precluded effective oversight. Nearly two billion claims are reviewed each year for citizens' health insurance, and reviewers spend an average of one second per claim. So they ignore most bills and focus on bills for more than ¥800,000 a month.[18] A special review committee for claims over ¥4,200,000 targets hospitals and physicians with reputations for billing for unjustified services and physicians in their first two years of practice.[19]

In theory, even limited insurance claims review can deter physicians from supplying inappropriate services. However, it is standard practice for physicians to list four or five diagnoses without indicating which treatments are paired with which diagnoses, making it difficult to tell whether treatment is appropriate. Reviewers do not typically assess patient care with clinical guidelines or examine medical records.

The MHLW is moving toward record keeping that will facilitate utilization review. To implement the Information Technology Strategy Initiative, in 2006, the MHLW planned to process all insurance claims electronically by 2011. By August 2010, 92 percent of medical claims were submitted electronically.[20] Some policy makers anticipate that even without legislation to change claims review, insurers will use protocols and preestablished criteria to screen and analyze claims, as already occurs in Korea.

Quality assurance can also check inappropriate use of services. However, Japanese hospital records are much sparser than those in France and the United States and lack information necessary for quality assurance. Frequently, they include only billing codes. Physicians typically record this information at discharge and provide no details on patient history, diagnoses, or treatment. So it is impossible to compare quality across hospitals or even to assess quality within a hospital.

Dr. Kenzō Kikuni wrote in 1984 that "a system of quality assurance for medical care has not been formally established in Japan." In 1997, John Wocher, executive vice president of the Kameda Medical Center, found the situation unchanged. He wrote that, despite the enormous interest in quality improvement, quality circles, and continuous quality improvement in Japanese business, "there is no hospital model in Japan . . . as an example of success."[21] This absence is ironic in light of burgeoning quality improvement in American hospitals, which draws its inspiration from quality assurance in Japanese industrial production. Wocher attributes this gap to the lack of domestic competition for medical services and the inability to export them, which would create international competition. The result is that there are no "financial incentives to monitor and improve quality of care."[22] In 2010, Wocher reports some change but notes that a "system in which quality indicators, sentinel events and/or incident reports are collected and analyzed . . . is not widespread nor sophisticated."[23]

CHIPPING AWAY AT PHYSICIAN DISPENSING AND ANCILLARY SERVICES

Physician drug dispensing is at the root of what John Wocher calls an "unhealthy relationship" between physicians and drug firms. Anthropologist Margaret Lock reported in 1980 that patients believe physicians overprescribe and do not use many of the medicines they receive. Patients said it would be rude to complain or refuse to purchase drugs from physicians who dispense them.[24] An MHW survey found that, on average, physicians prescribed at least five medications per patient visit in 1994.

Japan exceeds most other nations in drug consumption and in 1995, 29 percent of medical expenditures were for drugs. The United States spent 16 percent, although its drug prices were much higher. Japanese physicians prescribe few generic drugs: 17 percent of the quantity prescribed compared to 53 percent the United States.[25] About 30 percent of the drugs sold in Japan are rarely used elsewhere. John Wocher believes they have dubious value and that physician incentives explain their use.[26]

More expensive drugs yield higher profits because there is a larger spread between the physician's purchase price and their reimbursement. When alternative drugs are available within a therapeutic class, physicians stock the higher cost one, which is more profitable. Payments for new drugs exceed the payments for older ones, which encourages physicians to choose them even when cheaper drugs are equally effective. Japan uses more third-generation antibiotics than other countries. Unfortunately, their rapid adoption contributes to the development of drug-resistant microbes, such as MRSA (Methicillin resistant *Staphylococcus aureus*), an infection that can be fatal.[27]

Since 1990, the MHLW reduced the proportion of physicians who dispense drugs. It cut dispensing profits, introduced incentives to prescribe without dispensing, and raised copayments to discourage prescribing multiple drugs. The MHLW progressively lowered physicians' earnings on drugs from 25 percent in 1990 to 2 percent in 2000.[28] The MHW also paid higher prescribing fees to physicians who do not dispense than to physicians who do dispense, although it was still advantageous to the physician to dispense medicine when income from the drug sale was over ¥440 (about $3.00) because the drug profits offset the lower prescribing fee.[29] Reducing the profit from dispensing each drug, however, does not eliminate the incentive to prescribe. One hospital manager estimated in 2002 that dispensing drugs yields about 14 percent of revenue from hospital inpatients and 20 percent of revenue from ambulatory patients.[30]

Government regulators usually remain a step or two behind those they regulate as entrepreneurs devise new approaches in response to new rules. Some physicians gamed the system by referring patients to a freestanding pharmacy they owned just outside their clinic or hospital and received both the higher prescribing fee and the dispensing income. The MHW responded by requiring pharmacies to be independent of any medical facility. In 1994, it prohibited physicians from directing patients to designated pharmacies or receiving kickbacks in exchange for referrals.[31] Nevertheless these practices persisted.

In 1996, the MHW started paying lower dispensing fees to pharmacies that receive over 70 percent of their prescriptions from a single facility. These pharmacies earned only ¥200 ($1.70) to dispense a drug, while others received ¥450 ($3.80).[32] However, some hospitals and clinics located near one another swapped some prescriptions so that their pharmacies received less than 70 percent of prescriptions from one source and earned the higher fee.

The MHLW estimated that the proportion of dispensing physicians declined from 81 percent in 1997 to 59 percent in 2008.[33] The real rate was higher, given physicians' hidden ties to pharmacies. Nevertheless financial incentives still encourage physicians to prescribe and/or dispense drugs, and this persistent conflict of interest has medical as well as financial consequences.

The volume of prescribed drugs has increased even while the number of prescribing physicians has declined. Prescription drug expenditures dropped from 29.5 percent of medical spending in 1993 to 19.3 percent in 2000 and to 16 percent in 2001.[34] Yet the overwhelming share of decline in spending came from lower reimbursements; drug expenditures per capita adjusted for inflation continued to rise. From 1984 to 1997, per capita drug expenditures increased 3.8 percent annually. Only .01 percent of this growth was from increased prices; the rest came from additional prescriptions.[35]

Physician incentives help to explain why Japan makes much greater use of diagnostic screening and drugs than other countries. Virtually anyone can be tested as a precaution, even if they have neither symptoms nor risk factors, and patients rarely object because most tests are not invasive. One hospital manager estimated that laboratory tests earned a margin that exceeds 25 percent and may be as high as 45 percent.[36] Since the 1950s, it has become popular for individuals to undergo diagnostic testing in a manner that is referred to as "a human dry dock." Like boats taken out of the water for inspection and repair, individuals without indications of disease enter a hospital for a battery of tests and screenings. Such comprehensive testing without evidence of problems is not medically necessary. Physician-owned clinics often provide these services.[37]

REFORMING HOSPITALS AND PROFESSIONALIZING PRACTICE

Physician-owned facilities are the core of physician entrepreneurship in Japan. A study of physician-owned clinics in the 1970s showed that they were profit driven and increased drugs and ancillary services to generate income.[38] Conflicts of interest will continue to compromise medical practice so long as physicians own facilities that allow them to prescribe services that boost their income.

Japan is trying to transform physician-owned facilities into institutions that resemble tax-exempt charitable hospitals in the United States. In the 1970s, the Ministry of Finance reduced the medical corporation tax rate from 37.5 percent to 27 percent if the facilities became *special medical corporations* and operated an emergency room.[39] Physician owners could still govern the hospital and set

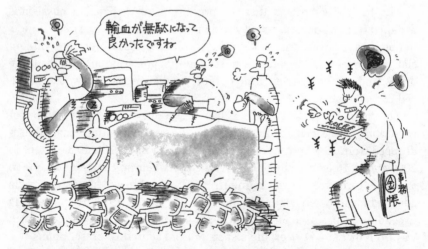

The surgeon is saying "Thank God, the transfusions are going to be wasted!" while the hospital administrator is calculating, in anguish, the cost of the transfusions purchased, which cannot be returned to the blood bank or reused in another patient.

Illustration by TRYANCE for article by Yasuda Nobuhiko. How much is your anesthesia? Blood transfusion. Life Support and Anesthesia (LiSA) *2, no. 11 (1995): 88.*

their salary and fringe benefits. However, they would relinquish ownership of capital and place it in a foundation. If the owners later liquidated the medical corporation, the capital would revert to the state. Most of these institutions have very low profits because they compensate their owners through salaries, fringe benefits and perks, so the reduced tax rate is not a strong incentive to convert. By 2007, only seventy-nine hospitals were organized as special medical corporations, and 55 percent of clinics were owned by sole proprietors.

In 2004, the MHLW proposed allowing medical corporations to be taxed at 22 percent and to issue tax-exempt bonds if they became *designated medical service organization systems*. To qualify, they would have to meet standards for financial and management transparency, allow public auditing, and follow rules on use of any surplus. The board of trustees would have to include community representatives.[40] The government stopped authorizing the creation of new special medical corporations in 2007 and required that all those existing convert into designated medical service organization systems by 2012.

The Diet enacted a major reform in 2007 by amending the Medical Service Act to stop the creation of new physician-owned medical corporations. It only allows new medical corporations organized as foundations. Existing physician-owned medical corporations can continue. But when they dissolve, the proceeds "shall be distributed to the government, local governments or other medical corporations specified by MHLW."[41]

Even if physicians convert their medical corporations into designated medical service organization systems, that will not end physician entrepreneurship, since physicians can still set their salaries and benefits. Unless regulations cap salaries and benefits and require physician owners to work enough hours to justify their income, physician owners will have entrepreneurial incentives.

Many physicians or their medical corporations own for-profit medical service corporations that sell medical supplies and hospital-related services.[42] These entities can distribute profits through dividends. Physician-owned facilities purchase medical supplies or services at high prices through corporations or subsidiaries nicknamed *tunnel companies*. The practice allows physicians to distribute some income through the tunnel corporation's dividends. To control these practices, the government established rules that require hospitals to make certain purchases through licensed local distributors.[43]

Accreditation, Certification, and Continuing Medical Education

The MHLW has countered conflicts of interest by reforms that professionalize practice, create standards to evaluate performance, and encourage accreditation. Since 2004, it promotes voluntary clinical laboratory and hospital accreditation. So far, accreditation does not affect reimbursement and there are no government or insurance sanctions for not being accredited. As of 2007, only 30 percent of hospitals were accredited.[44] In 2004, the MHLW began to certify continuing medical education (CME). Previously, providers called *gakkai* organized CME without credentials or oversight. The MHLW does not require physicians to participate in CME. It hopes that patients will prefer accredited hospitals and physicians with certifications.

To make use of market incentives, the MHLW permits hospitals to advertise their accreditation. Those that are MHLW-certified CME providers can issue certificates to graduates, who can advertise their credentials. In the future, the MHLW and professional organizations will probably require hospitals to be accredited and physicians to obtain CME credits.

Until 2003, Japan lacked mandatory postgraduate medical education. Then the MHLW required two years postgraduate training through internships and residencies. This reform may change Japan's unusual pattern of relations between medical schools and hospitals. In the past, physicians relied on their medical school networks (*Ikyoku*) for employment; indeed, hospitals had difficulty hiring or firing physicians without the network leader's consent. Graduate training and professional certification may reduce the Ikyoku's influence.[45] A new system to match medical school graduates to residency programs provides an alternative to the Ikyoku network.

While these changes do not directly address physicians' conflicts of interest, they promote the development of hospitals as independent institutions and of hospital standards and practice norms that constrain physicians' discretion and limit the power of their connections with their peers, which may compete with their responsibilities to their employers and patients.

OVERSIGHT OF GIFTS AND COMMERCIAL FUNDING

Three main statutes affect relationships between physicians and third parties including medical device and drug firms: the Physicians' Act, the Medical Service Act, and the Health Insurance Act. These laws make kickbacks, bribes, and gifts to publicly employed physicians a violation of civil and criminal law, but they do not apply to physicians in private practice.

In the 1990s, the state prosecuted several publicly employed physicians for receiving kickbacks in return for influencing hospital purchasing. Kickbacks thrived in the pacemaker industry because prices were unregulated, allowing manufacturers to pass on their cost. In 1992, seven physicians in public hospitals and twenty-four representatives of American pacemaker manufacturers were prosecuted. Among those convicted were the head of cardiology at Tokyo Metropolitan Hospital and a professor at Tokyo University Medical School. In response, the MHW took measures to lower the prices of pacemakers.[46] Other kickback prosecutions concerned purchase of laboratory equipment, radiology machines, anesthesia machines, and radiology equipment.[47]

Kickbacks can have adverse medical consequences for patients, as well as raising costs overall. The problem is clearest in studies of drug safety and effectiveness that are funded by drug companies. The testing of Lacidipine, a calcium channel blocker used to treat hypertension, illustrates the risk when drug firms sponsor clinical trials without adequate controls. Japan Glaxo, a subsidiary of GlaxoSmithKlein, recruited 100 hospitals and collected 540 cases in phase II and III trials. Sales representatives paid $17,000 in bribes to each of two civil servant physicians. Evidence in the trial showed that they falsified clinical data to improve results.[48] Drug firms often paid physicians to participate in post-marketing trials by reporting information on patients who used their products. These studies were a means to pay physicians for each patient to whom they prescribed the drug, promoting sales rather than research.[49]

Gifts are important in Japanese culture and business.[50] The boundary between acceptable gifts and illegal kickbacks has shifted over time. So have the kinds of relationships that exist between independent firms. Many supplier-purchaser relationships are termed *Tachiai*, a relationship of mutual dependence. Rather than selling products in individual impersonal transactions, suppliers include extensive support. The purchaser depends on the seller, and it is hard to distinguish the purchased product or service from additional tie-ins. There is no clear line between what is purchased, product support that is provided for free, gifts, favors based on a personal or business relationship, and kickbacks.

Medical device suppliers often bring their product to the surgeon at the time of surgery and sometimes prepare it for use and assist the physician. The hospital benefits because it does not have to stock supplies and keep inventory. The physician receives expert troubleshooting if problems arise. The practice creates loyalty since physicians need the seller's services. The seller obtains information on the physician's practice and can recommend additional materials to a responsive purchaser. In this sort of relationship, which often involves multiple products, it is difficult for the physician to choose a lower cost option from another company.

Similarly, medical equipment firms sometimes lend equipment to physicians. In return, the borrower pays for supplies and services needed to operate the equipment, or purchases other equipment. Firms tread a fine line when making loans: they earn less revenue from loans than sales, but they also want to attract and keep customers. These loans and services can be construed as kickbacks.[51]

Despite prohibitions, some firms pay cash gifts to publicly employed physicians as well as private practitioners. One drug firm executive reported in 2002 that drug firms used to give medical representatives cash in envelopes to pay physicians.[52] However, when firms independently asked physicians how much they received, they found it was less than the cash placed in the envelopes, indicating that representatives pocketed part of it, so firms searched for other means to make payments.

Firms carefully select physicians with whom they have a good relationship, to avoid making gifts to individuals who may report them. Firms frequently offer gift certificates at prestigious stores, golf outings, and entertainment. One medical equipment sales representative reports that physicians typically ask for gifts rather than waiting for representatives to initiate offers.[53] When representatives discuss equipment features, the purchasing physician sometimes suggests that the representative add something to "sweeten the arrangement," such as a home computer. Firms often oblige to make the sale, even though the practice is frowned upon or actually illegal.

Some private hospital administrators acknowledge that drug firms still make gifts to physicians, but they tolerate it.[54] They say it would be difficult to stop the practice without offending both physicians and drug firms; all hospitals would have to act together to avoid adverse consequences. Moreover, the funds that physicians receive from outside companies reduce pressure for hospitals to increase physicians' salaries, giving administrators an interest in avoiding taking measures to end the exchange of gifts.

JAPAN FAIR TRADE COMMISSION REGULATION OF DRUG FIRMS

The Japan Fair Trade Commission (JFTC) promotes market competition by restricting unfair trade practices. Until 2009, its jurisdiction included enforcement of the 1962 Premiums and Representations Act, which restricts payment and in-kind benefits to induce sales.[55] Anti-monopoly and fair trade laws apply to drug company relations with physicians in private practice as well as publicly employed physicians.[56] Although the JFTC's mission is not to control physicians' conflicts of interest, it curbs drug firm practices that exploit physicians' conflicts of interest as a means to promote sales. The JFTC changed three long-standing marketing practices: wholesalers concealing real drug prices through rebates or gifts of drugs, manufacturers' control over wholesalers' sale prices, and gifts and grants to individual physicians.

Manufacturer Rebates and Control of Wholesale Prices

Drug wholesalers used to give private practitioners free drugs with each order, based on the volume they purchased. When physicians purchased 100 boxes of a drug, the wholesaler would add 25 boxes as a rebate or gift. These rebates/gifts inflated the reported wholesale price, which was a baseline used by public hospitals to pay for drugs and by the MHLW to set physician reimbursement.[57] Both physicians and drug firms benefited. Physicians earned more profit. Drug firms increased sales from such targeted incentives for physicians to purchase their product rather than a competitor's.

If, instead of tendering the rebate, wholesalers lowered their price by an equivalent amount, the average wholesale price would decrease. The true amount that physicians earned would be disclosed and, in response, the MHLW would reduce drug reimbursement, which would then lower physicians' profits. In 1991, the JFTC deemed wholesaler gifts of drugs with each purchase a prohibited premium.[58]

The second marketing practice consisted of drug firms setting drug prices for individual clinics and hospitals. The drug company's representative would tell the wholesaler at what price to sell its drugs to each purchaser, adjusting purchase prices to increase incentives for physicians to dispense its drugs in response to competition. In 1982, the JFTC issued its Unfair Trade Code that made clear that manufacturers' control over resale price violated the Anti-Monopoly Law.[59]

The third marketing practice consisted of gifts and financial support to individual physicians, physician associations, and hospitals used to develop relationships and influence prescribing. Gifts included performing chores and personal services for physicians; golf outings, meals, and gift certificates at expensive stores; cash; research assistance, slides, and photocopying; and financial contributions to medical societies and physician organizations for conferences, professional activities, and travel.

In 1984, the JFTC issued Guidelines on Pharmaceutical Manufacturers and Gift Giving that restricted certain gifts and payments to *all* physicians and it revised these periodically.[60] The JFTC delegates oversight authority to an industry self-regulatory organization named the Fair Trade Council of the Ethical Pharmaceutical Drugs Marketing Industry (FTCEPDMI). To promote compliance with the 1984 JFTC gift guidelines, the FTCEPDMI established an industry code of conduct in 1984 and revised this in 1997 and 2007.[61]

Drug Firm Gifts and Grants

To comply with JFTC and FTCEPDMI codes, in 1984 the Japan Pharmaceutical Manufacturers' Association (JPMA) revised its code of conduct, established new guidelines, and revised both in 1993.[62] The JPMA1993 guidelines allowed drug companies to assist physicians with research, photocopying, and presentations related to their products since the JFTC deemed that legitimate promotion. However, the guidelines limited assistance unrelated to their products to about ¥100,000 ($700) a year per institution. Still, drug firms could hire physicians to conduct research, write articles, give lectures, or participate in post-marketing trials and reimburse their conference expenses.

There were no reporting requirements, so it is hard to gauge the extent of compliance. Some pharmaceutical representatives claimed the guidelines leveled the playing field and they felt less pressure to perform chores for physicians. An article noted that physicians complained about having to do their own literature searches and photocopying. Drug firms reported lower promotion expenditures the year the guidelines went into effect. But payments continue in different forms. One physician said "year-end parties, group tours and golf competitions can safely be continued by soliciting donations from 30 to 40 companies" so that no firm offers more support than allowed.[63]

Even more important, the FTCEPDMI code and related guidelines changed the way drug firms supply funds to physicians rather than end their financial support. Around 1993 the JPMA organized its members to collectively make contributions to physicians through foundations of two regional pharmaceutical industry associations: the Pharmaceutical Manufacturers' Association of Tokyo (PMAT) and the Pharmaceutical Manufacturers' Association of Osaka (PMAO). Using these pooled funds, the foundations make grants to physicians and medical associations. Because no single firm makes a direct payment to an individual physician or association, the JFTC does not deem such funding an unfair trade practice.

The PMAT and PMAO request that each of its member firms contribute a percentage of the foundation's budget that is the same as the firm's market share of drug sales. The PMAT and PMAO report contributing over ¥2.17 billion ($19.1 million) to 94 medical associations for conferences, meetings, and other activities through their affiliated foundations in 2001, and ¥1.508 billion ($12.82 Million) to 150 medical associations in 2007. The funds go to national or regional medical societies that submit grant proposals. The foundations do not contribute to local medical societies, such as medical school alumni associations in small cities. Officials at the PMAT say that it would be unfair to ask all drug firms to contribute, since they may have no business in that locality or related to those associations.[64] Local medical societies typically request and receive support directly from companies that do business in the area.

The PMAT and PMAO foundations generally contribute no more than half the cost of any activity or event. Medical societies can seek additional funds from other firms, such as medical device manufacturers or construction companies that have ties to medical schools. Medical societies file a brief report stating how they used the funds. They are supposed to return

funds not spent for activities requested in their grant proposal. The foundations, however, do not audit grantees.

In theory, collective funding precludes individual firms from using
grants to help change physician prescribing. However, evaluating the effects
of collective funding requires scrutiny of foundations' practices, which are
not transparent. Can individual companies influence the funding decisions
of the foundations? Do the foundations allocate funds to support activities
and specialty groups that correspond roughly to the distribution of products
of contributing companies? We do not know.

The JFTC's regulation of pharmaceutical firms' support contrasts sharply
with French and American regulation. It promotes fair market competition,
rather than merely prohibit kickbacks, as in the United States, or to promote
physician ethics, as in France. Unlike in France, which relies on the Order of
Physicians to oversee commercial funding of medical activities, or the United
States, which draws on the American Medical Association's ethical guidelines as a standard for federal regulation, in Japan, competition law and
industry guidelines supply the standard; organized medicine plays no role.

The substance of Japan's policy also differs from those of France and the
United States. Only Japan restricts individual company funding to individual recipients. France places virtually no restrictions on individual company support for individual physicians or associations. In the United States,
the Office of Inspector General uses Medicare Anti-Kickback Act compliance guidelines to discourage certain pharma funding. It targets support
that appears to control or use CME to promote off-label drug uses and prohibits other funding that constitutes a kickback.

Drug firms employ university physicians to conduct research and sometimes as consultants or speakers. The Ministry of Education allows drug
firms to support medical researchers if funds pass through the university.[65]
Around 2002, drug companies supplied over half of medical research funds
at Japanese universities. They sometimes make unrestricted research
grants, which researchers can spend on professional activities. They can use
such grants to reward physicians who promote their interests. The Ministry
of Education requires that physicians employed in medical schools and university hospitals receive the university's permission to speak at meetings
sponsored by drug firms. In 2002, Tokyo University limited their honoraria
to ¥50,000 ($400) for a talk, which typically took an hour or two.

ORGANIZED MEDICINE'S NEGLIGIBLE OVERSIGHT

The JMA has not used ethical codes to regulate physicians, unlike organized
medicine in France and the United States. The JMA adopted its first ethical

code in 1951, which stated six principles in 150 words. The JMA revised these as Principles of Medical Ethics in 2002.[66] However, the JMA does not issue ethical opinions, and its code plays no role in medical policy discussions. Physicians do not turn to the code when faced with practice problems; indeed, most are unaware it exists. Courts and government agencies do not look to the code for guidance.

The JMA's ethical code and principles do not mention conflicts of interest. The 2002 code says, "The physician will not engage in medical activities for profit-making motives." Yet the JMA directs its condemnation of profit making against investor-owned hospitals rather than physicians, even when they own hospitals and clinics.[67] The JMA has not tried to mitigate the effects of conflicts of interest inherent in physician drug dispensing either. It lacks guidelines on gifts from drug firms or other commercial interests. In 2004, the JMA published a report on the social responsibility of physicians which said that "physicians should refrain from accepting gifts from patients" because that will suggest they treat patients more favorably "in exchange for such gifts, and it will jeopardize the confidence in the medical profession."[68]

The JMA does not oversee licensing or conduct professional discipline. Instead, the MHLW issues licenses to medical school graduates who pass national licensing exams and it oversees physician discipline.[69] However, the MHLW committee that must approve any sanction includes representatives from the JMA and Japan Dental Association. The MHLW can sanction physicians for (1) conduct unbecoming a physician, (2) violations of medical laws, (3) drug addiction or abuse, and (4) criminal convictions when penalties involve more than fines. It can issue a warning, suspend licenses temporarily (from one month to five years), or revoke licenses.[70]

Traditionally the MHLW revoked licenses for criminal activities, insurance fraud, or drug impairment rather than for incompetence or questionable ethics. Recently it has broadened its reach in some egregious cases of medical misconduct. In 2004, the regulatory reform and privatization promotion commission proposed that physicians be required to renew their medical licenses periodically and receive training and testing.[71] From 1971 to 1990, the MHLW sanctioned 324 physicians.[72] It revoked six licenses for offenses that included murder, arson, sexual exploitation, and harboring a terrorist. The other physicians received lesser sanctions.

Significantly, the MHLW disciplinary committee is not proactive. It lacks investigative powers and relies on reports of misconduct brought to its attention. There is no mandatory reporting of misconduct, but the MHLW asks public health centers to send them news accounts about physician misconduct. It is considering instituting a program to obtain information regularly from law enforcement agencies or courts.

Table 9.1. Physician Discipline in Japan, 1971–1990

	No.	%
Medical license-related	86	26.5
Drug-related	52	16.0
Fraud and abuse of health insurance claims (non-criminal, often by physicians supervising medical practice by non-medical personnel)	41	12.7
Tax evasion	40	12.3
Bribery	26	8.0
Fraud (criminal, not necessarily medically related)	22	6.8
Professional negligence resulting in death or injury (not necessarily medically related)	21	6.5
False documentation	8	2.5
Murder or injury	7	2.2
Obscenity	6	1.9
Other	15	4.6
Total (n)	324	

Source: Data from Ministry of Health Labor and Welfare, analyzed by Dr. Estuji Okamoto.

CONCLUSION

Private practitioners simultaneously prescribe and provide services, and this compromises their ability to make unbiased treatment decisions. Combined hospital and physician payment reinforce incentives to increase or decrease services. The overlap between these roles is a key reason that Japanese patients are prescribed more drugs and have longer hospital stays than patients in France and the United States. It also explains the higher use of diagnostic imaging and tests and drug consumption. The MHLW has controlled spending through strict price controls but has not addressed the inappropriate use of services that arise from conflicts of interest.

Since 1990, the MHLW reduced incentives to perform certain overused services by replacing fee-for-service with per diems or bundled payment, and it is now moving rapidly toward prospective payment for most acute care. In the past, providers benefited from increased spending while the MHLW tried to control expenditures. Payment reforms align providers' incentives with the MHLW's goal of limiting spending and generating conflicts of interest from incentives to reduce services.

Because a single payment reimburses institutional and physician services, the MHLW cannot employ different incentives for hospitals and physicians so that each counters biases of the other, an option available in the United States and France. However, it has blended different forms of payment, balancing incentives to provide certain services with incentives to use other services frugally. This sophisticated way of countering perverse incentives reduces the risk of undertreatment generated by using only incentives to cut services.[73]

The JMA portrays itself as protecting patients from cost cutting that reduces quality of care, yet it blocked the creation of mechanisms that promote quality by monitoring physicians. It opposed reporting information on patient care that would allow insurers, the MHLW, or others to oversee medical practice. It ensured that utilization review has little bite. Moreover, neither the JMA nor other physician organizations have developed their own peer review or quality assurance. Japan lacks another potential check on physicians' discretion because the health care consumer movement and patients' rights groups are generally weak.[74]

Physician drug dispensing remains a key source of conflicts of interest. Since 1990, the MHLW has reduced the profitability of dispensing and the number of physicians who dispense drugs has fallen. However, those who dispense still have conflicts of interest. The legacy of drug firms' close financial ties to physicians continues to distort prescribing decisions. The MHLW is better at containing spending than countering physicians' conflicts of interest that can reduce quality of care.

The JFTC has changed drug-company funding of physicians and medical societies so that they now supply most of their funds collectively through foundations rather than by having each firm make separate payments. This shift prevents direct links between individual drug firm funding and individual recipients. If it works as it is supposed to, it precludes kickbacks and physician incentives to prescribe drugs of particular firms.

Reforms at the beginning of the twenty-first century are changing medical practice. The MHLW is trying to convert physician-owned hospitals into institutions that resemble not-for-profit charitable hospitals in the United States. Reforms in medical education, hospital standards, accreditation, and certification may also transform private practice. In addition, current policy aims to make university hospitals—previously publicly financed and organized—quasi-independent.

University hospitals and physician-owned hospitals that convert into designated medical service organization systems could develop in very different ways. They might become akin to French mutual insurer-owned hospitals or American staff-model HMOs or not-for-profit hospitals. If that occurred, they would offer a model for private medical practice that is not entrepreneurial. Alternatively, they might become financially driven institutions that promote physician entrepreneurship, cater to patients who are financially better off than average, and market innovative technologies.

A key issue for the future is whether advocates of deregulating insurance and hospitals succeed in implementing proposals that permit investor-owned hospitals, supplemental insurance that pays for uncovered services, and balance billing. If they do, those changes will create new kinds of physicians' conflicts of interest, entrepreneurship, and market competition. Yet they might also make it possible for insurers and private hospitals to oversee medical practice in new ways.

Part V

IMPLICATIONS

10

Reforms

To shed light on how reforms can help address physicians' conflicts of interest, table 10.1 displays a typology of four key policy strategies: (1) prohibit individuals from entering situations that pose conflicts of interest; (2) require disclosure of conflicts of interest to allow individuals affected to take protective measures; (3) regulate conduct to reduce opportunities for physicians with conflicts of interest to breach trust or abuse discretion; (4) impose sanctions on individuals who violate trust and require restitution. The first two strategies occur *before* the existence of conflicts of interest to preclude it or warn the vulnerable party. The third regulates conduct *during* the conflicted relationship to reduce the risk of misconduct. The fourth provides remedies *after* misconduct.[1]

The organization of medical practice can prevent certain conflicts of interest from arising. It can ensure that physicians who prescribe services or products do not earn income by their sale, preclude certain employment and payment arrangements, and prohibit physicians from receiving gifts from drug and medical device firms and other commercial interests. Alternatively, disclosing physicians' conflicts of interest enables patients (or those acting on their behalf) to take protective measures that may mitigate

Table 10.1. Conflicts of Interest: Intervention Points

PREVENTION	REGULATION	SANCTIONS/RESTITUTION
Before physician acts	While physician acts	After physician acts
Prohibit	**Supervise**	**Penalize**
physicians from entering into situations with conflicts of interest	conduct of physicians and limit their discretion	physicians for violation of trust
Disclose		**Compensate**
conflicts of interest		patients for harm caused if physicians abuse their trust

their effects. They can monitor their physician's conduct, consult another physician, choose another provider for some medical care, or terminate the relationship.

The regulation of medical practice can reduce physicians' discretion and the risk that they may act inappropriately. Evidence shows that professional organizations do not discipline physicians effectively. However, insurers and the state, working with physicians and other professionals, can develop practice guidelines and review the treatment that physicians recommend to limit their provision of unnecessary services. They can deny payment for elective surgery or other procedures unless the treating physician demonstrates that it is appropriate. They can check inappropriate prescribing of drugs, ordering of tests, or referrals. In addition, financial, civil, or criminal sanctions can deter inappropriate conduct. Courts can provide restitution to patients harmed.

CHOOSING AMONG ALTERNATIVE RESPONSES

Conflicts of interest that arise from different sources can produce similar financial incentives for physicians to act inappropriately and thus create similar risks for patients. In that respect, it matters little whether a conflict of interest arises from physician ownership of medical facilities, selling of services, employment, payment, or ties with third parties. Moreover, within each category of conflicts of interest, incentives can range from weak and diffuse to strong and direct. For example, the strength of the financial incentive to refer patients to physician-owned facilities varies depending on the number of investors and the way the investment is organized.

Therefore, policy makers should consider the probability that particular conflicts of interest give rise to misconduct, and the extent of harm such misconduct can cause. It is reasonable to assume that the larger the financial incentive and the more directly it is linked to individual physician choices, the more likely it is to affect their behavior. However, as an activity's social value increases, it makes sense to bear greater risk from the conflicts of interest that it produces. Still, often there is more than one way to produce socially valuable services. It is therefore important to assess the feasibility of producing desirable benefits by alternative means that either have no or less serious conflicts of interest.

Even when there is little risk of harm, society may want to curb activities that create conflicts of interest if the activity has minimal social value. For example, a prohibition on commercial interests offering physicians gifts would curb inappropriate influence over physician prescribing, yet patients and society would lose little from such a ban. Similarly, there would be no significant social loss from prohibiting physician investment in freestanding facilities that supplied services that they prescribe because others will supply those services and investment capital to finance these facilities if there is legitimate demand for them.

The situation is more complex, however, when physicians supply these services in their own practice, since that offers convenience and speeds service for patients, even though the incentives to generate income may still induce physicians to prescribe those services inappropriately. The issue then becomes whether, in order to enjoy the convenience, society should incur the risks. If the increased convenience from physicians supplying ancillary services is minor, prohibition is appropriate.

Regulators have strong grounds to prohibit conduct that can produce great harm, particularly if it is hard to detect misconduct or if possible remedies for health risks are inadequate. In other circumstances it makes more sense to tolerate conflicts of interest but subject physicians to oversight because the risk from the conflicted behavior is small, the cost of precluding the existence of a conflict of interest is great, and the conflict can be addressed adequately and at lower social cost through oversight.

For example, both fee-for-service and risk-sharing payments create conflicts of interest. However, banning these payment arrangements would be overly restrictive, since rewarding production and encouraging physicians to consider costs can produce social benefits. It makes more sense to restrict and regulate the use of these payment incentives, encourage the use of blended payment, and oversee physician practice to check inappropriate over- and underuse of services.

When oversight would be very costly or would reduce the value of the work physicians perform, it may be preferable to prohibit certain transactions as a preventive measure. So many transactions take place between patients and physicians that regulating conduct through rules for specific transactions is cumbersome and expensive. Monitoring compliance with detailed rules is costly, as is reviewing physicians' performance to determine whether they made proper clinical decisions. Often it is more efficient to prohibit broad classes of conduct through legislation than to adopt policies that regulate the details of physicians' behavior or provide sanctions for misconduct.

When the costs and benefits of prohibiting conflicts suggest that a ban would not yield a net gain, requiring that physicians disclose the conflict can help patients and their proxies make informed decisions as to whether they want to follow the physician's advice or seek an alternative provider. However, it is an insufficient response to important conflicts of interest and sometimes physicians and organizations use disclosure in ways that make matters worse. Revealing conflicts of interest should not be used to create a system of caveat emptor where the parties disclosing information can act as they please.[2]

France contains physicians' conflicts of interest first by reducing the private medical sector's size, then by restricting the scope of physician entrepreneurship. It prohibits private practitioners from selling ancillary services, a key source of conflicts of interest. France has also regulated employer influence on physicians and restricted many commercial practices. However, it has neglected to oversee private practitioners through utilization review and managed care, or to develop alternatives to fee-for-service payment in private practice. It started but then stopped the growth of not-for-profit medical facilities that employ physicians, largely because it has not reduced the authority of organized medicine over the medical market.

The United States has empowered insurers to oversee physicians' conflicts of interest through utilization review, other oversight, and payment incentives. However, when insurers replaced fee-for-service payment, they sometimes created new payment conflicts of interest by introducing physician risk sharing. The United States has not reined in the private sector's growth. It did, however, promote the growth of lay-directed, not-for-profit health maintenance organizations (HMOs) that employ physicians. It also restricted some role conflicts—such as physician self-referral—but only for certain physicians, while treating some patients, for designated services.

Japan has addressed conflicts of interest by moderately reducing and countering fee-for-service incentives. Yet, since national health insurance (NHI) began, it neither restricted physicians' entrepreneurial roles nor capped the size of the physician-owned medical sector until 2007, when it stopped allowing new physician-owned medical corporations that operate hospitals and clinics. Japan has neglected oversight of physician practice through practice guidelines, utilization review, or managed care.

THE INADEQUACY OF CONVENTIONAL REFORMS

France, the United States, and Japan offer examples suggesting that six frequently proposed reforms are either ineffective or inadequate remedies:

- Replace investor-owned firms with physician or not-for-profit owned entities.
- Defer to professional self-regulation.
- Rely on market competition.
- Publicly employ all physicians.

- Hold physicians to fiduciary standards and increase their liability for patient injury.
- Disclose conflicts of interest.

Replace Investor-Owned Firms with Physician or Not-for-Profit Owned Entities

According to one popular idea, the profit motive of lay-owned, for-profit firms generates conflicts of interest while supplying medical services through physician-owned practices or physician-directed, not-for-profit organizations avoids them.[3]

The experience of Japan shows that physicians' conflicts of interest exist in the absence of investor-owned firms, in physician-owned or -directed facilities. In traditional Japanese medicine, physicians said they offered their services without compensation and patients reimbursed them for supplies, namely drugs. Physicians lived off what patients contributed, so this arrangement surely encouraged physicians to prescribe drugs. In contemporary Japan, physicians continue to dispense and prescribe more drugs than physicians do in other countries, and to select more expensive brands when there is a choice.

Since World War II, Japan has virtually precluded ownership of clinics and hospitals by dividend-paying firms. The law promoted ownership by physicians or physician-owned corporations that do not pay dividends. Studies reveal that these facilities behave like lay-owned for-profit firms.[4] They generate a high volume of services and dispense a high volume of expensive drugs. They do not generally engage in public service, provide charity care, conduct medical research, forge medical innovations, or promote public health. Even though physician owners earn no dividends, they set their salaries and receive company cars, expense accounts, and other perks.

A similar phenomenon occurred in the United States in the early twentieth century when many physicians owned hospitals. Later, some physicians converted their hospitals into not-for-profit organizations and sought tax-exempt status. The Internal Revenue Service (IRS) was rightly concerned when the former physician owners controlled the board of trustees and the hospital had a closed medical staff consisting mainly of its former owners. It thought that these physicians used the not-for-profit hospital to subsidize their private practice, and the IRS did not grant them a tax exemption.[5]

In the United States today, few not-for-profit hospitals are controlled by a small group of physicians. Nevertheless, not-for-profit hospitals subsidize private practice through access to hospital resources, including a hospital's building, equipment, laboratories, and the services of nurses, residents, and interns. Not-for-profit insurers, such as Blue Cross and Blue Shield, finance hospitals and allow physicians to maintain entrepreneurial practices with little oversight. Some not-for-profit HMOs, such as Kaiser Permanente, create entrepreneurial incentives for their physicians by allowing them to bear insurance risk and increase their income when it earned a surplus. Not-for-profit university hospitals often adjust physician salaries annually to reward them for generating patient fees. Replacing investor-owned firms with physician-owned or not-for-profit organizations is insufficient to eliminate physicians' conflicts of interest.

Defer to Professional Self-Regulation

Some physicians believe that only organized medicine should regulate conflicts of interest; others even favor allowing it to control the medical economy. Yet professional control can reinforce physicians' conflicts of interest and stymie more effective and stringent oversight.

Organized medicine has exercised greater regulatory authority in France than in the United States or Japan. Since World War II, the Order of Physicians has controlled licensing and discipline and overseen private practice. It governs relations among physicians and between physicians and patients, hospitals, employers, and providers. Before entering into a contract, physicians must seek its advice as to whether the terms follow the Order of Physicians' drafted Code of Medical Deontology (Medical Deontology). Medical Deontology restricts certain conflicts of interest. It does not permit insurers or employers to use financial incentives (aside from fee-for-service) that encourage physicians to increase or decrease services; and it prohibits physician dispensing.

Nevertheless, the Order of Physicians inhibited arrangements that reduce or check conflicts of interest. From 1930 on, it opposed mutual insurers that employed physicians—which eliminates fee-for-service conflicts—by claiming that employment violated Medical Deontology. It insisted that medical secrecy/confidentiality does not allow billing codes to specify services that physicians supply, preventing insurer oversight. Rather than control physician ties with pharma, it joined with the drug and medical device trade associations to oppose restrictions on industry funding. As a result, individual drug and other medical supply firms still pay physicians' personal expenses when they attend professional meetings.

In the United States, professional self-regulation also tolerated significant conflicts of interest. For much of its history, the American Medical Association (AMA) permitted physicians to dispense drugs, own pharmacies, and perform clinical tests; it opposed legislation to prohibit these practices. It fought prepaid group practice, HMOs, and physician employment, which can reduce entrepreneurial and payment conflicts. It opposed restrictions on commercial firms making gifts to physicians and financing continuing medical education (CME) in ways that compromise its integrity. Today, state medical societies, the AMA, and medical specialty societies depend heavily on financial support from commercial interests for many of their activities.

Sometimes organized medicine does not even address physicians' conflicts of interest. The Japan Medical Association (JMA) has not developed policies, ethical codes, or guidelines to restrict kickbacks or gifts from pharmaceutical firms. Nor has it developed policies to cope with physicians' entrepreneurial or payment conflicts. Furthermore, in all three countries, even though organized medicine plays a role in institutions that can suspend or revoke medical licenses, these controls have not been very effective even for addressing serious misconduct.[6]

Rely on Market Competition

Rather than eliminate physicians' conflicts of interest, unregulated medical markets increase them. The U.S. medical economy is more market oriented than that of France or Japan and today has fewer professional and legal restraints on medical commerce than existed previously. Federal and state governments do not control fees outside of Medicare and Medicaid and the federal government has ended hospital planning. Many medical firms are investor owned. Antitrust law and health policy promote markets. The result is that physicians have a greater variety of conflicts of interest than their counterparts in France or Japan. They can engage in the full spectrum of entrepreneurial activities, alone or jointly with investor-owned firms or not-for-profit organizations. Though many are paid fee-for-service, they sometimes bear financial risk and have payment conflicts of interest that do not affect French and Japanese physicians.

Market competition created new conflicts of interest for physicians and exacerbated existing ones. At the same time, it allowed the growth of HMOs and managed care, which can eliminate entrepreneurial and payment conflicts and can oversee physicians. Markets enabled insurers and lay-owned firms to become countervailing powers to organized medicine. Ending professional and regulatory restraints was like opening Pandora's box: it released numerous negative forces, but at the same time it freed a positive one.

Publicly Employ All Physicians

All three countries have some public facilities that employ physicians and avoid conflicts of interest from payment, entrepreneurship, and ties to insurers and other providers—a major achievement. But publicly employed physicians sometimes engage in part-time private practice or consulting, which produces conflicts from entrepreneurship, payment, and third-party ties. Still, public employment does not create these conflicts, and precluding private consultations eliminates them.

Similarly, in all three countries, commercial interests can support the research activities of publicly employed physicians. In France, publicly employed physicians can also receive funds from drug and medical device firms to participate in professional activities. Yet commercial support is not a characteristic of public employment; the state can prohibit or regulate it. Nevertheless, public authorities often allow commercial interests to supply these funds to reduce their financial burden.

One risk of universal public physician employment is that the state may impose ideological agendas, or pursue goals antithetical to patient care, or promote war aims. A more likely problem is that the state will supply insufficient funds. In France and Japan, even though the most prestigious research and teaching hospitals are publicly owned, many patients choose private hospitals for routine services because of the amenities available in them. These patients will want to maintain alternatives to publicly employed physicians. The U.S. public is even more predisposed toward privately supplied medical services. Moreover, organized medicine has consistently fought to maintain private practice. A public medical sector can help restrict physicians' conflicts of interest, yet we should not preclude all private means to supply medical care. Few countries are likely to eliminate private practice.

Hold Physicians to Fiduciary Standards and Increase Their Liability for Patient Injury

Courts could intervene when physicians with conflicts of interest cause harm to their patients. Proponents of this approach say that we should not preclude physician entrepreneurship and self-referral because they produce benefits, even though some physicians abuse these arrangements. Instead, they argue, society should penalize physician misconduct and compensate patients who are harmed. The penalties could apply when physicians act in bad faith, when they act negligently, or whenever their patients are injured.

Philosopher E. Haavi Morreim proposes that courts hold physicians to fiduciary standards of loyalty to counter inappropriate physician self-referral.[7] She suggests that if a patient shows that a physician acted in bad faith, courts should require that the physician compensate the patient for injuries, emotional distress, and attorneys' fees and perhaps even pay punitive damages. That would discourage bad faith self-referral, she maintains. Courts could use this approach for other conflicts of interest as well.

This proposal has many drawbacks. It requires patients to sue physicians, but many will not. Some may not know they suffered injuries due to their physician's conduct or that their physician had a conflict of interest. Others will not sue because they believe they are unlikely to prevail, or they lack funds to pursue litigation. In the United States, attorneys will not represent patients for a contingency fee unless there is a strong chance they will win and earn a high award. Moreover, while the remedy may compensate patients bilked of money, they are inadequate for patients who were injured or killed. Policies that reduce the risk of harm are almost always preferable.

Furthermore, patients will often be unable to prove that physicians acted in bad faith because physicians can point to medical uncertainty or differences of expert opinion. Patients will lack remedies when conflicts of interest subtly bias physicians' clinical decisions, prescriptions, and referrals. As a result, patients will file most suits alleging bad faith when they have independent grounds to sue physicians: for negligence, violation of the anti-kickback laws, or other illegal conduct. Suits based on physician bad faith will be least helpful when most needed—when other remedies are unavailable.

A more promising approach is to hold physicians *strictly liable* for patient injuries when physicians self-refer or have other conflicts of interest. In other words, physicians would be held responsible for bad outcomes, even when they were not negligent. That would give physicians an incentive to avoid activities that create conflicts of interest. Still, physicians who engage in highly profitable entrepreneurial activities might find bearing higher liability risk worthwhile since they can purchase liability insurance. And strict liability for patient injuries does not provide a remedy for patients' financial loss arising from unnecessary clinical or diagnostic tests that do not inflict physical injury.

Although courts or legislatures could develop strict liability rules, there is no reason to believe they will do so in the United States any time soon. The current trend is to propose malpractice reforms that protect physicians from liability or cap patient awards. Legislation to impose liability on physicians when they are not negligent is apt to be defeated.[8] Japan, however, has increased its criminal prosecutions for physician negligence in recent years, but mainly for gross negligence.[9]

Disclose Conflicts of Interest

Many reformers call for disclosure of conflicts of interest. Some claim that disclosure cures the conflict. Others say that it allows patients to protect their interests. They presume that if the public is informed, many physicians will not engage in compromising financial arrangements and those that do are unlikely to betray their patients' trust. They believe that disclosure is simple and inexpensive, that it preserves patients' and physicians' autonomy and increases patient choice. Disclosure is appealing because it appears to be cost-free, prohibit nothing and to require no oversight or change in the organization of medical practice. Policies that rely on disclosure assuage physicians' conscience, console the public, relieve policy makers from confronting difficult choices, and shift the burden to patients. But rather than resolve conflicts of interest, disclosure typically fails to address them effectively.[10]

It is far easier to write rules that require disclosure than to make it occur. Most patient-physician discussions are private, so how will public authorities monitor physician compliance without adding the burdensome oversight whose absence supposedly makes disclosure preferable to other approaches? Should there be sanctions for all failures to disclose, or only when patients are injured? What sanctions are appropriate?

One way to promote disclosure is to require physicians to have patients read and sign a form that reveals their conflict of interest. Hospital physicians already ask patients to sign forms to document that they have disclosed the risks and benefits of proposed treatment and obtained their informed consent. However, these forms protect physicians from liability more effectively than they inform patients, who usually read them just before surgery, long after they have decided to undergo it. Patients and physicians typically view the rapid reading and signing of these forms as a formality, not an opportunity for discussion.

The use of conflict-of-interest disclosure forms will be even less helpful and more burdensome than informed consent forms. Surgery is an infrequent, dramatic event that alerts patients to risk; patients may have time to reflect between the time a physician first discusses surgery and when it occurs. In contrast, situations that raise conflicts of interest occur much more frequently. Patients are likely to pay less heed than they do for surgical consent.

What, When, and How to Disclose?

Physicians could reveal their conflicts of interest at several points. Should they do so once, or routinely? Physicians could reduce their burden by having patients read and sign disclosure forms only at the beginning of the relationship. But that would diminish the information's value. Most patients cannot anticipate what services they will need and their relation to a physician's conflict of interest. Patients will not find conflicts of interest related to potential medical problems as meaningful as when they concern current treatment. By the time physicians make medical decisions colored by conflicts of interest, patients may have forgotten the information disclosed long ago.

Physicians might also present information in ways that do not help patients. Should we monitor what physicians say to ensure that they accurately and effectively disclose their financial interests? Studies of physician disclosure of the risks and benefits of medical treatment indicate that patients often do not understand the information provided. New information seldom leads patients to reconsider proposed treatments. Detailed written forms sometimes obscure understanding.[11]

If the aim is to give patients objective information and appraisal of their risk, a neutral party should disclose the conflict of interest. Empirical studies indicate that individuals often disclose information selectively in ways that promote their interests. Moreover, individuals' own perspectives affect how they report information. Studies show that individuals perceive their own motivations and behavior positively and believe that they are fairer than average.[12] Physicians with conflicts of interest rarely believe that they compromise their patients' care and will disclose their conflicts of interest in ways that support that conclusion.

Physicians can reveal their financial arrangements in ways that do not alert patients to the risks. They can portray their conflicts of interest as innocuous, or imply that because they supply the services that they recommend they have expertise and can ensure quality care. Discussing their conflict of interest in this way is akin to advertising. Rather than make patients proceed cautiously, it will encourage them to accept the arrangement. Indeed, if disclosure effectively alerted patients to the limits of physician loyalty and their biases, it might undermine trust and damage the relationship.

We know from psychological experiments that the framework in which people make choices affects their decisions and that the same information presented in contrasting contexts produces different decisions. It may be possible to regulate the written information that patients receive; but it will be much harder to regulate the context in which it is presented—the patient-physician relationship. Patients turn to physicians for advice and expect them to act on their behalf. The relationship requires trust, which means that most patients will follow their physician's advice. Moreover, people typically follow the requests of authority figures.[13] Studies also show that individuals prefer to agree with and say yes to people whom they know and like.[14] Transference increases these tendencies.[15]

Many people acknowledge that physicians might be affected by conflicts of interest, but few believe that their own doctors would be.[16] Patients are likely to downplay conflicts of interest that physicians disclose. Experiments reveal that individuals discount the risk of bias when warned and that they have difficulty ignoring information provided even when they are aware it is not reliable.[17] When physicians inform patients that their advice may be biased, this message clashes with patients' understanding of the relationship. Rather than ceasing to trust their physician, patients usually resolve this cognitive dissonance by discounting the conflict of interest.

Disclosure does not create satisfactory choices. How should a patient react when she learns that her physician has an incentive to prescribe a test because he supplies it? She can refuse to obtain the test, but that would interfere with her treatment and disrupt the relationship. She could obtain the test from another provider, but that might make both the patient and physician feel uncomfortable. A greater drawback is that obtaining the test from another provider does not resolve the problem. If the incentive leads a physician to recommend a test inappropriately, the patient still receives an unnecessary test if she obtains it elsewhere.

The patient could consult another physician regarding whether she needs the test. That costs time and money, delays treatment, and undermines patient-physician trust. Studies show that individuals are less likely to search for alternative products and services when time is important or they are ill equipped to assess the differences.[18] When time is crucial, patients are unlikely to exercise this option. Moreover, physicians who are consulted for a second opinion are reluctant to contradict the initial recommendation unless they have a different medical opinion on the whole problem. Patients could end the relationship with their conflicted physician. That, too, is costly, especially when patients have a chronic medical condition that requires continuing attention or have had a long-standing relationship with their physician.

If physicians routinely supply ancillary services that they prescribe, patients will be unlikely to question the practice. People tend to perceive behavior as appropriate if they see others following the same pattern.[19] When public policy allows physicians to recommend and supply services, merged roles become prevalent. Then patients who prefer physicians without financial conflicts of interest might not be able to find one.

Disclosure's Negative Effects

Disclosure may lull the public into believing that this response is sufficient, thereby encouraging medical practice with conflicts of interest. Physicians may conclude that they are relieved of further responsibility. That would shift the responsibility from physicians to patients. Is it fair to require individual patients to cope with this burden?

Disclosure sometimes protects physicians from liability and might reduce their obligation to act in their patients' interests. Physicians can argue that because they revealed their conflicts, patients should be barred from complaining about their effects. If courts accept this argument, disclosure will replace a fiduciary model of patient-physician relations with caveat emptor. Disclosure has sometimes had this effect. Cigarette manufactures used disclosure of health risk to limit their liability to smokers.[20] The U.S. Supreme Court held that the Food, Drug and Cosmetic Act regulation of medical devices preempts state tort laws, thereby barring patient liability suits against manufacturers.[21] Courts might similarly interpret rules that require the disclosure of conflicts of interest to preempt patients' suits against physicians.

Since disclosure does not end practices that create conflicts of interest or create effective means to oversee physicians, it is insufficient to protect patients. Still, it offers some benefit when the activity that creates the conflict of interest is valuable, there are no good alternative means to supply it, and the risk from the conflict of interest is small.

COPING STRATEGIES

The experiences of France, the United States, and Japan reveal six strategies that can help cope with physicians' conflicts of interest:

- Increase medical care outside of private practice.
- Restrict entrepreneurship within private practice.
- Oversee entrepreneurial physicians.
- Regulate payment incentives.
- Restrict and regulate ties with third parties.
- Protect professional judgment.

Let us examine how these strategies have been used to advantage in some countries and how others might develop them.

Increase Medical Care Outside of Private Practice

The *universal* public employment of physicians is a potentially effective but unattractive remedy that few nations are likely to adopt. Still, it makes sense to increase the number of physicians who practice in public facilities or in not-for-profit organizations where physicians lack entrepreneurial, employment, and payment conflicts of interest.

The United States has the smallest proportion of publicly employed physicians of the three countries. It could easily increase public employment while maintaining a vibrant private sector. Although it does not deliver extensive medical services through elite public institutions as in France and Japan, it has some first-rank public medical centers, such as the National Institutes of Health, which attract patients interested in participating in clinical trials. Despite public criticisms in the past when it was organized differently, the Veterans Administration (VA) health system today is a leader in medical quality, integrated care, and electronic medical record keeping.[22] Local governments often operate public hospitals, which serve as a safety net for the uninsured even though they typically are underfunded and overburdened. These examples demonstrate that the United States can expand the medical care supplied using publicly employed physicians.

Without ending existing options, the federal government could develop publicly owned medical centers in urban areas for individuals insured through Medicaid and perhaps other insurers as well. It could also subsidize public hospitals owned by local governments. If physicians were paid salaries comparable to those employed in the VA, private practitioners who serve many Medicaid patients might prefer this to private practice. They would avoid the economic risks and constraints they face in private practice relying on low Medicaid fees. Public facilities could attract patients by offering some advantages over existing options. For example, they could offer patients both a primary care physician of their choice and a twenty-four-hour walk-in clinic. Some Medicaid patients use emergency departments for after-hours ambulatory care. They might prefer a facility that offers twenty-four-hour service with shorter waits that is better tailored to their needs than emergency rooms.

Not-for-profit prepaid group practices (PPGP) and not-for-profit clinics offer another alternative. Both typically employ physicians and avoid entrepreneurial conflicts of interest. Dr. Arnold Relman advocates organizing medicine around not-for-profit group practices. Dr. Atul Gawande finds that the Mayo Clinic and some other not-for-profit centers have organizational cultures that avoid physician entrepreneurship and promote high quality medical care.[23] The American health reforms enacted in 2010 boosted funding for not-for-profit community health centers by eleven billion dollars over five years. The federal government could continue to expand funding so that they can play a larger role in the medical economy. Nevertheless, in both the United States and Japan some not-for-profit organizations have allowed physicians to maintain entrepreneurial, employment and payment conflicts of interest. We need greater governmental oversight to ensure that these organizations do not produce physicians' conflicts of interest when setting compensation.

France and Japan have fewer not-for-profit medical facilities than the United States and could develop these as an alternative to private practice or public employment. In France, physician unions stymied mutual-insurer medical facilities that employed physicians. Then, in the 1970s, the state brought most not-for-profit hospitals into the publicly funded hospital system. In 1971, the NHI Fund for Salaried Workers promised physician unions that it would not create or promote not-for-profit facilities. It should reverse this policy. The National Federation of Mutual Insurers is the logical entity to develop not-for-profit medical centers.

Japan's lay-directed, public service, not-for-profit medical facilities have not grown much since NHI began. The Ministry of Health Labor and Welfare (MHLW) could promote their expansion. Japan stopped the formation of physician-owned medical corporations in 2007, and the MHLW has offered tax subsidies to physician-owned medical corporations that become not-for-profit foundations. So far, however, few have pursued this option. The MHLW would have more success if it offered grants to create new not-for-profit medical foundations. Recent Ministry of Education reforms are transforming university hospitals into independent not-for-profit entities that may supply medical services without physicians' conflicts of interest.[24] However, there is insufficient oversight to ensure that this will occur.

Restrict Entrepreneurship within Private Practice

In France, insurers generally do not reimburse diagnostic and laboratory tests performed, or drugs and vaccines dispensed, by physicians or physician-owned facilities. Only a few physicians own hospitals or diagnostic imaging equipment. In the United States, in contrast, physicians can engage in a much wider range of entrepreneurial practices, including providing ancillary and hospital services, sharing financial risk, and owning captive insurance companies. Japanese physicians can offer the full range of ambulatory and inpatient medical services and are the main owners of private facilities.

The United States and Japan could restrict entrepreneurial opportunities in private practice as France does. To avoid disruption and political opposition, they could grandfather existing arrangements and implement the change incrementally. Initially, insurers could end reimbursement for the most expensive or overused physician-supplied tests. Alternatively, insurers could decrease the number of physicians who supply tests. There is precedent for this approach. Unable to prohibit physician dispensing, Japan has reduced the number of physicians who dispense by lowering their profits and increasing patient copayments. In the United States, physician office laboratories declined when Congress held them to the same quality standards as other laboratories and managed care organizations reviewed whether tests were appropriate. Similar policies could reduce other physician-supplied ancillary services.

Oversee Entrepreneurial Physicians

Public and private insurers can oversee physician entrepreneurs. They can deny payment for unnecessary services and screen referrals to specialists and elective surgery. They can control whether patients receive treatment in a hospital or an alternative setting and how long patients remain hospitalized. Their formularies can restrict what drugs are covered and require higher copayments for more expensive drugs. In the United States, insurers began utilization review in the 1950s and expanded it when managed care grew in the 1980s, but reduced its use after 2000. Yet they still exercise greater oversight than do insurers in France or Japan.

Since the 1930s, when French physician unions blocked the use of billing codes that reveal what services physicians supply, insurers have had little control over clinical practice. Reforms in 2004 introduced billing codes that indicate the services patients receive, making utilization review possible. In addition, the High Authority on Health (HAS) developed guidelines to limit inappropriate medical practices. But it remains uncertain whether insurers will exercise effective oversight, because organized medicine maintains that they cannot restrict physician choices.

In Japan, the JMA blocked the use of utilization review. Since 1961, it has opposed detailed insurer claims review. In the 1980s, it stalled electronic claims review. However, the MHLW introduced electronic claims review in 2004 and plans to phase out all paper claims by 2012. Still, Japan lacks carefully developed practice guidelines that the state or insurers could use to deny payment.

Regulate Payment Incentives

Self-employed physicians have conflicts of interest when paid fee-for-service and when they share financial risk for the cost of services they do not themselves provide or for the cost of drugs and tests. In the United States, payers often make physicians bear financial risk. Japan sometimes uses bundled or per-diem payment, which encourages physicians to skimp on supplies, medication, or services, but doctors bear much less financial risk than in the United States. In France, physicians do not bear financial risk for the cost of services.

All three countries inadequately regulate physician payment. They should limit the strength of financial incentives to increase or decrease services. One way to do this is to blend payment methods. Supplementing capitation payment with fees for certain services reduces the incentives to skimp. Supplementing fee-for-service payment with risk-sharing moderates the incentive to increase services. Financial rewards for physicians who provide higher than average quality of care can also reduce the distortions from other payment methods.

Restrict and Regulate Ties with Third Parties

Kickbacks

All three countries prohibit kickbacks to *publicly employed* physicians, but only France does so *for all* physicians. In the United States, the federal government prohibits kickbacks in private practice only for services paid by Medicare or Medicaid. A few states prohibit kickbacks for all physicians, but their enforcement and sanctions are weak. Japan prohibits drug firms from paying private practitioners premiums that constitute unfair competition.

The United States and Japan should ban kickbacks for all physicians as France does. Even private medical practice serves a public service mission, so legislatures should enact statutes that hold all physicians to the same standards used for publicly employed physicians. Kickbacks that encourage physicians to prescribe drugs or medical products or to refer patients to specific facilities or specialists should have no place in medical practice, whether public servants or private practitioners supply patient care and regardless of who pays physicians.

Anti-kickback laws are not valuable without systematic enforcement. U.S. law offers an effective model. The False Claims Act imposes fines three times the amount of kickbacks for individuals and firms prosecuted under the Medicare Anti-Kickback Act (Anti-Kickback Act). To encourage individuals to report misconduct, *Qui Tam* statutes award those who report false claims up to 25 percent of any court judgment or settlement. This provision facilitates prosecution. In the past decade, courts imposed numerous multimillion-dollar judgments. In addition, many firms paid multimillion-dollar fines to settle cases. These firms must then follow strict compliance programs and make all financial records available to the government. Federal sentencing law also encourages firms to adopt and follow government-approved compliance programs voluntarily by reducing their penalties if an employee pays kickbacks without corporate authority. Most large medical firms now have compliance programs that increase their oversight of practice. France and Japan lack a comparable system of oversight or incentives to report misconduct. They could improve their enforcement by using similar strategies.

In all three countries, pharmaceutical firms have used post-marketing clinical trials in order to pay disguised kickbacks to physicians who prescribe their drugs. There are legitimate uses of post-marketing trials, but current regulation is insufficient to deter abuses.[25] Each national legislature should empower its drug safety agency to regulate post-marketing clinical trials. These agencies should allow only well-designed trials that generate information on drug risks as part of a firm's plan to evaluate all its products; it is especially important that all the results be made public. A system of checks should ensure that trials are not a covert means of paying physicians to prescribe specific drugs.

Gifts

Providers and firms sometimes make gifts to physicians to influence their clinical choices. In all three countries, legislation restricts certain gifts for publicly employed physicians. New legislation should bar *all industry gifts* to self-employed and privately employed physicians with restrictions similar to those that currently apply to public employees.[26]

One way to restrict gift-giving in the United States is to require that physicians who participate in Medicare or Medicaid not accept any gifts and to prohibit any firm reimbursed by these programs from offering gifts to any physician. Other legislation could require that hospitals and other institutions that participate in Medicare and Medicaid prohibit their employees, medical students in training, and physicians with practice privileges from accepting gifts. Amendments to the Medicaid statute could require partici-

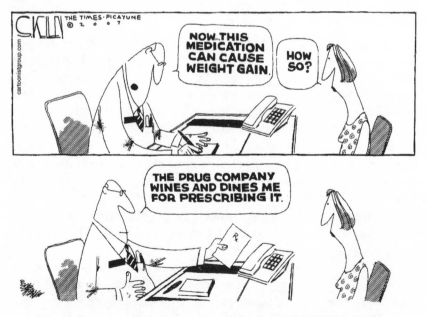

Cartoon by Steve Kelly. Source: CartoonStock.com. Published 27 April 2007.

pating states to enact legislation that revokes the license of physicians found to accept such gifts.

Financial Support from Pharma and Other Commercial Interests

To influence prescribing, promote sales, and foster physician reciprocity, pharma and other commercial interests fund CME, conferences and medical societies, and sometimes individual physicians. Each country addresses only part of the problem.

France allows commercial interests to reimburse all reasonable physicians' expenses incurred to participate in CME and professional meetings. They are only precluded from covering expenses unrelated to professional activities or for a physician's companion. Commercial firms can also support medical societies and CME providers. Today they fund much of the recently established accredited CME and sponsor their own unaccredited programs.

In the United States, Anti-Kickback Act compliance guidelines allow drug firms to underwrite CME and medical societies but prohibit their reimbursing individual physicians' expenses. The Accreditation Council for Continuing Medical Education (ACCME) guidelines for commercial support tries to control bias, holding that program planners and speakers must resolve conflicts of interest by having their programs peer reviewed; but the ACCME lacks means to enforce this policy. Moreover, commercial firms can slant curricula by only supporting programs related to their products.

Japan showed the direction reform should take when it severed links between individual donors and recipients. It restricts firms from individually supplying funds to physicians or medical associations. Instead, firms in the Japan Pharmaceutical Manufacturers Association (JPMA) supply collective support. Each JPMA member contributes a share of the JPMA grant budget that is proportional to their market share, and two foundations— each covering a separate region—disburse the funds.

In principle, individual firms do not control who receives funds. However, the funding process is not transparent. In addition, the JPMA can collectively influence the activities it supported. They appoint individuals who worked in pharmaceutical firms as foundation staff. Collective support can promote a class of drugs and off-label uses without favoring one firm's product. The foundations can support activities related to drugs rather than other medical issues or professional needs.

None of these countries eliminates the bias that arises from commercial interests choosing whom or what activities to support. Therefore, legislatures should prohibit industry financial support for accredited CME and other professional medical activities, both directly and through foundations or not-for-profit organizations. In its place, the government should provide funds for CME and other professional development, either directly or through an independent organization. The state could raise funds by taxing pharma, medical device firms, other medical suppliers, medical facilities, insurers, and physicians. In addition, just as each nation has authorities that set standards for medical school curricula, independent organizations unaffiliated with commercial interests should develop CME curricula based on assessments of problems that exist in medical practice and which activities are likely to have the greatest benefit to patients.

Firms and physicians would either pass along the tax through increased prices or absorb it and accept lower profits. Commercial interests already finance most CME and professional development. If they now pass on these costs in the prices they charge, then insurers and the public currently pick up the tab when they pay for their products. If the public bears this expense, it should choose how the funds will be used and avoid conflicts of interest that bias medical education. If commercial interests now absorb their CME spending, they can continue to do so.

Pharma could afford to absorb this tax, especially in the United States. Since the 1950s, the American pharmaceutical industry has earned higher profits than the average Fortune 500 companies have. Patents allow drug firms to enjoy exclusive sales and avoid price competition. High profit margins mean that prices do not necessarily reflect marginal increases or decreases in operating expenses. In France and Japan, in contrast, government agencies set drug reimbursement so firms cannot unilaterally raise prices.

Even if firms passed along the tax to consumers through higher prices, it would be worthwhile for the public to bear that cost. In all three countries, government or insurance pays for most medical care, and the additional expense for directly paying for professional development would be very small. In the United States, commercial interests contribute over $2 billion annually for CME. If commercial support for other professional activities also amounts to $2 billion, the $4 billion spent would be 0.0016 percent of national health care spending in 2008, about $13.16 per person.[27] The government could shoulder the cost of professional development without difficulty. Ending conflicts in CME would reduce inappropriate drug prescribing and improve quality of care, a significant benefit that might also lower drug spending.

Drug and medical device firms that seek government approval to sell their products must submit to regulatory agencies evidence that they are safe and effective based on clinical trials. Today, firms seeking approval supervise these trials, either directly or through contracts with clinical research organizations. They play a major role in designing the trial, formulating the questions asked, choosing the clinical researchers, overseeing the methodology, and interpreting and disseminating the results. This research is mired in conflicts of interest. The firms have an incentive to design and conduct the trial in ways that emphasize their product's benefits and minimize its risks.[28] Researchers who design the trial and report the results have an incentive to produce results that help the firm that pays them. Abuses are amply documented.

To avoid these conflicts of interest, legislation should require that government agencies oversee clinical trials. Firms that seek government approval to sell drugs or medical devices would still have to pay for clinical trials and could conduct initial trials independently. However, when firms were ready to conduct a phase III trial to be used in seeking approval to market a drug, a public agency would choose the researchers to design the study and conduct the clinical trials. These researchers should have no financial ties to firms related to products they evaluate or to products of the firm's competitors. The agency would also appoint an independent group to review the work of the evaluators.[29] The government drug agency should also oversee the design and administration of post-marketing (phase IV) clinical drug trials to ensure that they supply valuable information, that all the findings are reported, and that these trials are not used to promote products.

Protect Professional Judgment

Organized medicine has long sought to bar insurers and employers from restricting physicians' clinical discretion. However, it has also fought to maintain arrangements that entail entrepreneurial and payment conflicts of interest, inadvertently creating a need for third parties to oversee medical practice. Still, unless there are controls, insurers and employers might interfere with physicians' appropriate choices. We need institutions to oversee third parties to prevent that from occurring.

These institutions should require that employers and insurers justify their interventions based on independent clinical standards or guidelines and on studies of the effectiveness, risks, and cost of medical care, often called evidence-based medicine. These guidelines should not be developed by biased parties, such as insurers, pharma, or medical specialties, which now devise many existing guidelines. Nor should the state allow experts with conflicts of interest to participate in developing practice guidelines, as has France's HAS when it developed guidelines for diabetes and Alzheimer's.[30]

When disputes arise between insurers and physicians over what medical care is appropriate, physicians should be required to justify their medical decisions based on similar criteria. Insurers should not be permitted to overrule physicians when the weight of evidence is on the physician's side. When the balance of evidence suggests that physicians can supply appropriate medical care within the constraints of insurer and employer policies, the law should allow third parties to maintain their policies. In order to resolve disputes between physicians and third parties, the state should designate an independent entity to evaluate medical care, quality, effectiveness, and risk.

France's HAS started issuing practice guidelines in 2004. In the future, it may use guidelines to restrict practice discretion. The United States lacks authoritative national practice guidelines. Instead, professional associations, insurers, and other groups each create their own guidelines. There is no public oversight of privately created practice guidelines, and the process by which they are generated lacks transparency. Insurers and utilization reviewers frequently develop guidelines with the aim of controlling costs. Pharmaceutical firms and other commercial interests often have financial ties with physicians who have served on committees adopting guidelines. Critics charge that professional associations use guidelines to promote their income. Japan lacks guidelines to oversee practice or resolve disputes between insurers and physicians.

Neither France nor Japan has institutions to resolve disputes between insurers, physicians, and patients over what medical care is appropriate. In the United States, forty-seven states and Medicare and Medicaid allow patients to appeal insurers' refusal to supply medical services on the grounds that the service is not medically necessary or that it is experimental. The 2010 health reforms will extend independent medical review nationally. Outside of Medicare and Medicaid, typically, a private independent review organization (IRO) chooses a physician to evaluate the patient's medical record and medical request. If the reviewer decides that what the patient seeks is appropriate, the insurer must pay for the treatment.

The review process has significant drawbacks.[31] Frequently, the insurer can select the IRO, or nominate three IROs from which the patient then makes a choice. Conflicts of interest compromise this selection process. Frequently, the IRO also performs other work for insurers, such as conducting internal review, peer review, or utilization review. The IRO may depend on the insurer for this other work, which may prompt it to favor the insurer over the patient.

Furthermore, reviews treat patient appeals as individual grievances that have no bearing on policy. The insurer can deny these services for other patients similarly situated and force them to seek independent review. Each insurer chooses its own IRO and does not have access to the reviews obtained by other insurers that faced the same clinical issue. Reviewers typically rely on their personal knowledge rather than assess studies and literature evaluating medical practice.

All three countries would better protect appropriate physician clinical discretion if they combined authoritative practice guidelines with a system to review disputes between payers, physicians, and patients. A single physician reviewer should not resolve disputes; it makes more sense to rely on the weight of medical opinion. Nor should insurers be able to choose the IRO. Instead, a national organization, answerable to the state, should oversee such reviews. The basis for decisions should be transparent and public.

CONCLUSION

Nations can adopt some combination of these six coping strategies to mitigate physicians' conflicts of interest. Adoption or rejection of one strategy has implications for the use of others. For example, if a country employs all physicians in public medical centers or carefully regulated not-for-profit firms, that would eliminate entrepreneurial conflicts of interest and make it unnecessary to oversee physician decisions for these conflicts of interest. On the other hand, nations that lack publicly-owned and lay-owned, not-for-profit medical facilities have a plethora of entrepreneurial conflicts of interest and must regulate practice to cope with them.

Authorities can use various strategies to address conflicts of interest within private practice. Restricting physicians from dispensing drugs and supplying tests and ancillary services that they prescribe would curb many of their conflicts of interest. Utilization review can reduce inappropriate medical decisions. Regulation of physician payment can reduce the incentive for physicians to engage in these activities.

Factors beyond physicians and other groups advocating for their self-interest can impede the adoption of effective policies. The public and policy makers rarely perceive physicians' conflicts of interest as a crucial problem. More often they focus on other goals, such as controlling spending, increasing access to health care, or promoting productivity. When governments adopt policies to advance these goals, they affect how society copes with physicians' conflicts of interest, yet policy makers usually neglect to consider these effects. Even when policy makers do take this problem into account, they often sacrifice measures to curb conflicts of interest if it helps advance other goals.

Policies that address physicians' conflicts of interest often require changes in the organization of medical practice, the rules within which the medical economy operates, and the relationship between the medical profession, the market, and the state. The philosophical and ideological commitments that influence policy makers' views on these matters often take precedence. As a result, policy that affects conflicts of interest is often an incidental result of more general struggles over health and social policy.

In the future, international organizations—such as the World Health Organization (WHO), the United Nations, international development banks as well as international non-governmental organizations—might promote international norms on conflicts of interest in medical care. So too might international courts. Several factors are likely to encourage this development.

The pharmaceutical and medical device industries operate globally, yet national differences in how they conduct clinical trials and market drugs raise troubling ethical issues. Advocates argue that the rights of patients and human research subjects are a human rights issue, and international law has supported this trend.[32] The WHO advocates international registration of clinical trials to promote transparency and international norms. As the same time, critics have charged that WHO guidelines for flu vaccine and immunization were biased toward purchasing certain products because they relied on experts with financial ties to firms that produced the products.[33] These developments have thrust medical conflicts of interest onto the international stage.

Other aspects of medical care are also going global and encourage international norms. Firms sell insurance and operate medical facilities cross nationally. Patients and medical personnel now move across borders. International standards are emerging for hospital accreditation. International trade policies influence national policies on corruption, fair trade practices, and the scope of market competition, all of which shape business and governmental practices that bear on physicians' conflicts of interest. Equally important, many physicians and others argue that medical professionalism should transcend local law.

11

Professionalism Reconsidered

> Perhaps the most important [parts of professional codes of ethics] . . . are those that deal with . . . conflicts of interest. . . . This is the critical test of professionalism in that in order to justify a monopoly over practice it must be assumed that it will not be used for selfish advantage.[1]
>
> —Eliot Freidson, 2001

Regardless of how society organizes medical care, it cannot preclude all conflicts of interest; and third parties have limited ability to oversee conflicts of interest because physicians need some discretion to perform their work. Moreover, regulation imposes costs. Controls and bureaucratic rules can demoralize professionals and interfere with their performing well. Whatever institutions and rules society uses to cope with conflicts of interest will be more effective if physicians not only respect them but are also guided by an ethos of public service, fidelity to patients, and commitment to knowledge and excellence. Here, professionalism can play an important role. This chapter explores its potential, limits, and relation to public policy, focusing on the United States.[2]

Contemporary American professions, sociologist Eliot Freidson explains, exhibit distinctive characteristics: they perform specialized work and are granted privileged labor force status based on knowledge and skill; require formal training for employment that is controlled by the occupation; inhabit a sheltered position in the labor market based on credentials created by the occupation; exercise exclusive jurisdiction over a designated division of labor; perform a service mission; and through socialization, are committed to quality over profit.[3] Freidson, like a dozen earlier leading Anglo-American social thinkers ranging from Beatrice and Sidney Webb, writing in 1917, through Talcott Parsons and Everett Hughes, writing in 1971, argued that professional control is an alternative productive and economic framework to the usual capitalistic organization.[4] These thinkers portray professions as promoting the public good and the pursuit of knowledge and excellence.

In a similar vein, French sociologists have observed that in France, professions were imbued with public service norms due to their historical ties to the church and the state. French professions originated in medieval corporations created by the state and linked to the church. These corporations were imbued with a moral and spiritual dimension and their members possessed an *esprit de corps*. When the state abolished medieval guilds and corporations it created publicly controlled and funded professions that were public servants. Since then, the state has organized, coordinated, and integrated professional groups in the private sector through centralized institutions so that they serve a public function.[5] In addition, there arose new entities that performed the functions of corporations: associations for mutual aid were organized around employment groups.

Some thinkers, however, dissented from this positive portrayal. As early as 1911, social critic George Bernard Shaw wrote, "Every profession is a conspiracy against the laity." Shaw was debunking the idea that professions were different from other occupations or economic enterprises. His turn of phrase recalls Adam Smith's criticism of self-serving collusive behavior in his 1776 book, *The Wealth of Nations:* "People of the same trade seldom meet together, even for merriment and diversion, but the conversation ends in a conspiracy against the public."[6]

From the Progressive era through the post–World War II period, however, the prevailing American view was that professional expert judgment was more enlightened and disinterested than that of laypersons. Beginning in the 1960s, many people criticized that assumption and questioned authorities and institutions. Critiques of expertise challenged professions in general and medicine in particular. Since then, critics have sustained their attack on the beneficent image of professionalism.

One school of critics objected to physician paternalism and championed patient rights. They argued that patients should have autonomy and be able to decide what medical treatment they receive. In their view, physicians routinely preclude patients from participating in decisions where the choice of treatment involves important value choices rather than solely technical matters. They advocated that patients should be *partners* in decision making. Disability rights advocates articulated this spirit in their rallying cry: *Nothing about us, without us.*[7] Philosophers, lawyers, and courts promoted the idea that patients must give their *informed consent* prior to medical interventions. That required that physicians tell patients of the risks and benefits of treatments that they proposed and explain alternatives to their proposed treatments.

A second group of critics objected to *medicalization* of problems and argued that medicine was often used as a form of *social control* that had replaced legal and religious authority over individuals. These critics argued that many issues were framed as medical problems with the assumption that physicians and medical institutions should oversee them when in fact patients or public policy should determine the choices. They maintained that physicians ignored the views and insights of patients and people with disabilities and chronic illnesses. The women's rights and women's health movement showed that physicians often promoted stereotyped social roles for women.[8]

Several writers criticized professional power.[9] Julius Roth wrote that many sociologists were "apologists . . . justifying the professionals' control over their work . . . clientele, . . . public policy, or public service." Other writers documented divergence between professional interests and the public interest and questioned whether professions promoted the public interest. In France, critics charged that organized medicine allied itself with the state, a form of corporatism antithetical to democratic values; succumbed to commercialism; and was compromised by conflict of interest.[10]

Market proponents claimed that in suspending competition, professions protected themselves rather than promoting the public interest. Milton Friedman and other economists argued that organized medicine restricted entry into practice and competition to extract profits. Freidman even called for an end to medical licensing. Other critics noted that policies that allowed patients to select any physician precluded important consumer choices, particularly access to a system of coordinated care, such as prepaid group practices (PPGPs) and staff-model health maintenance organizations (HMOs). Jeffrey Berlant, a sociologist and physician, argued that organized medicine used ethical codes to restrict price competition, advertising, and alternative health care organizations. Legal scholar Clark Havighurst argued that antitrust law should apply to physicians; in 1975 the U.S. Supreme Court ended the professional exemption to antitrust.[11]

Still others argued that changes in financing compromised the ability of physicians to serve as patients' agents. Starting in 1980, Dr. Arnold Relman called attention to the commercialization of medicine, a new medical-industrial complex, and the rise of investor-owned medical firms. These, he argued, created physicians' conflicts of interest. In the mid-1980s sociologist David Mechanic described an "era of rationing and commercialization" that changed physicians' role from "sole agent of the patient's welfare to a role of balancing the patient's wants and needs against the aggregate population and a fixed budget." Now "the physician . . . role . . . is transformed from advocating to allocating."

Managed care organizations (MCOs) became a more significant part of medical care and developed means to oversee physicians' clinical care that used financial incentives to change their clinical choices. As managed care grew in the United States, William Sullivan warned that it "threatened to preempt professional judgment" and the "identity of the medical profession." He asked, "What is left of professionalism after managed care?"[12]

In his 1994 book, Steven Brint argued that professions had been transformed from *social trustees* to *experts* purveying technical services. "The essential characteristics of professions have nothing to do with public service, ethical standards or collegial control, however often these . . . grow up in support of the professions' claims to distinction." The idea that the professions were social trustees, he wrote, was now an ideology. Nevertheless, when professionals embraced the expert model, they lost "their distinctive voice in public debate" because they lacked a sense of public or social purpose. Yet Brint did not regret this change, because "claims to representing 'the public good' can lead to excesses of self-interest legitimated in the name of professional authority."[13]

Despite these criticisms, advocates of professionalism as a moral ideal persist. Freidson, a poignant critic of professional power and professional dominance, also saw professionalism's potential. In his two recent books, Freidson argued that professional norms could be a source of moral authority that counter bureaucratic norms and market pressures. While professionals "should have no right to be proprietors of the knowledge and techniques of their disciplines, they are obligated to be their moral custodians." He argued that "there is still . . . foundation for the professional's claim of license to balance the public good against the needs and demands of the immediate clients or employers. Transcendent values add moral substance to the technical content of disciplines." Freidson did not seek to reestablish a professional ideology but thought that professional norms should promote more than technical goals.[14]

In 2004, William Sullivan summarized the ideal of professionalism.

> The structure of professions embodies the proposition that . . . human or intellectual capital ought to be treated as a public trust, rather than simply an individual possession to be traded upon without regard of the consequences to others. Consequently, the professions are organized so that individuals must submit to the corporate organization in order to acquire their specialized skills and . . . can only benefit personally from the employment of this "human capital" by applying it according to standards that are established and . . . monitored for the public benefit. . . . Professions operate within an explicit contract with society as a whole. . . . The basis of these contracts is a set of common goals shared by the public.
>
> These are public values. In economic parlance, they are public goods . . . values from which all benefit and which depend on everyone's cooperation, but to which no individual market actor has a strong incentive to contribute. The professions . . . are . . . public occupations even when they work outside government . . . supported institutions.[15]

Some economists gave credence to this ideal by arguing that professional ethics can supplement markets and government. Nobel laureate Kenneth Arrow, a decade after publishing his classic 1963 article on market failure in medical care, wrote that professional norms can help correct that problem. When Victor Fuchs surveyed economics in his 1996 American Economics Association presidential address, he asserted that "one of the greatest errors of health policy-makers today is their assumption that market competition or government regulation are the only instruments available. . . . There is . . . need for a revitalization of professional norms as a third instrument of control."[16] Like Arrow, Fuchs argued that professionalism can shape conduct in socially beneficial ways when markets and state controls cannot or do not.

PROMOTING PROFESSIONALISM: THE CONTRIBUTIONS OF THE STATE AND MARKET

Freidson and other advocates of professionalism believe that it promotes very different values than do markets or bureaucracies, because it uses a different organizing principle and follows a different logic.[17] Yet this conventional wisdom overlooks the contribution of the state and markets to fostering professionalism's values. The experiences of France, the United States, and Japan reveal that the state, market, and lay organizations can foster medical professionalism's core values.

Public Service

Sociologists contrast the development of public professions (called *professions of office*) in continental Europe with the growth of professions in protected private labor markets (called *free professions*) in the United States and the United Kingdom (UK). In Europe, the church and the state organized professional training, certification, and employment. Professions received status and economic security by attending elite state-sponsored educational institutions and through public employment.[18] In the United States and the UK, the civil service was smaller and played a less directive role in the economy. Instead, the state supported certain occupations within the private sector by designating them as professions, protecting them from competition and allowing them to control the training and certification of their members.[19] Neither model prompted physicians to develop a robust public service role on their own. The state and lay charities created the conditions necessary for physicians' work to become a public service.

In medieval France, public service values emanated not from medical guilds but from the Catholic Church, which provided charity for those who were unable to care for themselves in institutions known as houses of God (*Hôtel-dieu*) or hospitals. During the French Revolution, the state assumed the church's charitable responsibility, nationalized hospitals, and made them medical institutions for the poor. Leaders proposed that the state provide medicine as a service for all the public by employing a physician in every canton, but that was beyond the state's means. Nevertheless, over the next century and a half, the state expanded medical access through public hospitals and publicly employed physicians. The state also facilitated self-employed physicians' pursuit of public service by subsidizing private practice and restricting certain opportunities for private gain. Thus charities and the state were a key source of the public service ideal, in addition to the funds and institutions through which physicians performed public service.

France's public hospital and private medical sectors became less distinct over time. The state expanded public hospitals' mission, first to individuals who could make only partial payments, and eventually to all citizens. It financed medical care outside hospitals by paying self-employed physicians to treat designated populations, such as rural agricultural workers and military veterans. Furthermore, the state promoted lay-directed mutual aid associations, which financed medicine for the middle class, and often supplied medical care with employed physicians in their facilities. Organized medicine, however, supported increasing access to medical care only if it was done in a manner that promoted private practice.

In the United States, medicine also developed two spheres: a private sector in which self-employed physicians served those who could pay; and a public service sector in which charities and the state funded dispensaries and hospitals for the poor. Charities and the state were the source of public service ideals that we now associate with medical professionalism. Private practitioners complained that these institutions improperly supplied medical care to individuals who were able to pay physicians.

In the twentieth century, hospitals developed technology that made them better sites for surgery and many treatments than physicians' or patients' homes. It also offered some advantages to women undergoing high-risk deliveries. Hospitals then began to recruit paying patients to subsidize their charitable work. Physicians lost fee-generating patients, so some started private hospitals. Eventually not-for-profit hospitals allowed self-employed physicians to treat and bill middle-class patients. Physicians referred paying patients to not-for-profit hospitals, which in return subsidized their private practice.

Thus, American hospitals blurred the distinction between the public and private sectors. The state subsidized not-for-profit hospitals through grants and exemptions from taxes and requirements of other private firms; in return, these hospitals reduced the state's need to supply medical care through public facilities. But private practice remained at odds with public service and depended on state subsidies to serve those without means. Significantly, organized medicine opposed national health insurance (NHI) and private insurance arrangements that broadened access to medical care.

In Japan, medicine emerged with self-employed physicians providing ambulatory care and medication. But Japan lacked a developed tradition of religious charities or hospitals before the state adopted Western medicine, created public hospitals, and employed physicians. In the late nineteenth and early twentieth centuries, private and public efforts extended access to medical care. Some rural cooperatives employed physicians, and the state mandated that industrial employers provide their workers medical care. However, the Japan Medical Association (JMA) opposed medical coops and employer-sponsored clinics because they offered medical care at lower prices than self-employed practitioners.

Japan developed community-based health insurance during World War II, and after the war the state tried to make public hospitals the center of its health system. However, the JMA opposed this approach and insisted that it subsidize physician-owned hospitals. Self-employed physicians supported extending medical care to a larger public only when state financing supported their private practice.

Prior to insurance, private practitioners in all three countries customarily adjusted fees based on the patient's resources. Public service norms might motivate this behavior, but economists say that price discrimination maximizes income. Furthermore, organized medicine's fee schedules set *minimum* fees. In France, the Code of Medical Deontology (Medical Deontology) even prohibits reducing fees as unfair competition. French and American medical ethical codes prohibited physicians from advertising fees, which could lower prices. Organized medicine opposed PPGPs and mutual insurance clinics, which supplied medical services at lower cost than traditional private practice.

Medical Knowledge and Training

Professionals determine their patients' needs based on knowledge; but the production, dissemination, and application of medical knowledge rely on states and markets.

France has nurtured medical knowledge through state medical schools since its revolution and, after World War II, by making public hospitals centers for research and training. Physicians and organized medicine could not finance this training and research. In the late twentieth century, despite opposition from physicians, the state began to promote continuing medical education (CME). It required NHI funding to compensate private practitioners for the time they spent in CME to induce them to participate.

In the United States, initially, individuals could practice after interning with a practitioner or graduating from a medical school. Both modes of training proved inadequate. Physician-owned medical schools neglected clinical training and laboratory science and granted degrees to those who paid, regardless of proficiency. Medical education improved after states passed licensing laws that limited practice to graduates of schools they approved and required that they pass state exams. Physician-owned schools folded, and medical education shifted to state universities and state-subsidized not-for-profit medical schools.

The federal government spurred the growth of medical knowledge after World War II by funding scientific and medical research and expanding academic medical centers. Federal funds also developed other fields— epidemiology, social science, applied statistics—that transformed medical knowledge. The 1962 Food, Drug and Cosmetic Act Amendments required that drug firms demonstrate the effectiveness and safety of products using controlled clinical trials before they can be sold. This regulation transformed pharmaceutical and medical knowledge. It set a standard that the medical profession had not developed; indeed, the American Medical Association (AMA) opposed this reform when Congress held hearings on the legislation.

The legal requirements to demonstrate efficacy and safety in clinical trials became the model for evaluating clinical practice that is now called *evidence-based medicine*. It goes beyond individual or aggregate clinical experience to draw on statistics, survey research, and experimental design, epidemiology, and randomized controlled clinical trials. Today the state, third-party payers, and private institutions develop practice guidelines to encourage practice based on knowledge and on evidence and outcomes research.[20]

In Japan, the state, rather than the medical profession, spurred the adoption of Western medical knowledge. State schools trained physicians in Western medicine and state hospitals employed them. Since the late 1990s, the state has promoted graduate medical education and CME. Lay-owned commercial firms saw opportunities in the accreditation of clinical laboratories and hospitals. They developed private accreditation organizations as well as firms to help reorganize practice to meet the standards. Soon the state supported them and promoted voluntary laboratory and hospital accreditation. Neither the JMA nor other physician organizations played a significant role in developing practice standards, laboratory or hospital accreditation, or quality standards.

Markets spurred innovation in technologies and new products and encouraged the transfer of basic science into clinical practice. Particularly since World War II, pharmaceutical, medical device, and diagnostic imaging firms transformed medical care. The development of drugs, medical devices, and other medical products goes beyond clinical medical expertise and requires capital and markets. At the same time, in the United States, market incentives encouraged insurers and hospitals to cut costs. They shortened hospital stays, shifted patients to ambulatory settings, and challenged traditional practices unsupported by solid evidence. Medical outcomes often improved.

Fidelity to Patients' Interests

Both the state and market can support as well as compromise physicians' loyalty to patients. Public and private employment challenge physicians' fidelity to patients in different ways.

Public employment usually promotes fidelity to patients by insulating physicians from financial concerns. Nevertheless, if public authorities inadequately fund medical facilities and underpay physicians, doctors will sell their services through an illegal market, which compromises that commitment. In eastern European states during the Soviet era, patients often needed to make under-the-table payments to publicly employed surgeons and other specialists to receive treatment, and the practice continues today.[21] Japanese patients, too, make monetary gifts to physicians employed by prestigious public hospitals, a practice that encourages better service to patients who pay the most. Similarly, French public hospital physicians can boost their income by offering private consultations at higher fees than regular consultations, which encourages them to give preferential treatment to patients who pay private fees. These practices counter the principle that physicians serve all the public equally, a value their public employment is intended to enshrine.

Self-employed physicians, in contrast, are never free from financial concerns. They must generate patient revenue and control practice costs to ensure their financial security. Today, however, self-employed physicians have less risk that patients will not pay them than previously because state-supervised compulsory insurance covers all French and Japanese patients, and public and private insurance cover most American patients. That reduces financial uncertainty and its threats to fidelity. Still, self-employed physicians also have numerous opportunities for compromising financial ties with other providers and commercial interests that publicly employed physicians lack.

The state may compromise physician loyalty to patients by using medicine as a means of social control. Totalitarian regimes pose the most risk. The German Third Reich used physicians to further genocide and eugenics. State-employed physicians in the Soviet Union experienced structural strain between state goals and the welfare of patients. Aided by physicians, the state placed some dissidents in asylums and controlled them with drugs. In France, the Vichy régime restricted Jews from medical practice and restricted access to medical care by Jews.[22] Public hospitals enforced these policies most readily, but the Order of Physicians also enforced these exclusions in private practice. Even democratic states may use physicians to violate patients' rights. Physicians employed by the U.S. armed forces helped oversee torture in the name of gathering intelligence in the Guantanamo prison during the presidency of George W. Bush.[23]

If government policies attempt to restrict specific medical services or services for certain groups, they have greater leverage over publicly employed than self-employed physicians. However, government policies can also impose such policies on private practitioners. The U.S. Medicaid program, for example, restricts abortions by not reimbursing private practitioners for performing them.[24]

On the other hand, the state has promoted fidelity to patients through law. A key example is the law of informed consent. Although medical norms sometimes encouraged physicians to consult patients, a very strong tradition of paternalism led physicians to make decisions without consulting patients even when there were important choices that involved value trade-offs rather than merely technical issues. It required either court decisions or legislation in these three countries to change medical practice norms and promote informed consent and patient choice as well as other patient rights.

Implications

The interplay of markets, the state, and professionals yields a more robust form of professionalism than unfettered professional control would. Ironically, professionalism requires a medical economy under mixed rather than professional control, and it functions best when the medical profession, the market, and the state have overlapping authority, each with checks on the others.

There are national differences in the manifestations of professionalism as well as the extent to which physicians and medical organizations promote practice based on professional standards, medical knowledge, and the pursuit of excellence. Physician organizations in the United States have played a leading role in the development of medical education, oversight of practice, and the development of clinical standards, while physicians in France and Japan have not. The American College of Surgeons (ACS) developed professional standards for hospitals. The AMA took the lead in developing standards for medical schools and graduate medical education and oversaw the marketing of drugs for the first half of the twentieth century. Numerous specialty medical societies have developed clinical practice guidelines. Physicians developed group practices that fostered cooperation and systems of peer review.

What explains the lack of similar physician initiatives in France and Japan? The reason is uncertain but it is not due to the absence of professional power. In France, during the medieval era, physicians were protected by monopolies and granted authority over membership and power over practice through guilds. Starting in the mid-nineteenth century, physicians organized unions that negotiate fees with insurers, allowing them to exercise collective market power on behalf of self-employed practitioners. Physicians' unions continue today. Since the Second World War, the state has granted physicians authority over private practice through the Order of Physicians, an organization whose leaders are elected by all licensed physicians.

Japanese physicians have been granted significant authority as well. The state promoted the growth of medical societies and the JMA as privileged civil society organizations in the early twentieth century. In the postwar era, physicians were granted a privileged position as owners of hospitals and clinics and protected from competition by investor-owned firms and lay-directed not-for-profit hospitals. The JMA is represented on government commissions that set fees and on local governmental bodies that control the expansion of public and private hospitals. Nevertheless, the JMA waited for the state and lay organizations to develop standards for medical education, graduate medical education, accreditation for clinical laboratories and hospitals, and even ethics guidelines for physician relations with commercial interests.

PROFESSIONALISM AS A MEANS TO COPE WITH CONFLICTS OF INTEREST

Professionalism can help mitigate conflicts of interest. But our case studies reveal that conflicts of interest can compromise professional norms and conduct. Therefore, it is insufficient to rely *exclusively* on professionalism.

A key problem with relying on individual practitioners to draw on professional norms and avoid conflicts of interest or effectively cope with them is that often they do not recognize their conflicts of interest. Professional organizations may be able to identify conflicts of interest that individual physicians fail to see and address them through overseeing physicians and disciplining them when they violate norms. However, professional organizations are ultimately dependent on their members and are responsive to them, and this compromises their ability to oversee physicians. Moreover, professional organizations have their own conflicts of interest that compromise their oversight role. In the United States, the AMA and specialty medical societies depend on funds from pharmaceutical firms and other commercial interests. In France, the Order of Physicians promotes having commercial firms supply funds for professional medical activities. In Japan, too, many professional medical associations rely on funds from pharma.

Professional self-regulation as a substitute for legal oversight has major drawbacks. While professional norms can influence conduct, the medical profession today lacks an effective means to enforce its norms. The Order of Physicians, to which all French physicians must belong, can sanction physicians, but it has limited resources for oversight. The evidence suggests it has not disciplined physicians for most activities involving conflicts of interest; rather, it focuses on misconduct that is also penalized through criminal or civil law.

In the United States, to practice medicine physicians need not be members of the AMA and today less than a third of physicians join. Since 1979, antitrust law has barred the AMA from sanctioning members for engaging in competitive activities. When exercised, collegial and professional oversight is often sorely deficient. As Freidson summarizes his study of medical group practice, "Obedience to the rules of etiquette discouraged critical attitudes toward colleagues, the communication of critical information to others about the performance of colleagues, the discussion of critical evaluation with colleagues, and the undertaking of collective social control."[25]

Even more important, professional guidelines might be weaker than standards that legislatures and courts develop, so using them exclusively precludes more effective responses. For example, the AMA has often developed ethical guidelines on conflicts of interest as a substitute for legal oversight. It opposed congressional legislation to prohibit physician drug dispensing by invoking its own code of ethics, which allowed the practice. Since the 1970s, it has opposed legislation that would restrict physicians from receiving gifts and funding for professional activities from pharma. It sought to block legislation that would prohibit physician self-referral by invoking its own guidelines, which set weaker standards and were unenforceable.

Similarly, the AMA opposed the Medicare Anti-Kickback Act (Anti-Kickback Act) compliance guidelines drafted by the Office of the Inspector General (OIG), arguing that its own weaker standards were sufficient. The OIG proposed that to avoid the risk of legal liability, physicians should at a minimum comply with the AMA's guidelines on gifts from drug firms, and the OIG suggested other criteria that physicians should also meet. The AMA argued that the OIG should not adopt standards stricter than the AMA guidelines and that it should assure physicians that as long as they followed the AMA guidelines they would not be prosecuted for violating the Anti-Kickback Act. In France, when legislation appointed the Order of Physicians to oversee industry funding to physicians, the Order interpreted the law to ensure the continued ample flow of funds instead of strictly overseeing grants. Rather than demonstrating that professionalism can promote noble ideals, these are examples of professionalism that is self-serving.

Professional norms play a useful role when they are stronger or broader than existing legal standards and third-party oversight and do not discourage the state or third parties from strengthening their own standards. Then, rather than shield physicians, professional organizations and professional norms can encourage a higher standard of conduct.

Physicians and physician organizations can help cope with conflicts of interest without restricting other forms of oversight. Drs. Arnold Relman, Marcia Angel, and Jerome Kassirer, all of whom served as editors of the *New England Journal of Medicine*, have advocated that professional societies and medical schools develop policies to avoid financial conflicts of interest. They and others promoted reform by making the study of physicians' conflicts of interest a respectable scholarly enterprise.

A number of physician researchers on medical school faculties used their skills to investigate the effect of conflicts of interest on medical practice. Since the 1990s, studies of this problem have burgeoned. My search of articles in the Medline database found that the phrase *conflict of interest* was in the title or abstract of only 20 articles from 1970 to 1980 and 41 articles from 1981 through 1990, but rose to 124 articles from 1991 through 2000 and to 238 articles from 2001 through November 2010.

In France, a group of physicians founded *Prescrire*, a medical journal that reviews medical practice and accepts no advertisements or corporate funding. It offers unbiased evaluations and offers a model for medical journals free from conflicts of interest that arise from ties to pharma.[26] Other physicians founded *Formindep*, an organization that promotes the independence of physicians and medical education from pharmaceutical industry influence.[27] About a decade ago, a few physicians in the United States founded *No Free Lunch*, which advocates that physicians not accept gifts from drug and medical device firms and other commercial interests.[28] It disseminates studies on the risks of physicians' conflicts of interest. Another group, *Healthy Skepticism*, disseminates studies on pharmaceutical issues and conflicts of interest.[29]

Since 2002, several American medical schools have adopted policies that restrict pharma detailers from supplying meals or other gifts to physicians, residents, or interns. In recent years, Dr. Relman and others have proposed that physicians not participate in CME funded by grants from commercial interests. Two leading medical organizations in the United States and Europe adopted a charter in 2002 which declares that professionalism requires "collective efforts to improve the health care system for the welfare of society," commitment to "a just distribution of finite resources," and "managing conflicts of interest."[30] The Open Society Institute program on Medicine as a Profession, later succeeded by the Columbia University Institute on Medicine as a Profession, are among the new groups spurring these efforts.[31]

Physicians can advocate legal and policy changes that help address physicians' conflicts of interest. For example, in the 1940s the ACS proposed that the Internal Revenue Service (IRS) not allow kickbacks and fee splitting as tax-deductible business expenses. The ACS lobbied for state anti-kickback legislation, and the AMA initially joined this effort. In the 1990s, Dr. Relman and other physicians advocated legislation that prohibited physician self-referral and other practices that create conflicts of interest.

Physicians can employ another strategy to cope with conflicts of interest if necessary: protest and/or resistance to policies that require them to violate their obligations to patients or that create serious conflicts of interest. Eliot Freidson anticipated this issue when he wrote, "professionals claim the moral as well as the technical right to control the uses of their disciplines so they must resist economic and political restrictions that arbitrarily limit its benefits."[32] Professionalism should lead physicians employed by the state or private firms to oppose policies that induce them to act in ways that conflict with their obligations toward their patients. Global Physicians and Lawyers for Human Rights have drawn on medical ethics to counter governmental programs from using physicians and lawyers to violate human rights and to support physicians who resist authority to avoid cooperating with abuses.[33]

FUTURE PROSPECTS

David Mechanic argues that there is a disjuncture between traditional concepts of medical professionalism and changing structures in the American medical economy. Physicians used to expect that professionalism meant they would be trusted, have autonomy, and exercise control over all facets of practice. With the growth of managed care, however, organizations, particularly for-profit firms, exercise control over practice, compensation, division of labor, use of technology, and even clinical standards. Mechanic argues that we need a new professional ethic in which physicians have responsibility to allocate resources but also to advocate on behalf of patients and have some discretion. Advocacy, he says, should occur within the emerging structures used to organize practice, using a framework that assures the allocation of resources is subject to norms of procedural justice and a medical culture that supports evidence-based medicine and promotes population health.[34] He explains that such structures may require a regulatory framework and that professionalism requires that physicians adapt to "changes in organizational, technological, economic, and cultural influences."[35]

How can we promote professionalism as a positive force in medicine? There are competing challenges. Over-regulation of physicians can stunt professionalism; at the same time, economic and organizational arrangements that create physicians' conflicts of interest corrode it. Reorganizing medical practice to minimize physicians' conflicts of interest would promote professionalism in two ways: it would remove a corrosive influence on professional norms and judgment; and it would reduce the need to mitigate physicians' conflicts of interest by using intrusive measures that diminish professionalism, most notably detailed oversight and rules that reduce physicians' clinical discretion.

Today, by performing entrepreneurial roles rife with conflicts of interest, physicians reduce their moral authority and credibility as experts. If physicians want to control their work and influence practice and policy in a robust way, they need to assure the public that their judgment, advice, and advocacy are not compromised. That will require physicians to curb many of their entrepreneurial activities. If they do not, then the state or private entities—spurred by patients, other professionals, and various economic interest groups—probably will.

Medical practice draws on the knowledge of other healing professionals, as well as scientists, clinical investigators, epidemiologists, social workers, economists, sociologists, anthropologists, and even lawyers. In addition, physicians depend on firms that produce drugs, medical devices, diagnostic equipment, and other sophisticated tools. They frequently work in hospitals and other institutions or rely on them to supply and coordinate a vast array of clinicians and services. Patients and society count on these institutions and organizations to create an environment in which professional values flourish for all those who work there, not only physicians.[36]

Society should ensure that these organizations and other professionals act in the interest of patients. It will probably have to create legal obligations for them to do so. A good place to start is by creating such obligations for pharmaceutical and medical device firms, managed care organizations, and other insurers and hospitals. Since these organizations also have obligations to serve owners and other parties, public policy will need to address their conflicts of interest. The law should ensure that these organizations cannot easily trump their new duties to patients to fulfill their other obligations. Likewise, the law must ensure that obligations of employees in these organizations to serve their employers do not overrule their obligations to serve the interests of patients.

It is unnecessary for the law to define these organizations or their employees as fiduciaries to patients; it only needs legislation to impose certain legal obligations for them to act in patients' interests—or to not harm their interests—that are strong enough to limit their pursuit of some corporate interests. Then society can develop institutional and legal means to oversee their conflicts of interest. With a renewed professionalism, physicians can play an important role in holding these organizations accountable and helping to ensure that they do not compromise patients' interests.

Conclusion

The Way Forward

Over the last century, American reformers advocated the adoption of policies that would insure all the public, manage medical spending, and improve the quality of medical care. As they continue their efforts they should add a new goal: reducing the presence of physicians' conflicts of interest where feasible and mitigating those that cannot be eliminated.

How should we deal with physicians' conflicts of interest in the future? I propose the following. Individual physicians and organized medicine should restrict activities that create conflicts of interest for practitioners and physician organizations. Physicians can change the way they conduct their own medical practice as well as participate in broader change through professional organizations and civic engagement. Physician organizations can develop ethical standards and policies for medical practice, continuing medical education (CME), and other medical activities. Even more important is another step that many physicians will find difficult. Physicians should accept the authority of federal and state government and laymen to reform the medical economy in ways that reduce and regulate physicians' conflicts of interest.

Physicians ought not claim that only they should oversee their conflicts of interest since they have not done so effectively. Indeed, organized medicine promoted a medical economy that creates conflicts of interest and physicians have often fought to maintain them. Third-party payers and organizations directed by laymen should also oversee physicians' conflicts of interest. These organizations should be publicly accountable and their policies transparent to ensure physicians and the public that their oversight serves patients' interests rather than their own.

The public should also reform federal health policy. Medical care is an essential public service and we must grant public officials authority to oversee its delivery. We should acknowledge the interests of individuals and firms that supply medical services, but not guarantee them entrepreneurial freedom. Markets are an important means to supply medical care but must be structured and overseen to ensure fidelity to patients, the integrity of medical knowledge and practice, and prudent use of public funds. That requires significant change.

The most important checks on conflicts of interest are structural. We should reduce the size of the physician- and lay-owned entrepreneurial medical sector and expand the public and not-for-profit sectors. When publicly owned medical facilities are properly organized, the physicians they employ are free from financial conflicts of interest that compromise practice. Not-for-profit organizations that employ physicians can also remove financial incentives that compromise physicians' clinical choices, but they have allowed conflicts of interest more often than public employers. The government should regulate not-for-profit medical practices to ensure that they are not operated for the benefit of their physician and lay employees. It is important to regulate payment incentives for both self-employed and employed physicians. Moderate incentives to encourage physician productivity and discourage unnecessary expenditures have their place, but we need greater oversight to control their negative effects.

To ensure that public medical facilities provide excellent care and become centers of innovation, the federal governments must make public employment more financially attractive. But, it should not rely on, or allow, physicians to earn money from part-time private practice or consulting for commercial interests. The federal government should regulate the size of the entrepreneurial medical sector (physician- and lay-owned) and subsidize the growth of not-for-profit practices to ensure alternatives to the public and entrepreneurial sectors. Congress should also extend its regulations of kickbacks, false claims, and gifts in the Medicare and Medicaid programs so that they apply universally. Tax subsidies and grants subsidize much of the medical care supplied today, and all medical care has a public service aspect. Graft and corruption should have no place.

We should also curb conflicts of interest *within* private practice that arise when physicians supply the drugs, laboratory and diagnostic tests, and other ancillary services that they prescribe. Nearly all ancillary services that physicians prescribe should be supplied by independent providers and organizations. We can move in this direction in steps and allow exceptions—for example, allowing physicians to dispense vaccines while inoculating patients. Government policy should subsidize the formation of independent entities that are owned by public or regulated not-for-profit organizations to supply laboratory and diagnostic tests and ancillary services. Restricting entrepreneurial opportunities would allow physicians' greater discretion than controlling their conflicts of interest by oversight of their clinical choices. Utilization review is most appropriate when physicians are entrepreneurs.

Practice guidelines must not be developed by individuals biased toward promoting the income of drug and medical device firms, medical facilities, insurers, or particular practice specialties. They should be created under public auspices and the professionals who perform this work should be free of financial ties to commercial firms or groups that have a financial interest in the outcome. We should change the system used to review disputes between insurers and patients regarding whether a particular treatment is necessary or experimental. These decisions should be overseen by public authorities, not by insurers who contract with individual reviewers.

We now fund crucial medical activities through discretionary contributions from commercial interests that grant funds to promote their products. The price we pay is compromised knowledge and education, lower quality, and increased spending. Instead, public authorities should raise and allocate these funds. If Congress does not want to draw on general revenue, it can assess commercial medical firms, insurers, and medical facilities. A federal agency should allocate these funds to not-for-profit entities that would distribute them. Public policy should preclude practitioners, clinical researchers, and medical organizations from accepting funds from pharma, medical device firms, and other commercial interests.

Most states require that a physician earn credits for CME to maintain his or her license but do not specify the curriculum or oversee what is taught. Commercial interests choose what CME covers because they supply most of the funds. Accredited CME should be entirely publicly funded, with revenue derived from a tax on the industry, medical institutions, and physicians. Commercial interests should not be allowed to donate funds for accredited CME unless they channel it through public authorities that decide how it is used.

Today, the United States allows drug and medical device firms to oversee studies that the Food and Drug Administration (FDA) relies on to evaluate whether their products are effective and safe enough to be sold. Yet these firms often skew the findings through flawed experimental design, biased or incomplete data collection, and misleading reporting. Legislation should require that the evidence used to evaluate applications for marketing products come from studies conducted independently of firms that patent, develop, or sell the product and that the studies are conducted under FDA oversight. When firms wish to conduct phase III clinical trials, they should supply the funds to a subsidiary of the FDA, which would contract with independent firms to design and conduct the evaluation. Individuals and firms who help design, oversee, conduct, and interpret these studies should have no financial ties to commercial interests. Individuals who perform this work should be barred from employment with affected commercial interests for several years.

Many Americans believe that self-regulation, disclosure, and minor tweaking of legal rules are adequate safeguards for physicians' conflicts of interest. That faith is comforting, but unsupported. Structural and institutional reforms are necessary to curb corrosive influences. In order to ensure patient safety, preserve the integrity of medical practice, and promote professionalism we must control physicians' conflicts of interest. That requires fundamental reform of how we finance, organize, and oversee medical practice.

Appendix

The Idea of Conflicts of Interest: Its Origins and Application to Physicians

Rules for dealing with financial conflicts of interest were developed in other professions long before they were in medicine, in part because civil servants, bankers, and lawyers traditionally handled significant sums of money, whereas medical practice did not until recently. Yet the law generally regulates conflicts of interest in relationships that strongly parallel to patient-physician relations. Usually one party is delegated powers to serve another, the relationship requires dependency, and it is socially beneficial to impose obligations on the party granted authority.

Typically, professionals first viewed conflicts of interests as an ethical issue that individuals should address themselves. Then professions developed group norms, often set forth in ethical codes.[1] Subsequently, the state developed policies, laws, and regulatory tools to oversee professionals. First it developed sanctions to prohibit and penalize misconduct. Later, given the difficulties of monitoring, detecting, proving misconduct, and of finding adequate remedies for injury, the state found ways to reduce the risk of misconduct through rules that address conflicts of interest.

Conflict-of-interest principles developed most fully in fiduciary law, which has its origins in the Roman law *fiducia,* a legal institution used to transfer property. The term means trust, faith, confidence, assurance, credit. Oddly enough, although Roman law gave rise to civil code legal systems, most of them did not incorporate the fiducia. However, English law incorporated Roman law ideas and drew on the fiducia to develop fiduciary principles in trusts and agency and then disseminated these ideas, first to other areas of private law and later to public law for government officials. Some rules prohibit fiduciaries from performing roles or engaging in activities that create conflicts of interest; others reduce the fiduciary's discretion; still others require fiduciaries to account for their actions or supply remedies when they breach their trust.

In contrast, France and most other civil law countries initially developed conflict of interest principles in public law without reference to the fiducia or fiduciary. France later introduced these ideas in private law and often drew on Anglo-American financial law, which included fiduciary principles. Japan adopted ideas about conflicts of interest from both civil law and American law. Today, courts and legislatures in all three countries some-times regulate the conflicts of interest of individuals who are not fiduciaries or public servants but occupy positions of trust, have authority over a depen-dent party, or exercise delegated powers.

The rules used to regulate fiduciaries and public officials often lack a precise equivalent for physicians because their situations are not identical. However, while serving patients, physicians can perform other roles that give rise to conflicts of interest. As a result, physicians might make treat-ment decisions, prescribe drugs and therapy, or refer patients in ways that promote their own interest over that of the patient.

Public policy and insurers can prevent physicians from engaging in roles or activities that create conflicts of interest by prohibiting them from dispensing drugs and administering tests or referring patients to facilities in which they have a financial interest. Alternatively, they can reduce physicians' discretion or oversee their conduct and insist that they account for their choices. For example, they can create practice guidelines, employ utilization review to monitor clinical choices, and either restrict certain choices or insist that physi-cians justify them. Furthermore, public policy can oversee conflicts of interest by setting constraints on the finance and organization of medical practice.

FROM ROMAN LAW TO CIVIL LAW

In Roman law, the *fideicommissa* was a means by which a person leaving a will (the testator) transferred goods upon his death to a party who would hold them for the beneficiary. The fiducia was a means of separating posses-sion from ownership of property in relationships similar to modern mort-gages.[2] These legal categories established relationships where one party served another and had moral obligations to act in that party's interest. Roman law regulated these relationships.

In the seventeenth century, Roman law concepts were widely used in southern France and the fiducia and fideicommissa were part of ancient French law. The 1804 Napoleonic Code incorporated many Roman law concepts from ancient French law, but not the fiducia and fideicommissa. The Napoleonic Code became the model for continental European civil law and spread to over seventy countries. Unlike France, Germany, Austria, Switzerland, Netherlands, and Liechtenstein incorporated the Roman law fiducia into their civil codes. They later used them to form Anglo-American style trusts and fiduciary obligations.

Despite the absence of the fiducia in France's civil code, French judges and legal commentators referred to the fiducia because they were familiar with its presence in five European civil codes and in Roman law. When Japan adopted Western institutions during the Mejei Restoration (1867–1912), it formed a civil code modeled on the German law which included the fiducia, and on French law.

In medieval France, the Catholic Church followed Roman law and defined the public good as occupying a sphere distinct from individual interests that were governed by private law. Jean-Jacques Rousseau developed the idea of a general public interest that is not reducible to the sum of individual private interests. After the French Revolution, public law was premised on the idea of a public good different from private interests.[3] Individuals who perform public roles are obligated to promote the public good, but they sometimes engage in activities that compromise fulfilling their duty; these activities constitute conflicts of interest. For this reason, France first developed conflict of interest rules in public law to prevent public servants from using their power or their position to further private interests.

Contemporary French law has numerous rules that govern the duties of public officials or agencies involved in government purchasing and planning. They frequently require that the public actors have no conflicts of interest. Individuals serving as experts on pharmaceutical and other issues for government agencies typically must disclose their financial ties to private parties potentially affected by their advice.[4]

When France revised its law that governs publicly held companies in 1966, it used American law as a model and transplanted a legal framework with fiduciary obligations and conflict-of-interest rules.[5] Still, attempts to add the fiduciary to the French civil code failed in 1937, 1992, and 1995, and succeeded only in 2007.[6] The 2007 reform harmonized French law with European Community law that incorporated the fiduciary under the 1985 Hague convention.

In French law today, the fiduciary is an instrument to transfer property, hold property, or allow operation of a surety created by explicit contacts or by actions that the law holds create a fiduciary by default. Unlike Anglo-American trusts, ownership is not divided between title and equitable enjoyment. French fiduciaries are not held to a higher standard of conduct than other commercial actors, or subject to explicit conflict-of-interest rules. In Anglo-American law, courts created such rules, so such obligations may later emerge in French law.

ANGLO-AMERICAN LAW

In the United Kingdom's common law, judicial decisions include principles and rules that are precedents which courts follow in subsequent cases. Britain developed its native law but incorporated some Roman law from Catholic Church canon law and from commentaries on Roman and English law.

Early Medieval English law was formal and rigid, so aggrieved parties would often appeal to the King's Chancellor to use his equitable powers to create remedies where no legal recourse existed. The Chancellor, a representative of the Catholic Church, was trained in canon law—which included Roman law maxims and equitable principles—and often also in Roman law.[7] Roman law equitable principles were a fertile source for the Chancellor's remedies.[8] Over time the Chancellor's decisions grew into equity jurisprudence and a parallel judicial system arose. Law and equity each had their own courts, jurisdiction, and principles. Later, legislation merged law and equity into a single system.

Equity law created the trust, drawing on the Roman law fideicommissa and fiducia.[9] It designated trustees and agents as *fiduciaries,* held them to high standards, devised means to hold them accountable, and crafted remedies for breaches of trust. Courts created rules to oversee fiduciary conflicts of interest. Over time, fiduciary principles and conflicts of interest rules spread to other areas of law.

Trusts are used to convey or control property. The grantor transfers property to the trustee for the exclusive benefit of a beneficiary. The trustee holds the legal title, while the beneficiary has equitable entitlement to its use. Trustees cannot use trust property for their own benefit. Their powers are to be exercised exclusively for the beneficiary's benefit. Trustees may not consider the interest of third parties or themselves. Trustees may not compete with the trust, or enter into personal financial transactions with a trust, except in unusual circumstances, and then only if they disclose their arrangement and the beneficiary gives knowing and intelligent consent. Trustees may receive previously agreed-upon, reasonable compensation for their services.

Courts typically deter trustees from entering into situations that create conflicts of interests. They can take preventive measures that limit the trustees' discretion without demonstrating past harm to beneficiaries or unjust enrichment of the trustee. Courts can declare void any transaction between the trust and trustee acting in his or her personal capacity if the transaction is not fair. They may also declare any benefits received by a trustee to be held in a constructive trust for the beneficiary. If a trustee enters into a transaction that violates fiduciary obligations of loyalty, the beneficiary can object after the fact, the action will be void, and the beneficiary can receive restitution. If a trustee is disloyal, courts can remove the trustee or prevent the trustee from being paid.

Anglo-American law often treats delegated powers as property and deems parties delegated authority to be fiduciaries. The prime example is the agent, a person who agrees to act for, represent, and be controlled by a principal.

An agent's duty is to give single-minded attention to the principal's affairs and to subordinate personal interests, except with the principal's consent. Agents must not act for their own benefit, help other parties to compete with their principal, or disclose a principal's confidential information.

Agents must not take advantage of their position or use for their personal benefit information or opportunities acquired as a result of their position. If an agent violates his obligations, the principal can disavow any agreement the agent has made, thereby shifting responsibility to the agent. Agents who breach their duty of undivided loyalty may be liable even if there is little risk of harm to the principal. Payments to an agent from third parties are suspect and may indicate a violation of loyalty. Principals can terminate agency relationships if the agent misbehaves and often can do so without cause.

Anglo-American law also regulates as fiduciaries bankers, corporate officers and directors, money managers, pension fund managers, and others who hold property for or exercise powers on behalf of others. Similarly, it holds lawyers to fiduciary standards because they manage the legal affairs of others and represent them. It also treats as fiduciaries parents acting for children and guardians acting for their wards.

As late as the seventeenth century, public offices were sold in Great Britain.[10] The idea of government as a *public trust,* popularized by John Locke in the eighteenth century, grafted the fiduciary idea onto government functions. It articulated a basis for removing leaders and made it possible to speak of conflicts of interest of public officials and regulation of public officials to ensure that they do not use their public powers for private purposes.[11]

JAPANESE LAW

When Japan adopted Western institutions in the 1860s, it developed its law based on the German and French civil codes and on American law for finance, trusts, and agency. Its civil code included fiduciary principles from German and American law. Its corporate law used fiduciary principles to regulate corporate officers and directors. After World War II, legislation imposed on corporate officers and directors a fiduciary duty of loyalty. The Commercial Code uses fiduciary principles to regulate self-dealing by directors. The Commerce Act establishes a duty of loyalty and prohibits executives in investor-owned corporations from accepting bribes that jeopardize the corporate interest.[12]

The Trust Act and Civil Code include special obligations for trustees, agents and other fiduciaries, which scholars call *Jūtakusha* (trustee) and *Jūninsha* (fiduciary) or *Shin-nin Kankei* (trust relationship). Agents are prohibited from entering into certain role conflicts (*Rieki-Sōhan*).[13] Public servants are regulated as fiduciaries. The criminal code includes penalties for breaching fiduciary obligations (*Hainin*). It prohibits public employees, including physicians, from accepting bribes or gifts. The Lawyers Act does the same for lawyers.[14]

In the 1990s, Japan promoted transparency (*tōmeisei*) and passed a Freedom of Information Act. This was similar to France's efforts to promote an open and fair government process under the rubric of *transparence*. To protect purchasers and consumers of financial services, Japan required greater disclosure of financial ties; they were less stringent than American Securities and Exchange Commission requirements on which they were modeled. [15]

CIVIL LAW MANDATE RELATIONS

The French and Japanese civil codes developed the Roman law *Mandatum*, contracts in which one party acts for another. One party, the mandatary, transacts activity for the benefit of the principal or mandant.[16] Mandate contracts resemble common law agency relations but require consent of both parties.

Agents are fiduciaries and are required to act in the exclusive interest of the principal. Mandate contracts can serve the common interest of mandatary and mandant, or a third party. If both the principal and mandatary have an interest in the subject of the contract, there may be conflict of interest. Mandataries are required to act in good faith, but need not act exclusively for the principal. Thus mandataries have fewer conflict-of-interest restrictions than agents.[17]

In Japanese law, there is no duty of accounting during the mandate contract, only after completion. In addition, the duty of loyalty is weaker than in fiduciary relations because the mandate party is expected to have some benefits from the contract and can act in its own interest in performing this role.[18] In Japanese law, patient-physician relations are a mandate relationship.

Acronyms

ACCME	Accreditation Council for Continuing Medical Education (U.S.)
ACS	American College of Surgeons
AFSSAPS	Agence Française de Sécurité Sanitaire de Produits de Santé (Drug and Medical Product Safety Agency, France)
AGMF	Association Générale des Médecins de France (General Association of French Physicians)
AMA	American Medical Association
ANAES	Agence Nationale d'Accréditation et d'Evaluation en Santé (National Agency for Accreditation and Evaluation of Health, France)
ASCs	ambulatory surgery centers (U.S.)
CCMC	Committee on the Cost of Medical Care (U.S.)
CEJA	Council on Ethical and Judicial Affairs of the American Medical Association
CLIA'88	Clinical Laboratory Improvements Amendments of 1988 (U.S.)
CME	continuing medical education
CMS	Center for Medicare and Medicaid Services (U.S.)
CNAMTS	Caisse National d'Assurance Maladie des Travailleurs Salariés (NHI fund for salaried workers, France)
CNFMC	Conseils Nationaux de la Formation Médicale Continue (National Councils for Continuing Medical Education, France)
CRR	Council for Regulatory Reform (succeeded by the Council for the Promotion of Regulatory Reform, Japan)
CSIMC	Central Social Insurance Medical Council, or Chūikyō (Japan)
CSMF	Confédération des Syndicats Médicaux Français (Confederation of French Medical Unions)
CT	computer tomography
DGCCRF	Direction générale de la concurrence, de la consommation et de la répression des fraudes (Bureau of Competition, Anti-Fraud and Consumer Affairs, France)
DHFL	Democratic Health Federation League of Japan
DHHS	Department of Health and Human Services (U.S.)
DPC	diagnostic procedure combinations (Japan)
DPJ	Democratic Party of Japan
EC	European Community

ECJ	European Court of Justice
ERISA	Employee Retirement Income Security Act (U.S.)
FDA	Food and Drug Administration (U.S.)
FDCA	Food, Drug and Cosmetic Act (U.S.)
NMF	National Federation of French Mutual Insurers
FNMF	*Fédération nationale de la mutualité française* (National Federation of French Mutual Insurers)
FNOSS	Fédération Nationale des Organismes de la Sécurité Sociale (National Federation of Social Security Organizations, France)
FPMAJ	Federation of Pharmaceutical Manufacturer Associations of Japan
FTC	Federal Trade Commission (U.S.)
FTCEPDMI	Fair Trade Council of the Ethical Pharmaceutical Drugs Marketing Industry (Japan)
GAO	General Accounting Office/ Government Accountability Office (U.S.)
HAS	Haute Autorité de Santé (High Authority on Health, France)
HIB	Health Insurance Bureau (Japan)
HMO	health maintenance organization (U.S.)
IGAS	Inspection Générale des Affaires Sociales (Inspector General for Social Affairs, France)
IPA	independent practice associations (U.S.)
IRO	independent review organization (U.S.)
IRS	Internal Revenue Service (U.S.)
JCAHO	Joint Commission on Accreditation of Healthcare Organizations (U.S.)
JCQHC	Japan Council for Quality in Health Care
JFTC	Japan Fair Trade Commission
JMA	Japan Medical Association
JPMA	Japanese Pharmaceutical Manufacturers Association
Kemporen	National Federation of Health Insurance Societies (Japan)
LDP	Liberal Democratic Party (Japan)
LEEM	Les Entreprises du Médicament (Medication Enterprises, the pharmaceutical industry trade union and successor to SNIP, France)
MCO	managed care organization (U.S.)
MH	Ministry of Health (France)
MHLW	Ministry of Health, Labor and Welfare (Japan)
MHW	Ministry of Health and Welfare (Japan)
MRI	magnetic resonance imaging
MSA	Medical Service Act (Japan)
NHI	national health insurance
OECD	Organization for Economic Cooperation and Development
OGC	Organisme Gestionnaire Conventionnel pour la Formation Professionnelle Conventionnelle des Médecins (Organization for Management of Continuing Medical Education Under Negotiated Accords, France)

OIG	Office of Inspector General (U.S)
PBMs	pharmaceutical benefit managers (U.S.)
PhRMA	Pharmaceutical Research and Manufacturers' Association (U.S.)
PMA	Pharmaceutical Manufacturers' Association (U.S.)
PMAO	Pharmaceutical Manufacturers' Association of Osaka
PMAT	Pharmaceutical Manufacturers' Association of Tokyo
PPGP	prepaid group practice (U.S.)
PPMs	physician practice managers (U.S.)
PPO	preferred provider organization (U.S.)
PRO	peer review organization (U.S.)
PSRO	physician standard review organization (U.S.)
QIO	quality improvement organization (U.S.)
SCAP	Supreme Commander for the Allied Powers in Japan
SMC	specified medical cost (Japan)
SNIP	Syndicat National de l'Industrie Pharmaceutique (National Pharmaceutical Industry Union, France)
SNITM	Le Syndicat National de l'Industrie des Technologies Médicales (Medical Device Manufacturers' National Trade Association, France)
USMF	l'Union des Syndicat Médicaux Français (Union of French Physician Syndicates, France)
WHO	World Health Organization
WLF	Washington Legal Foundation (U.S.)

Glossary of French Terms in English

English	French
Accords negotiated between NHI funds and physician unions	*Convention*
Common Classification for Medical Procedures	*Classification Commune des Actes Medicaux (CCAM)*
Compulsory practice guideline	*Références médicales opposables (RMO)*
Council of Accounts	*Cour des comptes*
Direct relationship	*Entente directe*
Law on hospitals, patients, health and Regions	*Loi HPST, Hôpital, patients, santé, et territories*
Medical Charter	*Charte de la médicine libérale*
Medical information system	*Programme de médicalisation des systèmes d'information (PMSI)*
National Agency for Accreditation and Evaluation of Health	*Agence Nationale d'Accréditation et d'Evaluation en Santé (ANAES)*
National spending goals	*Objectifs nationaux de dépenses d'assurance maladie (ONDAM)*
NHI funds / mutual insurance funds	*Caisses*
Organisation for the Management of CME under Physician Accords	*Organisme Gestionnaire Conventionnel Formation Professionnelle Conventionnelle des Médecins (OCE)*
Point system	*Indice synthétique d'activité*
Public health officer	*Officier de santé*
Regional Hospital Planning Agency	*Agence Regionale d'Hospitalisation (ARH)*
Treating physician gatekeeper	*Médecin traitant /Médecin referant*

Acknowledgments

My principal research funding was a year-long Abe Fellowship from the Japan Foundation though the Social Science Research Council. I also received a German Marshall Fund fellowship in 2000 and a Fulbright Fellowship in France, 2001. I was supported as a visiting professor at the faculté de droit de l'Université de Rennes in 2001, where I was also a researcher at the Centre de Recherche Juridique de l'Ouest (CRJO) funded by the Centre National de Recherche Scientifique (CNRS). I also worked as a consultant for the Fédération Nationale de la Mutualité Française (FNMF) and wrote several reports on related issues. The FNMF provided numerous contacts, offered intellectual support, and shared their archives. I was a consultant for the Accreditation Council for Continuing Medical Education and wrote memos on how conflicts of interest are addressed in various sectors outside of medicine and on conflicts of interest in continuing medical education. Suffolk University Law School has supported my work and provided summer research funding. I am also grateful for the outstanding work of Suffolk's librarians, particularly Scott Akehurst-Moore, Ellen Beckworth, Rick Buckingham, Diane D'Angelo, Ellen Delaney, Jeanie Fallon, Sabrina Holley-Williams, Betsy McKenzie, Susan Sweetgall, and Susan Vaughn. Kuniko Yamada McVey of the Harvard-Yenching Library also offered valuable assistance.

In his review of my manuscript for *Medicine, Money and Morals: Physicians, Conflicts of Interest*, Dan Fox suggested that I compare the United States with other countries. There were limits on adding national comparison in that book, but his idea challenged me to me to undertake this comparative study.

In France, Jean de Kervasdoué supported the project from start to finish and shared his own considerable knowledge of French health policy. Brigitte Feuillet-Liger, Phillippe Pierre, and other colleagues at the l'Institut de l'Ouest: Droit et Europe (IODE-CNRS) and its department, the Centre de Recherche Juridique de l'Ouest (CRJO), and the faculté de droit de l'Université de Rennes played a crucial role in the study and remain colleagues and friends. I benefited from the library and the knowledge of my colleagues at the Institut d'Etudes des Politiques de Santé de l'Université de Paris VI, particularly Laurent Degoss, Isabelle Durand-Zaleski, Dominique Jolly, and Bernard Tessiere. Several French scholars collaborated with me in exploring conflicts of interest in French law, its medical economy and beyond, and continue to work with me: they include Joël Moret-Bailly, Jean-Paul Demarez, François Eisinger, and Dominique Thouvenin. Lionel Benaiche helped me understand French and European Community drug law and policy and served as an entree to the AFSSAPS, the French drug agency. Philippe Duneton, APSSAPS's director, also supported my work. I am grateful for the cooperation of Caisse National d'Assurance Maladie des Travailleurs Salariés, l'Ordre des Médecins, Agence Française de Sécurité Sanitaire de Produits de Santé, and the journal *Préscrire*.

While living in Japan in 2002 I was a Visiting Research Scholar at Tokyo University Law School, assisted by Norio Higuchi, Hisakazu Hirose, and Yoshi Nomi. I met Estuji Okamoto while a visiting scholar at Cho University Law School in 1993, and we co-authored an article on physicians' conflicts of interest in Japan in the United States in 2000. He has continued to collaborate with my research. Robert Leflar has also helped me with contacts and insights for the last decade. In addition, I benefited from the Abe Fellowship retreats and assistance from the Japan Foundation staff.

I was assisted by an advisory board in each country: in the United States, Hank Greely, Timothy Jost, and Rosemary Stevens; in France, Bernard Glorion, Martin Hirsch, Gilles Johanet, Jean de Kervasdoué, Claude Le Pen, and Dominique Thouvenin; in Japan, Estuji Okamoto, Norio Higuchi, and Naoki Ikegami.

Grey Osterund was a brilliant editor. I also benefited from comments on drafts by numerous people. In the United States they included Lawrence Brown, Dan Fox, Peter Jacobson, Tim Jost, John Lantos, David Mechanic, James Morone, Michael Millenson, Wendy Parmet, Justin Silverman, Rosemary Stevens, and Kenneth Wing. French reviewers included Joël Moret-Bailly, Pierre Chirac, Jean-Paul Demarez, Isabelle Durand-Zaleski, François Eisinger, Pierre-Jean Lancry, Hervé Maisonneuve, Philippe R. Mossé, Phillippe Pierre, Gérard de Pouvourville, Monika Steffen, Dominique Schmidt, and Renaud Tamisier. Reviewers of material on Japan included Christa Altenstetter, John Campbell, Naoki Ikegamai, Gregory Kaza, Robert Leflar, Ryozo Matsuda, Reed Mauer, Philippe Mossé, Yoshi Nomi, Estuji Okamoto, Mark Remeseyer, Barbara Starfield, John Wocher, and Nobuhiko Yasuda.

Many people also helped me along the way. In France they included Gilles Bardelay, Jean-Martin Cohen-Solal, Etienne Caniard, Philippe Foucras, Jean Pierre Gallet, Nicolas Gombault, Gilles Johanet, Noëlle Lenoir, Christine

Meyer-Meuret, Rémy Nizard, Christian Poimboeuf, Dominique Polton, Jean-Louis Portos, Christophe Rateau, Philippe Ravaud, Louis Serfaty, Agnes Schmitz Schweitzer, Jean-Dominique Tortauyaux, and Elsa Passer. In Japan they included Mark A. Colby, Eric Feldman, Koichi Kawabuchi, Hirobumi Kawakita, Rihito Kimura, Yasushi Kodama, Isao Mori, Ryu Niki, Lawrence Repeta, Hideaki Shiroyama, Paul Talcott, and Naruo Uehara. I am also grateful to the numerous public officials, doctors, hospital administrators, pharmaceutical company employees, and scholars who took time to answer my questions and explain how things work in practice and how that differs from the written rules and policy. Several students worked as research assistants for me over the years; among them were Kara Brown, Christopher Brooks, Hak Chang, Taya Furmanski Mashburn, Ryoko Hatanaka, Mai Naitō, Eileen Nee, Naitō Rei, Charlotte Sailly, David Spielberg, Patricia Tarabelsi, Sophie Wernert, Danielle White, and Sarah Wilton. Anthony Ruggiero assisted with the index.

My thinking on professionalism was stimulated by serving on the Advisory Board of the Open Society Institute, Program on Medicine as a Profession directed by David Rothman. I learned much from my many colleagues including David Blumenthal, Norman Daniels, Eli Ginsberg, Jerome Kassirer, Robert Lawrence, Wendy Levinson, Susana Morales, Kenneth Shine, James R. Tallon, Jr., and Gerald Thomson. I was also enriched by my continuing dialogues with colleagues in the Robert Wood Johnson Foundation's Investigator Award program, ably administered by Sol Levine, Al Tarlov, David Mechanic, Robin Osbern, and Lyn Rogut. In addition to supporting my earlier work on Accountable Health Care, its meetings and fellow awardees have been a center of my intellectual growth. Over the years I have also benefited from the support and collegiality of George Annas, Edward Beiser, Thomas Bergin, Troy Brennan, Dan Brock, Alan Buchanan, Alexander Capron, Christine Cassel, Steve Crane, Barry Furrow, Tamar Frankel, Eliot Freidson, Deborah Freund, Leonard Glantz, Tim Greaney, Mark Hall, Joel Handler, Sandra Johnson, Eleanor Kinney, Fran Miller, Sol Levine, Wendy Mariner, Philip Quinn, Robert Schwartz, Mark Schlesinger, Deborah Stone, Sol Touster, Arnold Weinstein, Sidney Wolf, Calvin Woodard, and Irv Zola.

My father, Lloyd, and brother, Victor, nurtured my interest in and provided models for comparative and international research. Victor also shared his own knowledge of and contacts in France. My wife, Wendy Schoener, offered perspective, critique, and support throughout the project. Nina Rodwin wondered if it would ever end. But as Benjamin Rodwin said, referring to the Eiffel Tower, "C'est nest pas si grand que ça."

Notes

FOREWORD

1. Douglas R. Waud, Pharmaceutical promotions—a free lunch?" *NEJM* 327, no. 5 (1992): 351–53. Dennis F. Thompson, Understanding financial conflicts of interest, *NEJM* 329, no. 8 (1993): 573–76. Marc A. Rodwin, *Medicine, money and morals: Physicians' conflicts of interest* (New York: Oxford University Press, 1993).

2. Marc A. Rodwin, Conflicts of Interest: The limitations of disclosure. *NEJM* 321, no. 20 (1989): 1405–9.

INTRODUCTION

1. George Bernard Shaw, Preface, *The doctor's dilemma: A tragedy* (Baltimore, MD: Penguin, 1988). The play was first performed in 1906 and published in 1913.

2. Kurt Eichenwald and Gina Kolata, Hidden interest—when physicians double as entrepreneurs, *New York Times*, 30 November 1999, 1.

3. Interviews by the author with François Eisinger and Pierre Chirac, fall 2001.

4. Jean-Yves Nau, Justice: Les premières suites judiciaires de l'affaire des prothèses. Une trentaine de chirurgiens orthopédistes libéraux sont mis en examen pour escroquerie à l'encontre de la sécurité sociale, *Le Monde*, 22 November 1994.

5. *Maiinichi newspaper*, 22 September 1992.

CHAPTER 1

1. Eliot Freidson, Identifying professions. In Freidson, *Professional powers: A study of institutionalization of formal knowledge* (Chicago: University of Chicago Press, 1988), 20–40.

2. For a review of how the challenges to medical authority played out in bioethics, see David J. Rothman, *Strangers at the bedside: A history of how law and bioethics transformed medical decision making* (New York: HarperCollins, 1991). On changing ideas in the sociology of professions, see the review essay by Charles L. Bosk, Avoiding conventional understandings: The enduring legacy of Eliot Friedson, *Sociology of Health & Illness* 28, no. 5 (2006): 637–53.

3. For market critiques, Milton Friedman and Simon Kuznets, *Income from independent professional medical practice* (New York: National Bureau of Economic Research, 1945); Elton Rayack, *Professional power and American medicine: The economics of the American Medical Association* (Cleveland, OH: World Book, 1967); Jeffrey Lionel Berlant, *Profession and monopoly: A study of medicine in the United States and Great Britain* (Berkeley: University of California Press, 1975), 64–127; Charles Weller, "Free choice" as a restraint of trade, and the counterintuitive contours of competition, *Health Matrix* 3, no. 2 (1985): 3–23. For patients' rights, George J. Annas, The hospital: A human rights wasteland, *Civil Liberties Review* 1, no. 4 (1974): 9–29; George J. Annas, *The rights of hospital patients* (New York: Avon, 1975). For voice, Marc A. Rodwin, Consumer voice and representation in health care, *Journal of Health Law* 34, no. 2 (2001): 223–72; Marc A. Rodwin, Exit and voice in American health care, *Michigan Journal of Law Reform* 32, no. 4 (1999): 1041–67.

4. The concept of conflict of interest originates in fiduciary law, has been used to govern professionals who exercise power or authority for a designated party. The appendix examines the concept's development and dissemination. See also Marc A. Rodwin, Strains in the fiduciary metaphor: Divided physician loyalties and obligations in a changing health care system, *American Journal of Law and Medicine* 21, nos. 2 & 3 (1995): 241–57; Peter Jacobson, *Strangers in the night: Law and medicine in the managed care era* (New York: Oxford University Press, 2002), 222–49; Francis H. Miller, Secondary income from recommended treatment: Should fiduciary principles constrain physician behavior? In *The new health care for profit: Doctors and hospitals in a competitive environment*, ed. B. Gray, 153–69 (Washington, DC: National Academies Press, 1983); Maxwell J. Mehlman, Dishonest medical mistakes, *Vanderbilt Law Review* 59, no. 4 (2006): 1137–73.

5. Marc A. Rodwin, *Medicine, money and morals: Physicians' conflicts of interest* (New York: Oxford University Press 1993), 9–11 and 253–55.

6. David Blumenthal, The vital role of professionalism in health care reform, *Health Affairs* 13, no. 1 (1994): 252–56.

7. Public Law 111–148,124 Stat.119 (2010).

8. For an assessment of the law, see Marc A. Rodwin, Why we need health care reform now, *Journal of Health Politics, Policy and Law*, 36, no. 3 (in press), along with the other contributions to the theme issue on the health care reform.

CHAPTER 2

1. In 2000, France had 197,224 physicians; 56,206 were employed in publicly funded hospitals; *Annuaire des Statistiques Sanitaires et Sociales*, 1998. M. Duriez, P. Lancry, D. Lequet-Slama, et S. Sandier, *Le système de santé en France* (Paris: Presses Universitaire de France, 1999). For a contemporary analysis of French health policy, see Jean de Kervasdoué, *Très chère santé* (Paris: Perrin, 2009). Monika Steffen, The French health care system: Liberal universalism, *Journal of Health Politics, Policy and Law* 35, no. 3 (2010): 336–69. For a comparative analysis of French and American

health policy and history, see Paul V. Dutton, *Differential diagnoses: A comparative history of health care problems and solutions in the United States and France* (Ithaca, NY: Cornell University Press, 2007).

2. David Wilsford, *Doctors and the state: The politics of health care in France and the United States* (Durham, NC: Duke University Press, 1991), portrays organized medicine as weak compared to the state.

3. Matthew Ramsey, *Professional and popular medicine in France, 1770–1830* (Cambridge: Cambridge University Press, 1988), 20.

4. Corporations could represent members in court, provide mutual aid, and exempt members from military service and taxes. Trades sought corporate status to reduce competition and the Crown conferred it to garner political support. Laurence Brockliss and Colin Jones, *The medical world of early modern France* (New York: Oxford University Press, 1997), 9; Jacques Le Goff, Les métiers et l'organisation du travail dans la France médiévale. In *La France et les français*, ed. M. François (Paris: Gallimard, 1980), 310–37

5. William H. Sewell, Jr., *Work and revolution in France: The language of labor from the old regime to 1848* (Cambridge: Cambridge University Press, 1980).

6. Laurence Brockliss and Colin Jones, *Medical world of early modern France* (New York: Oxford University Press, 1997), 21, 186–89.

7. Lamy, *Droit de la Santé*, Editions Lamy, Paris, paragraphes 238–5–238–8. Partie 2, Acteurs de Santé. Titre 2.

8. Ramsey, *Professional and popular medicine in France*, 30; Brockliss and Jones, *Medical world of early modern France*, 622–69.

9. Michele Harichaux, *La rémunération du médecin* (Paris: Economica, 1979).

10. Brockliss and Jones, *Medical world of early modern France*, 534, 544–45.

11. Ramsey, *Professional and popular medicine in France*, 63, 118–19.

12. Paul Delaunay, *Le monde médical parisien au dix-huitième siècle* (Paris: Jules Rousset, 1906).

13. Maurice Rochaix, *Les questions hospitalières: de la fin d l'ancien régime à nos jours* (Paris: Berger-Levrault, 1996); Christian Maillard, *Histoire de l'hôpital de 1940 à nos jours: Comment la santé est devenue une affaire d'état* (Paris: Dunod, 1986), ch. 1, 5–12; Thomas McStay Adams, *Bureaucrats and beggars: French social policy in the age of the enlightenment* (New York: Oxford University Press, 1990).

14. George Rosen, Mercantilism and health policy in eighteenth-century French thought. In Rosen, *From medical police to social medicine: Essays on the history of health care* (New York: Sciences History Publications, 1974), 201–19; R. Sand, *Vers la médecine sociale* (Liège, Belgique: Baillere, 1948), 187–88.

15. John Frangos, *From housing the poor to healing the sick: The changing institution of Paris hospitals under the Old Regime and Revolution* (Madison, WI: Associated University Presses, 1997), 25.

16. Jean-Jacques Rousseau, *The social contract and discourses*, trans. G. D. H. Cole (1762; Mineola, NY: Dover, 2003). E. J. Sieyès, *What is the third estate?* trans. M. Blondel, ed. S. E. Finer (1789; New York: Praeger, 1964).

17. These competing conceptions of the public interest are explored in Steven Kelman, *Making public policy: A hopeful view of American government* (New York: Basic Books, 1987), 265–76.

18. Claude Dubar et Pierre Tripier, La catégorisation professionnelle en France: l'État et les professions. In Dubar and Tripier, *Sociologie des professions* (Paris: Armand Colin, 1998), ch. 7, 141–55; Alain Desrosieres, Éléments pour l'histoire des nomenclatures professionnelles. In *Pour une histoire de la statistique*, Tome 1 (Institut National de la Statistique et des Etudes Economiques (INEE), 1977); Alain Desrosières et Laurent Théveont, *Les catégories socio-professionnelles* (Paris: La Découverte, 2002); Pierre Rosanvallon, *L'État en France de 1789 à nos jours* (Paris: Seuil, 2008).

19. There was no adequate replacement for the 12 percent to 30 percent of the population needing public assistance.

20. Although this system spread to Haut-Rhin, Vosges Haute-Saône, Moselle, and Saône-et-Loire, it did not extend across France. Alsace had a distinct public culture; like Switzerland and some small German states, it had strong local governments. It remained mostly under French control until the Franco-Prussian war in 1871, but many Alsatians fought against France during the Napoleonic wars.

21. Ramsey, *Professional and popular medicine in France*, 114–15.

22. Ann E. La Berge and Mordechai Feingold, *French medical culture in the nineteenth century* (Amsterdam: Edition Rodopi B.V., 1994), 215–32.

23. Timothy B. Smith, *Creating the welfare state in France: 1880–1940* (Montreal: McGill-Queen's University Press, 2003).

24. Henri Hatzfeld, *Du paupérisme à la sécurité sociale, 1850–1940* (Paris: Armand Colin, 1971).

25. Mutual aid societies were supervised by municipal authorities and limited to 2,000 members. Alan Mitchell, The function and malfunction of mutual aid societies in nineteenth century France. In *Medicine and charity before the welfare state*, ed. J. Barry and C. Jones, 172–89 (New York: Routledge, 1991). For data on their growth, see Pierre Guillaume, *Mutualistes et médecins: Conflits et convergences, XIXe-XXe siècles* (Paris: Editions de l'Atelier/Editions Ouvrières, 2000), 16.

26. Louis-Napoléon Bonaparte was elected president of the Second Republic in 1848; a coup in 1851–1852 elevated him to emperor. He grew up in Germany, spent time in England and the United States, and was also influenced by French socialists.

27. Mitchell, Function and malfunction of mutual aid societies, 181. French population data are from Massimo Livi-Bacci, *A concise history of world population* (Malden, MA: Wiley-Blackwell, 2001).

28. Pierre Guillaume, *Le rôle social du médecin depuis deux siècles: 1800–1945* (Paris: Association pour l'Etude de l'histoire de la Sécurité Sociale, 1996), 118. David

Wilsford, 1993. The state and medical profession in France. In *The changing medical profession: An international perspective*, ed. F. W. Hafferty and J. B. McKinlay, 124–37 (New York: Oxford University Press, 1993).

29. Chevandier Act, Loi du 30 novembre 1892. Jacques Léonard, *La médecine entre les savoirs et les pouvoirs: Histoire intellectuelle et politique de la médecine française au XIXème siècle* (Paris: Aubier, 1981), especially chapters 12, 14, and 18. Membership statistics are from Guillaume, *Le rôle social du médecin*, 120.

30. Guillaume, *Le rôle social du médecin*, 147–48, quoting from *Le Médecin Syndicaliste*, Bulletin de l'Union des syndicats médicaux, Décember 1919: "Chacun construit suivant sa structure. Le patron veut faire du médecin un salarié. L'Etat veut en faire un fonctionnaire."

31. Monika Steffen, Régulation, politique et stratégies professionnelles: Médecine libérale et émergence des centres de santé (Thèse de science politique, Institut d'Etudes Politiques, Université des Sciences Sociales de Grenoble, 1983), 239–41. Monika Steffen, The medical profession and the state in France, *Journal of Public Policy* 7, no. 2 (1987): 189–208.

32. Guillaume, *Mutualistes et médecins*, 70–74.

33. The term *secret médical*, literally, medical secret, has different connotations from the English term *confidentiality*. Regarding opposition to insurer oversight, see Paul V. Dutton, *Origins of the welfare state: The struggle for social reform in France, 1914–1947* (New York: Cambridge University Press, 2002), 112. Pierre Theil, *Le corps médical devant la médecine sociale* (Université de Paris X; Paris: Librairie Bailliere, 1943).

34. For mutual insurer pharmacies, see Guillaume, *Mutualistes et médecins*, 72–73. For free choice of physicians, see Guillaume, *Le rôle social du médecin*, 108. Physician unions also asked that self-employed physicians be allowed to treat private patients in public hospitals.

35. In response to physician lobbying, Paris and Lyon also paid some private practitioners to supply medical care. Martha L. Hildreth, *Doctors, bureaucrats, and public health in France, 1888–1902* (New York: Garland, 1987), 216–17.

36. *Loi sur l'Assistance médicale gratuite, 1893* (15 July 1893). Martha L. Hildreth, Medical rivalries and medical politics in France: The physicians' union movement and the medical assistance law of 1893, *Journal of the History of Medicine and the Allied Sciences* 42, no. 1 (1987): 5–29. Physician unions also lobbied to amend the Law on Workplace Accidents to raise state-set fees, allow patients to choose their own physician, and ensure physician freedom to prescribe. Amendments in 1895 met these demands.

37. Jules Romains. *Knock: Ou, le triomphe de la médecine: comédie en trois actes* (Paris: Gallimard, 2000); *Doctor Knock: A comedy in three acts*, trans. Harley Granville-Barker (London, Sidgwick & Jackson, 1935).

38. Timothy B. Smith, The social transformation of hospitals and the rise of medical insurance in France, 1914–1944, *Historical Journal* 41, no. 4 (1998): 1055–87, at 1079, 1081–82, 1062.

39. Loi du 21 décembre 1941. This legislation governed hospital administration until the formation of the Fifth Republic in 1958.

40. Smith, Social transformation of hospitals, 1080. Starting in 1901, the FNMF also operated dispensaries.

41. Guillaume, *Le rôle social du médecin*, 149–78. However, a regional medical union worked with an industrial consortium of Roubaix-Tourcoing.

42. Léon Bourgeois, *Solidarité* (Paris: Armand Colin, 1896). See also Paul Weindling, The modernization of charity in nineteenth-century France and Germany. In *medicine and charity before the welfare state*, ed. Jonathan Barry and Colin Jones, 190–206 (New York: Routledge, 1991), 202; J. E. S. Haward, The official social philosophy of the French third republic: Léon Bourgeois and solidarism, *International Review of Social History* 6 (1961): 19–48; Michel Dreyfus, *La mutualité. Une histoire maintenant accessible* (Paris: Mutualité Française, 1988), 42.

43. See Patrick Hassenteufel, *Les médecins face á l'état: Une comparaison européenne* (Paris: Presses de Sciences Po, 1997), 95.

44. J. E. S. Haward, Solidarity: The social history of an idea in 19th century France, *International Review of Social History* 4 (1959): 261–64. The Radical Party was part of the wartime government and its leader, Georges Clemenceau, headed the cabinet from 1917 to 1919. After 1919, the Radical Party moved toward the center as it supported private property against socialists and communists.

45. Alain Chatriot, *La démocratie sociale à la française: L'expérience du conseil national économique 1924–1940* (Paris: Éditions La Découverte, 2002).

46. Henry C. Gallant, Origines historiques du plan français de sécurité sociale In Gallant, *Histoire politique de la sécurité sociale française 1945–1952* (Paris: Cahiers de la Fondation Nationale des Sciences Politiques, 1955), ch.1, 9–26; Paul Douglas, The French social insurance act, *Annals of the American Academy of Political and Social Science* 164 (1932): 2549.

47. The Medical Charter was adopted November 30, 1927, and published in *Le Médecin Syndicaliste*, 1 January 1928, 37–39. See Pierre Laroque, ed., *The social institutions of France* (London: Taylor and Francis, 1983), especially the contribution by Roy Evans. Paul V. Dutton, La médecin libérale rencontre le médecin syndicaliste (1920–1930), *Bulletin de l'Histoire de La Sécurité Sociale* 49 (2004): 79–98.

48. Paul Cibrié, *Syndicalisme médical* (Paris: Confédération des Syndicat Médicaux Français, 1954), 68.

49. La loi du 30 Avril 1930 modifiant et complétant la loi du 5 Avril 1928 sur les assurances sociale. *Journal Officiel* 1 May 1930. *Journal Officiel* 29 Novembre 1931. *Journal Officiel* 24 Mars 1940.

50. Harry Alvin Millis, *Sickness and insurance: A study of the sickness problem and health insurance* (Chicago: University of Chicago Press, 1937), 112.

51. Medical secrecy often protected physicians rather than patients. Dominique Thouvenin, *Le secret médical et l'information du malade* (Lyon: Presses Universitaires de Lyon, 1982).

52. Isadore Sydney Falk, *Security against sickness: A study of health insurance* (Garden City, NY: Doubleday, Doran, 1936), 110.

53. Romain Lavielle, *Rapport sur le fonctionnement des CCMs presenté au nom de la Section Permanente du Conseil Supérieur des Sociétés de Secours Mutuel* (Centre des Archives Contemporaines in Fontainebleau, CAC Dossier 1991 0085/2 Caisses Chirurgicales Mutuelles, 1932). Thanks to Paul Dutton for this information.

54. Guillaume, *Le rôle social du médecin*, 226.

55. William Sullivan, *Work and integrity: The crisis and promise of professionalism in America* (New York: HarperCollins, 1995), 29–61.

56. Individuals had proposed such organizations since the 1845 National Congress of Physicians. See Pierre Guillaume, La préhistoire de l'Ordre des médecins. In Guillaume, *L'exercice médical dans la société: Hier, aujourd'hui, demain. Contributions au colloque organisé par l'Ordre national des médecins les 29 et 30 Septembre 1995 à Paris* (Paris: Masson, 1995), 273–84; F. Raoux, Naissance de la corporation médicale 1879–1943 (Thèse de médecine, Faculté de St. Antoine, Paris, 1979), 32.

57. The government refrained from issuing the Senate bill as a decree in 1939 because a single physician union, *Syndicat des médecins de la Seine*, objected that a commission in which physicians were not the majority decided appeals. Hassenteufel, *Les médecins face à l'État*, 42–43.

58. Physician unions, which promote their members' interests, operated the Family Council, which conflicts with their mediating patient-physician disputes. Guillaume, La préhistoire de l'Ordre des médecins, 273–85.

59. On 18 October 1943, the provisional French government of Algeria suppressed the Order of Physicians and created a parallel structure. Physicians then elected representatives. P. Chevit, L'ordre des médecins (Thèse de Médecine, Faculté de Médecine de St. Antoine, Paris, 1978).

60. Jean-Jacques Dupeyroux, Michel Borgetto, and Robert Lafore, *Droit de la sécurité sociale*, 16ème ed. (Paris: Dalloz, 2008).

61. Claudine Herzlich, The evolution of relations between French physicians and the state from 1880 to 1980, *Sociology of Health and Illness* 4, no. 3 (1982): 241–53. Ellen M. Immergut, *Health politics: Interest and institution in Western Europe* (Cambridge: Cambridge University Press, 1992), 34–79; Donna Evleth, La bataille pour l'Ordre des médecins, 1944–1950, *Le Mouvement Social* no. 229, October-Decembre (2009): 61–77.

62. Joël Moret-Bailly, *Les déontologies* (Aix-en-Provence: Presses Universitaires d'Aix-Marseille, 2001), 114–25. In 2004, the government incorporated Medical Deontology into the Public Health Code.

63. The Order of Physicians also lobbies on behalf of physicians, functions as a learned society, and issues reports on medicine and ethics.

64. *CJCE (Cour de justice des communautés européennes) Affaire C-292/92*, 15 December 1993, *Ruth Hunermund e.a. contre Landesapothekerkammer Bader-Württemberg*. However, they cannot discriminate between professionals from different states.

65. Joël Moret-Bailly, *Les déontologies*. Jöel Moret-Bailly, Déontologie. In *Dictionnaire de la justice*, ed. L. Cadiet, 316–30 (Paris: Presses Universitaires de France, 2004). Joël Moret-Bailly, Règles déontologiques et fautes civiles, *Recueil Dalloz* (2002), 2820–24.

66. Evleth, La bataille pour l'Ordre des médecins, 209.

67. *Arrêt Teyssier*, 16 may 1946, 113. The reference to social insurance taking preference was in Article 5 of the Code of Medical Deontology. The Order of Physicians removed it in the next revision. Jean-Louis Morgenthaler, La Mutualité Française de 1945 à 1976: De la tradition au modernisme (Thèse présentée pour le doctorat au troisième cycle de sociologie, Université de Nancy II, 1981).

68. Decision of 18 January 1949, reprinted in *Bulletin Federation Mutualité* 9 (1949): 12.

69. *Conseil d'Etat, arrêt Rousset*, 6 January 1950; *Conseil d'État, arrêt Privat*, 27 April 1951; *Conseil d'Etat, arrêt Chaigneau*, 29 January 1954; *Conseil d'État, arrêt Costier*, 1 October 1954.

70. Jean De Kervasdoué, La politique d'état en matière d'hospitalisation privée (1962–1978), analyse des conséquences contradictoires, *Les Annales Economiques* 16 (1980): 25–26.

71. Immergut, *Health politics*, 121, note 94, citing 24 February 1960, SAN 7517, Archives.

72. Henri Hatzfeld, *Le grand tournant de la médecine libérale* (Paris: Les Éditions Ouvrières, 1963).

73. Cyrille Dupuis, Honoraires: les spécialistes dépassent, les caisses tolèrent, *Le Quotidien du Médecin*, 24 October 2002. In a poll, 48 percent of practitioners acknowledged charging more than the fee schedule.

74. Antoinette Catrice-Lorey, *La dynamique interne de la sécurité sociale, du système de pouvoir à la fonction personnelle* (Paris: Economica, 1982).

75. *Journal Officiel*, 31 October 1971. Article L162–2; la loi du 3 Juillet 1971. This became articles 257–265 of the social security code. Geneviève Rebecq, *Protection sociale* (Paris: Editions du Juris Classeur, 2007).

76. A few court decisions have held that charging more than two or three times the negotiated fees violates the tact and moderation norm. Simone Sandier, Valérie Paris, and Dominique Polton, *Health care systems in transition: France* (Copenhagen: European Observatory on Health Systems and Policies, 2004).

77. Lamy, *Droit de la santé*, Editions Lamy, Paris, Etude 256 (for clinical laboratories), Etude 238 (for laboratories and pharmacies) Loi n. 75–626 du 11 juillet 1975. *Code de la santé publique*, art. L. 6211–8, 1. The rules only prevent NHI reimbursement.

78. The *clinique* was renamed Alphamed in 1990 and Hexagone Hospitalization in 1993, when it had fifteen facilities.

79. Nicolas Tanti-Hardouin, *L'hospitalisation privée: Crise identitaire et mutation sectorielle* (Paris: La Documentation Française, 1996); Nicolas Tanti-Hardouin, Le

système de santé: La recomposition de l'offre hospitalière, *La santé: Cahiers Français* 324 (2005): 61–62. Physician ownership statistics from Europe stratégie analyse financière (EUROSTAF), *Les cliniques privées: Perspectives stratégiques et financières* (Paris: EUROSTAF, 1996), 133. For hospitalization and surgery, Sandier, Paris, and Polton, *Health care systems in transition*, 73. For imaging equipment, *Statistique annuelle des établissements de santé* (Paris: Direction de la recherche, des études, de l'évaluation et des statistiques, 1996).

80. See Discours de Alain Juppé, 15 November 1995, reprinted in *Droit Social* 3 (1996): 221–37. The cap on spending for private practitioners is called Objectifs nationaux des dépenses d'Assurance maladie (ONDAM). The compulsory practice guidelines are called *Reference Medicales Opposables* (RMO). The national hospital accrediting agency was *Agence Nationale d'Accréditation et d'Evaluation en Santé* (ANAES).

81. Jean De Kervasdoué, ed., *Le carnet de santé de la France en 2000* (Paris: Dunod, 2002), 89–90.

82. *Plan Hôpital 2007*, available at http://www.sante.gouv.fr/htm/dossiers/hopital2007 (accessed 13 November 2009). The model for the payment system was the prospective payment system used by Medicare in the United States, which uses diagnosis-related groups. The medical information system was called *Programme de medicalisation du systeme d'information* (PMSI).

83. Ministère de la santé et des sports. *Rapport 2009 au Parlement sur les missions d'intérêt général et l'aide à la contractualisation des établissements de santé*, 26.

84. Victor G. Rodwin and Claude Le Pen, Health care reform in France: The birth of state-led managed care, *NEJM* 351, no. 22 (2004): 2259–62. Claude Le Pen, *Les habit neufs d'Hippocrate* (Paris: Calmann-Lévy, 1999); V.G. Rodwin, R. J. Launois, B. Majnoni d'Intignano, and J. C. Stéphan, Les réseaux de soins coordonnés (RSC): propositions pour une réforme profonde du système de santé, *Revue Française des Affaires Sociales* 1 (January/March 1985): 37–61. In 1997, CNAMTS negotiated an accord with the physician union MG France that allowed physicians to coordinate medical care for participating patients. The Order of Physicians initiated but then dropped disciplinary proceedings against participating physicians.

85. Loi no. 2004–810 du 13 août 2004 relative à l'assurance maladie, *Journal officiel*, no. 190, 17 August 2004, http://www.legifrance.gouv.fr/texteconsolide/SSEAFI.htm.
Physicians can charge patients without referrals 17.5 percent more than negotiated fees. Patients do not need referrals to consult pediatricians, gynecologists, ophthalmologists, psychiatrists, or dentists.

86. Institut de Recherche et documentation en Economie de la Santé, Sickness funds reform; new governance: France Survey no. 4:2004. *Health Policy Monitor* (International Network Health Policy & Reform Bertelsmann Stiftung Foundation, 2004), available at http://www.healthpolicymonitor.org/index.jsp.

87. Recent reforms affecting private health insurance in France, *Euro Observer* 6, no. 1 (spring, 2004): 4–5.

88. Loi 2009–879, portant réforme de l'hôpital et relative aux patients, à la santé et aux territoires, *Journal Officiel*, no. 0167, 22 july 2009, p. 12184, Article 59. Jean de Kervasdoué, La loi "Bachelot," innove, étatise et s'arrête en chemin, in Jean de Kervasdoué, ed., *Carnet de santé de la France 2009—Economie, droit et politiques de santé* (Paris: Dunod, 2009), 29–38. The regional hospital planning agency is called *Agence Regionale d'Hospitalisation*

89. Académie National de Pharmacie, *Rôle des pharmaciens dans les établissements hospitaliers pour personnes âgées dépendantes* (EHPAD) (Decembre 2009).

90. Supplemental insurance typically covers copayments, deductibles, and physician charges that exceed the fee schedule. Some policies pay for private hospital rooms and other amenities. Mutual insurers supply nearly 60 percent, for-profit insurers 21 percent, and provident and commercial insurers 19 percent. Agnès Couffinhal and Valérie Paris, *Utilization fees imposed to public health care system users in France* (2001), available at http://www/irdes.eu/EspaceAnglais/Publications/OtherPubs/UtilisationFeesImposed France.pdf (accessed 10 November 2009). Agnès Couffinhal and Valérie Paris, Cost sharing in France, Working Paper, 2003, available at http://www.irdes.fr/english/wp/CostSharing.pdf (accessed 10 November 2009).

91. J. F. Chadalat, *La répartition des interventions entre les assurances maladies obligatoires et complémentaires en matière de dépense de santé* (Paris: Commission des comptes de le sécurité sociale, 2003). Ryoji Fuji, The reform of health care system and complementary health insurance in France, *The Japanese Journal of Social Security Policy* 8, no. 2 (2009): 57–67.

92. Monika Steffen, Privatization in French health politics: Few projects and little outcome, *International Journal of Health Services* 18, no. 4 (1989): 651–61.

93. Monika Steffen and Wolfram Lamping, European union and health policy: The "chaordic" dynamics of integration, *Social Science Quarterly* 90, no. 5 (2009): 1361–79. Monika Steffen, *Health governance in Europe: Issues, challenges, and theories* (London: Routledge, 2005).

94. Thomas C. Buchmueller and Agnès Couffinhal, Private health insurance in France. OECD Health, Working Paper No. 12 (2004), 19. ESLSA/ELSA/WD/HEA (2004) 3, available at http://www.oecd.org/dataoecd/35/11/30455292.pdf (accessed 10 November 2009).

95. Rémi Pellet, ch. 2, L'Europe et la Sante, 39–118, in J. de Kervasdoué, *Carnet de santé de la France 2009* (Paris: Dunod, 2009). Scott L. Greer, *The politics of European Union health policies* (Maidenhead, Berks, England: Open University Press, 2009). Scott L. Greer, *Becoming European: How France, Germany, Spain and the UK engage with European Union health policy* (London: Nuffield Trust, 2008), http://www.nuffieldtrust.org.uk/ecomm/files/Becoming-European-191108.pdf (accessed 12 May 2010).

CHAPTER 3

1. Elisabeth Zoller, *Introduction to public law: A comparative study* (Koninklijke Bill: Martinus Nijhoff, 2008), 1–21.

2. Claude Dubar et Pierre Tripier, La catégorisation professionnelle en France: l'État et les professions. In Dubar and Tripier, *Sociologie des professions* (Paris: Armand Colin, 1998), ch. 7, 141–55.

3. Yves Mény, *La corruption de la république* (Paris: Fayard, 1990). See also Sylvain Burmeau and Yves Mény: La confusion des pouvoirs produit les conflits d'intérêts, *Mediapart: le journal* (6 July 2010). Yves Mény, France: The end of the republican ethic? In *Democracy and corruption in Europe*, ed. D. D. Porta and Y. Mény (Paris: La Découverte, 1997), 7–21.

4. Physicians employed in public hospitals are governed by rules different from those that govern civil servants. Jean-Marie Auby, Jean-Bernard Auby, Didier Jean-Pierre, et al., *Droit de la fonction publique* (Paris: Dalloz, 2009), 1191, 1192.

5. Décret 47.945 du 25 Novembre 1987, Art. 2. The user fee that physicians pay hospitals for services is called *la redevance.* For medical research centers the user fee rate is 25 percent for consultations and 40 percent or 60 percent for most surgeries. For other hospitals the user fee is 15 percent for consultations and 20 percent for surgery.

6. Loi du 27 juillet 1989.

7. Décret d'application R-614–28–10 du code de la santé publique. Loi du 30 Octobre 2002. Loi de financement de la sécurité sociale pour 2003. Each hospital has a committee to oversee private consulting, but they typically rely on the physicians' reports.

8. These hospitals set physicians' salaries through their negotiations with unions, subject to state approval.

9. Physicians are more likely to treat fewer patients rather than reduce the number of services their patients receive. They reduce their workload without lowering their quality of care.

10. La Loi n. 83–634 du 13 juillet 1983 portant droits et obligations des fonctionnaires (dite loi Le Pors). Serge Salon and Jean-Charles Savignac, *La fonction publique et ses problèmes actuels* (Paris: Sirey, 1967), 233–42. John A. Rohr, Ethical issues in French public administration: A comparative study, *Public Administration Review* 51, no. 4 (1991): 283–97.

11. The principal statutes are: Code de la Santé Publique Article L-6115–8, L-6117–2, R-710–17–4; Code de la Sécurité Social, D-162–2-5. In addition, numerous criminal law statutes govern health care and health products. See also Lionel Benaiche and Marie-Laure Godefroy, *Droit pénal des produits de santé* (Paris: Litec, 2003); Joël Moret-Bailly, Les conflits d'intérêts des experts consultés par l'administration dans le domaine sanitaire, *Revue Droit Sanitaire et Social* 4 (2004): 855–71.

12. Décret no 83–1025 du 28 Novembre 1983 concernant les relations entre l'administration et les usagers, article 13. *Code de santé publique,* art. L 5323–4. Joël Moret-Bailly, Le rôle des experts au sein des agences de sécurité sanitaire, *Annales de la Régulation,* LGDJ 2: (2009): 327–43.

13. Agence Française de Sécurité Sanitaire des Produits de Santé, *Charte déontologique: Responsabilité de l'expert et sécurité juridique* (2002).

14. The literal translation is "Conflicts confessed, conflicts forgotten (Conflits avoués, conflits oubliés)." *La Revue Prescrire* 16, no. 168 (1996): 891.

15. Lionel Benaiche, *L'expertise en santé publique et principe de précaution.* Report for the Ministry of Justice and the Ministry of the Economy, Finance, and Industry, August (2004): 12.

16. The legal pleadings are available at http://formindep.org/le-Formindep-saisit-le-Conseil-d.

17. Maladie d'Alzheimer et autres démences: Un guide HAS biaisé, des affirmations hasardeuses, *La Revue Prescrire* 29, no. 304 (2009): 150.

18. HAS discusses its change in HAS Rapport annuel du Groupe Déontologie et Indépendance de l'expertise pour l'année 2009, May, 2010. http://www.hassante.fr/portail/upload/docs/application/pdf/2010-07/rapport_activite_2009_synthese.pdf.

The new HAS process for addressing conflicts of interest may be found at Haute Autorité de Santé, Guide des déclarations d'intérêts, et de gestion des conflits d'intérêts. http://www.has-sante.fr/portail/upload/docs/application/pdf/guide_dpi.pdf. The director of HAS discussed these changes and the law suit in Senate hearings. See http://videos.senat.fr/video/videos/2010/video5340.html AC20100616-03-h1n1-degos.flv; http://http5.senat.yacast.net/senat/VOD/commission/2010/AC20100616-03-h1n1-degos.mp3.

19. Lamy, *Droit de la santé*, Editions Lamy, Paris, Etude 256, Laboratoire d'analyse de biologie médicale.

20. Monika Steffen, Régulation, Politique et stratégies professionnelles: médecine libérale et émergence des centres de santé (Thèse de science politique, Institut d'Etudes Politiques, Université des Sciences Sociales de Grenoble, 1983); Jean-Louis Morgenthaler, La mutualité Française de 1945 à 1976: De la tradition au modernisme (Thèse présentée pour le doctorat au troisième cycle de sociologie, Université de Nancy II, 1981).

21. Geneviève Rebecq, *Protection sociale* (Paris: Editions du Juris Classeur, 2007), Fasc. 430–25.

22. Jean-François Chadelat, *La répartition des interventions entre les assurances maladies obligatoires et complémentaire en matière de dépensés de santé* (Paris: Commission de comptes de le sécurité sociale, 2003), available at http://www.sante.gouv.fr/htm/actu/chadelat.pdf (accessed 13 November 2009).

23. Dominique Thouvenin, *Le secret médical et l'information du malade* (Lyon: Presses Universitaires de Lyon, 1982).

24. The French term for compulsory practice guidelines is *reference medicales opposables* (RMO).

25. Michel DeSaint, *L'exercice en groupe de la médecine: Aspects juridiques, fiscaux, comptables* (Paris: Librairies techniques, 1981); Société civile professionnelle Art. 14, Loi 66–879 du 29 novembre 1966 modifiée par la loi 90–1258 du 31 décembre 1990

relative à l'exercice sous forme de sociétés des profession libérales soumises à un statut législatif ou réglementaire dont le titre est protégé.

26. My review of contracts in one lawyer's practice in 2000 revealed user fees ranging from 5 percent to 17 percent.

27. I interviewed more than a dozen private hospital physicians and managers in 2000–2001.

28. Interviews by author, 2000–2001.

29. The *Clinique Tonquin* in Lyon was organized in this way.

30. Jean-Pierre Alméras and Henri Péquignot, *La déontologie médicale* (Paris: Litec, 1996); Conseil National de l'Ordre, *Commentaires du code de déontologie médicale* (Paris: Ordre National des Médecins, 1996). The code and commentaries on it are available at http://www.conseil-national.medecin.fr/?url=deonto/rubrique.php; http://www.conseil-national.medecin.fr/?url=deonto/rubrique.php (accessed 13 November 2009).

31. No sharing group practice income, Articles 22, 87. In addition, unlike that in the United States, one of the three French versions of the Hippocratic Oath precludes secret fee splitting. "I will not participate in any secret fee splitting (*Je ne participerai à aucun partage clandestin d'honoraires*). It also prohibits dispensing or prescribing for profit, Articles 21, 26; remuneration for productivity, Article 97; advertising, Articles 80–81, 97; commercial practice, Articles 19, 25; practicing where medical are products sold, Article 25; reviewing insurance claims, Articles 100, 105; and maintaining a second office, Article 85.

32. CE, 17 November 1969. CE sect. 14 February 1969, Association syndicale nationale des médecins exerçant en groupe ou en équipe, Rec. 96 et CE 13 main 1987, syndicat national professionnel des médecins du travail.

33. All hearings were closed until the European Court of Human Rights required that disciplinary hearings be open to the public in 1981. But no information is published.

34. In 2000, the disciplinary bureau included two full-time lawyers, one person to document the work, and five secretaries. Volunteer physicians and a member of the Council of State review appeals from departmental disciplinary decisions. The Order of Physicians regional chapter, departmental chapter, or national office can initiate complaints. So can the physician's union; the Minister of Health, the Minister of Social Security; the regional and public prosecutors; the regional and departmental directors of *affaires sanitaires et sociales*. For analysis of recent administrative changes, see Jean De Kervasdoué et Rémi Pellet, *Carnet de santé de la France 2006: Economie, droit et politiques de santé* (Paris: Dunod, 2006), 71–101.

35. Joël Moret-Bailly, L'accès à la justice disciplinaire (Paris: Mission de recherche droit et justice, 2002). See also Joël Moret-Bailly, L'organisation juridique des compétences des professionnels de la santé. In *Modalités et conditions d'évaluation des compétences professionnelles des métiers de la santé. Rapport au ministre de l'éducation et au ministre de la santé*, ed. Y Matillon (Paris: Ministre de la santé et des solidarités,

2003), 57–86; F. Perret-Richard, F. 2007. Les contentieux des juridictions disciplinaires des professions de santé. In *Vers un droit commun disciplinaire?* ed. Pascal Ancel and Joël Moret-Bailly, 261–74 (Saint-Etienne: Press Universitaire de France, Saint-Etienne, 2007).

36. There were six suspensions for one to three years; eight for six to nine months; twenty-three for three to four months; and sixteen for two to three months.

37. In 2000, the Order of Physicians decided twenty-three administrative appeals for public safety. It suspended ten physicians' licenses between four months and three years and dismissed thirteen complaints.

38. The text of the decisions was provided by the Order of Physicians. The most frequent category for discipline (ten physicians) was for medical incompetence/malpractice. Four physicians were sanctioned for having improper sexual relations with their patients. Five were disciplined for various financial crimes: two for social security billing fraud, two for financial misconduct with another physician, one for other fraud. Another eight were for various problems including not keeping medical records, charlatanism, violation of businesses regulation, using nonapproved tests, issuing a medical certificate in violation of the law, and violating medical confidentiality rules. Three were subject to discipline based on information that does not reveal the nature of the misconduct.

39. One of these physicians had his license suspended for a year; three had suspensions for four months, and four had suspensions for three months.

40. Hervé Maisonneuve, Les conflits d'intérêts en formation médicale continue. In *La formation médicale continue*, ed. P. Gallois (Paris: Flammarion Médecine Sciences, 1997), 88–92.

41. The 1953 law includes prohibition on receiving commissions or having other interests for prescribing (*intérêt ou ristournes*), Article 549; prohibition on fee splitting (*compérage*), L-365. Décret du 24 Septembre 1987. *Journal Officiel*, 30 janvier 1993. This became Article L-365–1 of the public health code, later recodified as Article L-4113–6.

42. This event has been reported to me by dozens of practicing physicians, health policy scholars, and personnel who work for Merck. I have found no written confirmation.

43. Jean-Yves Nau, Des prothèses en or: une importante escroquerie à la sécurité sociale révèle la gabegie pouvant exister dans le secteur des implants orthopédiques, *Le Monde*, 19 June 1994; Jean-Yves Nau, L'entrée en application de la loi "anticadeaux," *Le Monde*, 29 November 1994; Jean-Yves Nau, Justice: Les premières suites judiciaires de l'affaire des prothèses, *Le Monde*, 22 November 1994; *Le Canard Enchaîné*, 22 June 1994.

44. Anonymous interviews, 2000 and 2001.

45. Code of Public Health L-4113–6. Physicians convicted of violating the law face penalties including up to two years' imprisonment, €75,000 in fines, limits on the right to practice medicine for up to ten years, and additional criminal prosecution. See Jean Pierre Gribeauval, La répression des pots-de-vin dans les professions de

santé, *La Revue Prescrire* 13, no. 130 (1993): 333–36; Isabelle Lucas-Baloup, *Médecin/ Laboratoires: 30 questions sur les avantages en nature* (Paris: SCROF, 1993).

46. Christian Millau, Médecins, Étoiles et folies, *Gault & Millaut* (1993): May, 9.

47. Prise de position et premiers commentaires concernant l'article 47 DMOS du 27 Janvier 1993. Nouvel Article L. 365–1 du Code de la santé publique. Conseil National de l'Ordre des médecins, Conseil National de l'Ordre des pharmaciens, Syndicat National de l'industrie pharmaceutique. 21–04–1993. 21 March 1993.

48. "C'est bien parce que les médecins ne peuvent plus assumer les frais de participation aux congrès et aux manifestations scientifiques, qu'une sorte de partenariat, de mécénat s'est organisé entre médecins et industrie pharmaceutique." Interview in *Quotidien du Médecin*, 22 March 1993.

49. Directive 92/28/CCE, du 31 mars 1992, article 9. Concernant la publicité faite a l'égard des médicaments à usage humain. *Journal Officiel des Communautés Européennes*, 30 April.

50. The law was introduced under socialist prime minister Pierre Bérégovoy. On 29 March 1993, after the center-right won legislative elections, Edouard Balladur was appointed prime minister. Circulaire du 9 juillet 1993 relative à l'application de l'article L.365–1 de Code de la santé publique. *Journal Officiel*, 6 août 1993. 11051–11053.

51. Translation by the author.

52. My distinction is inspired by Charles Bosk's and Eliot Freidson's distinction between normal and abnormal errors: normal errors are technical errors that any physician can make; abnormal errors have a moral component that call the physician's character and judgment into question. Charles Bosk, *Forgive and remember: Managing medical failure* (Chicago: University of Chicago Press, 1979); Eliot Freidson, *Doctoring together: A study of professional social control* (Chicago: University of Chicago Press, 1984).

53. Mme Colette Nouvel-Rousselot, president of Laboratories Doms-Adrian, commented: "We are all accomplices in this affaire [medical gifts to doctors] including public authorities that cover up the actions of the pharmaceutical industry." Les cadeaux des labos: Le grand débat. *Le Généraliste*, 13 April 1993, 1422–46, at 1444.

54. Association loi de 1901. These associations play an important informal role in hospital finance. Some medical school research departments get private funding from industry and use part of these funds to subsidize the clinical work of physicians who perform both research and clinical care. Hospital administrators are reluctant to ask questions because they know that the funds sometimes bring direct benefits to the hospital.

55. Anonymous interview. AFSSAPS also turns a blind eye. It receives data from every pharmaceutical manufacturer listing the physicians involved in trials for each drug, yet it has never analyzed these data to see what it might reveal about payments to physicians to start patients on drugs.

56. Interview with Dr. Daniel Grunwald and Pierre Fernandez, November 2002.

57. Loi du 4 mars 2002, L. 4113–13. For other changes, see L. 4163–1; L. 4113–6; L. 4113–8; L. 4113–13; L. 4113–105

58. Décret n. 2007–454 du 25 mars 2007 relatif aux conventions et aux liens unissant les membres de certaines professions de santé aux entreprises et modifiant le code de la santé publique (dispositions réglementaires).

59. L. 4113–6 Code Santé Publique. R 4113–104. See also *Modalités d'application de l'article L 4113–6 du CSP après la parution du décret 2007–454 du 25 mars 2007.*

60. LEEM, Mise en œuvre de l'article L.4113–6 du CSP, 26, November, 2009.

61. Cinq ans d'observation et un constat: Rien à attendre de la visite médicale pour mieux soigner, *La Revue Prescrire* 26, no. 272 (2006): 383–89, at 384, note c; J. Bignall, Monitoring reps in France, *Lancet* 344 (1994): 536; La Directive Européenne 92/28 CEE 31 mars 1992. Loi N. 94–42 du 18 janvier 1994. R. 5122–11, Code de la santé publique; Décret no 96–531 du 14 juin 1996 relatif à la publicité pour les médicaments et certains produits à usage humain et modifiant le code de la santé publique; deuxième partie: Décrets en Conseil d'Etat, *Journal Officiel*, 16 June 1996, 8962–67.

62. Charte de la visite médicale, 22 Decembre 2004, Loi N. 2004–810 du 13 août 2004 relative à l'Assurance Maladie. *Journal Officiel*, 17 August 2004, 14598–626.

63. Cinq ans d'observation et un constat, 386.

64. J. Pascal, F. Riou, and J. Chaperon, Difficultés de mise en place et enjeux institutionnels de la formation continue des médecins libéraux, *Santé Publique* 12, no. 2 (2001):177–89. For 2005 participation statistics, see Yves Matillon, Dominique LeBoeuf, and Hervé Maisonneuve, Defining and assessing the competence of health care professionals in France, *Journal of Continuing Education in the Health Professions* 25, no. 4 (2005): 290–96, 96; Hervé Maisonneuve, Medical education and the physician workforce of France, *Journal of Continuing Education in the Health Professions* 25, no. 4 (2005): 289.

65. La loi 13 aout 2004 relatif à la reforme de 1'Assurance Maladie, Art. L. 4133–1–1. L.4133–2 du Code de la Santé Publique.

66. Loi no. 2009–879 du 21 juillet 2009 portant réforme de l'hôpital et relative aux patients, à la santé et aux territoires, *Journal Officiel* 22 July 2009, p. 12184, Article 59.

67. Christine d'Autume and Daniel Postel-Vinay, Mission relative à l'organisation juridique, administrative et financière de la formation continue des professions médicales et paramédicales. Paris: Inspection générale des affaires sociales, 2006. Rapport no. 2006–02. Available at http://www/ladocumentationfrancaise.fr.rapports-publics/0640001809/index.shtml (accessed 13 November 2009).

68. Ibid., 23–27.

69. Formation médicale continue organisée par un organisme agréé en partenariat avec des entreprises de santé. Code de Bonnes Pratiques.

CHAPTER 4

1. Hawaii requires employers to provide insurance to full-time employees.

2. Kaiser Family Foundation, State health facts online. (Accessed 7 December 2009, at http://www.statehealthfacts.org/)

3. The Patient Protection and Affordable Care Act, Public Law 111–148, 124 Stat. 119 (2010).

4. The four-stage categorization is my framework. For the classic history, see Paul Starr, *The social transformation of American medicine* (New York: Basic Books, 1982). For an alternative history, see Donald W. Light, Ironies of success: A new history of the American health care "system," *Journal of Health and Social Behavior* 45, extra issue (2004): 1–24. For distinctions between different kinds of markets, see Neil Fligstein, *The architecture of markets* (Princeton, NJ: Princeton University Press, 2001).

5. Frederick Evert Kredel and John Hampton Hoch, Early relation of pharmacy and medicine in the United States, *Journal of the American Pharmaceutical Association* 28, no. 10 (1939): 706.

6. John Morgan, *A discourse upon the institution of medical schools in America* (Baltimore, MD: Johns Hopkins University Press, 1937).

7. Richard Harrison Shryock, *Medical licensing in America, 1650–1965* (Baltimore, MD: Johns Hopkins University Press, 1967), 23. The states that repealed laws were Ohio (1826), Alabama (1831), Mississippi (1836), South Carolina, Maryland, and Vermont (1838), Georgia (1839), New York (1844), and Louisiana (1852).

8. Starr, *Social transformation of American medicine*, 42. Between 1875 and 1900, 114 medical schools were opened.

9. Even university medical schools typically divided tuition among faculty. Harvard medical school operated on this basis until the 1890s. Starr, *Social transformation of American medicine*, 114–16.

10. Henry E. Sigerist, *A history of medicine* (New York: Oxford University Press, 1951). By 1900, there were roughly 100 dispensaries; their numbers decreased as hospitals grew and public hospitals began providing the poor ambulatory care. Charles Rosenberg, Social class and medical care in nineteenth-century America: The rise and fall of dispensary, *Journal of the History of Medicine and the Allied Sciences* 29, no. 1 (1974): 32–54.

11. "Many a struggling young city physician is deprived of the opportunity of earning a living because patients, who are amply able to pay ordinary fees, stultify themselves by accepting hospital alms." Hospital and dispensary abuse, *JAMA* 48, no. 7 (1907): 613–15, reprinted *JAMA* 297, no. 6 (2007): 651.

12. National Medical Convention, 1847. Code of Medical Ethics. *Archives of the American Medical Association, Proceedings of the National Medical Conventions held in Philadelphia, 1846, and New York City, 1847*, 83–106. Chicago: AMA. Reprinted in *Ethics in medicine: Historical perspectives and contemporary concerns*, ed. Stanley J. Reiser, Arthur L. Dyck, and William J. Curran, 26–34 (Cambridge: MIT Press, 1977).

In 1873, the AMA established a Judicial Council to interpret the code and to decide appeals from members disciplined by local and state medical societies. Morris Fishbein, *A history of the American Medical Association: 1847 to 1947* (Philadelphia: W. B. Saunders Company, 1947), 949.

13. Code of Medical Ethics, 1847, Article 1, Section 4, Duties for the support of the professional character.

14. Perry H. Millard, The propriety and necessity of state regulation of medical practice, *JAMA* 9, no. 16 (1887): 491.

15. Lawrence M. Friedman, Freedom of contract and occupational licensing 1890–1910: A legal and social study, *California Law Review* 53, no. 1 (1965): 487–534. *Dent v. West Virginia*, 129 U.S.14 (1889).

16. Abraham Flexner, *Medical education in the United States and Canada* (New York: Carnegie Foundation for the Advancement of Teaching, 1910).

17. Abraham Flexner, Medical colleges: The duty of the state to suppress bad ones and to support good ones, *The World's Work* 21 (1911): 1440.

18. Arthur Dean Bevan, Cooperation in medical education and medical services: Functions of the medical profession, of the university and of the public, *JAMA* 90, no. 15 (1928): 1173–77.

19. Kenneth Wing, *The law and American health care* (New York: Aspen Law and Business, 1998), 8.

20. David Rosner, *A once charitable enterprise: Hospitals and health care in Brooklyn and New York, 1885–1915* (Cambridge: Cambridge University Press, 1982).

21. Wing, *Law and American health care*, 3.

22. Hospital service in the United States, *JAMA* 84, no. 14 (1925): 961–67.

23. 1928 Income Tax Unit Ruling 2421, I.T. 2421, VII-2 C.B. 150 (1928). As recently as 1969, the IRS denied tax-exempt status to a not-for-profit hospital controlled by its previous physician owners; IRS Revenue Ruling No 69–545 (1969).

24. AMA, Medical economics: Private group practice, *JAMA* 100, no. 21 (1933): 1693.

25. Rosemary Stevens, *In sickness and in wealth: American hospitals in the twentieth century* (New York: Basic Books, 1989), 140–70.

26. P. Maxwell Foshay, Medical ethics and medical journals, *JAMA* 1(1900), quoted in Fishbein, *History of the AMA*, 198.

27. AMA, Secret nostrums and the journal, *JAMA* 34, no. 22 (1900): 1420. Fishbein, *History of the AMA*, 198.

28. James G. Burrows, *Organized medicine in the Progressive era: The move toward monopoly* (Baltimore, MD: Johns Hopkins University Press, 1977), 49–51.

29. Fishbein, *History of the AMA*, 197–233 and 870–86. The AMA trustees noted, "We have reason to believe that if the AMA requests it, a semi-official recognition of

this Council will be made by the government." Harry F. Dowling, *Medicines for man: The development, regulation and use of prescription drugs* (New York: Alfred A. Knopf, 1970), 169.

30. The AMA Council on Pharmacy rules are in Fishbein, *History of the AMA*, 870–72. See also AMA Council on Pharmacy and Chemistry. Report of the council. *JAMA* 40 (1905): 265–266. AMA Council on Pharmacy and Chemistry. The secret nostrum vs. the ethical proprietary preparation, *JAMA* 40, no. 8 (1905): 718–19.

31. Peter Temin, *Taking your medicine: Drug regulation in the United States* (Cambridge, MA: Harvard University Press, 1980), 38.

32. Pure Food and Drug Act of 1906, U.S. Statutes at Large (59th Cong., Sess. I, Chap. 3915, pp 768–72).

33. Samuel Hopkins Adams, *The great American fraud* (New York: P. F. Collier and Son, 1905).

34. Sherley Amendment to Pure Food and Drug Act, 1912.

35. See Sheryl Calabro, Breaking the shield of the learned intermediary doctrine: Placing the blame where it belongs, *Cardozo Law Review* 25, no. 6 (2004): 2241–316.

36. William Osler, Chauvinism in medicine. In Osler, *Aequanimitas, with other addresses to medical students, nurses and practitioners of medicine*, 2d ed. (Philadelphia: Blakiston, 1906), 277–306. Osler added: "To modern pharmacy we owe much, . . . but the profession has no more insidious foe than the large borderland pharmaceutical houses. No longer an honored messmate, pharmacy in this form threatens to become a huge parasite, eating the vital body of the medical."

37. Starr, *Social transformation in American medicine*, 34. Manufacturers continued to use medical personnel to market infant formula. Judith Richter, *Global strategy for infant and young child feeding* (Geneva: International Baby Food Action Network, 2005).

38. George H. Simmons, The Abbott Alkaloidal Company—high finance and methods of working the medical profession. *JAMA* 50, no. 11 (1908): 897.

39. Simmons, Abbott Alkaloidal Company, 897, 895, 900.

40. Chauncey D. Leake, The pharmacologic evaluation of new drugs, *JAMA* 93, no. 21 (1909): 1632–34. See also Ernest E. Irons, The clinical evaluation of drugs, *JAMA* 93, no. 20 (1929): 1523–24; W. A. Puckner and Paul Nicholas Leech, The introduction of new drugs, *JAMA* 93, no. 21 (1929): 1627–30.

41. Harry F. Dowling, The American Medical Association's policy on drugs in recent decades. In *Safeguarding the public: Historical aspects of medicinal drug control*, ed. J. B. Blake (Baltimore, MD: Johns Hopkins University Press, 1970), 123–31.

42. C. Rufus Rorem and Robert P. Fischelis, *The costs of medicine*. Committee on the Cost of Medical Care, No. 14 (Chicago: University of Chicago Press, 1932), 231.

43. U.S. FDA, Promulgation of regulations under the Federal Food, Drug, and Cosmetic Act *Federal Register* 3, no. 251 (1938): 3168. U.S. Senate, 100th Congress.

Subcommittee on the Health of the House Committee on Energy and Commerce, *Physician dispensing of drugs: Hearings on H.R. 2093*, 1st Session, 22 April 1987, 15.

44. For more detailed discussion, see Marc A. Rodwin, *Medicine, money and morals: Physicians' conflicts of interest* (New York: Oxford University Press, 1993), 19–52.

45. AMA, *Proceedings of the House of Delegates* (hereafter, *AMA Proceedings*) (June 1913): 12–15, 24–25.

46. Frank G. Lydston, The surgical commission man and surgical canvassing, *Philadelphia Medical Journal* 4, no. 1 (1899): 837–40.

47. For 1912 survey, see *AMA Proceedings* (June 1913): 12–15; for 1914 survey, see *AMA Proceedings* (June 1915): 12.

48. For Wisconsin, Rosemary Stevens, *American medicine and the public interest* (New Haven, CT: Yale University Press, 1971), 84; for other state laws, Loyal Davis, *Fellowship of surgeons: A history of the American College of Surgeons* (Springfield, IL: Charles C. Thomas, 1960), 435.

49. For defenders of fee splitting, see C. L. Evans, Sic vos non vobis, *Journal of the Missouri State Medical Association* 8 (April 1912): 405–6. For critics, see Lydston, Surgical commission man and surgical canvassing, 181; John G. Bowman, General hospitals of 100 or more beds, *Bulletin of the American College of Surgeons* 4 (1919): 66–69.

50. AMA, Association News, *JAMA* 38, no. 25 (1902): 1661. AMA, House of Delegates, *Principles of medical ethics*, 1903. Available at http://www.ama-assn.org/ama1/pub/upload/mm/43/1903principlesofethi.pdf (accessed 10 November 2009). Chapter 2, Article I, Section 8 states that it is derogatory to professional character to accept rebates, patent surgical instruments, or patent medicines. Article VI, Section 4 condemns giving, soliciting, or receiving commissions.

51. Fishbein, *History of the AMA*, 277 (1912 report); *AMA Proceedings* (June 1915): 12 (1914 report).

52. Davis, *Fellowship of surgeons*, 481, 414.

53. Greer Williams, The Columbus five-year cure for fee-splitting, *Modern Hospital* 78, no. 6 (1952): 67–69, 94–95.

54. Milton I. Roemer and Jay W. Friedman, *Doctors in hospitals: Medical staff organizations and hospital performance* (Baltimore, MD: Johns Hopkins University Press, 1971), 5.

55. Horace M. Alleman, Lodge practice, *Pennsylvania Medical Journal* 15 (December 1911): 223, quoted in Burrows, *Organized medicine in the progressive era*, 127.

56. Report of the Board of Censors, *Transactions of the Medical Association of the State of Alabama* (1890), 75–79; AMA, Medical economics: Contract practice, *JAMA* 49, no. 24 (1907): 2028–29; Burrows, *Organized medicine in the Progressive era*, 128.

57. AMA, Medical economics: Private group practice, *JAMA* 100, no. 21 (1933): 1698.

58. Ibid. The AMA survey included single and multispecialty groups, practices that pooled income, and those in which physicians kept their fees. The average size was five to six physicians. Rufus C. Rorem, *Private group practice clinics* (Chicago: University of Chicago Press, 1931), counted over 150 multispecialty groups in which physicians shared income, with the average having eleven physicians.

59. Helen Clapesattle, *The Doctors Mayo* (Minneapolis: University of Minnesota Press, 1941). Rorem, *Private group practice clinics*, 115–18.

60. Helen L. Johnston, *Rural health cooperatives*, Public Health Bulletin No. 308 (Washington, DC: Cooperative Research and Service Division, Farm Credit Administration, and Division of Medical and Hospital Resources, Public Health Service, 1951); Herman Miles Somers and Anne Ramsay Somers, *Doctors, patients, and health insurance* (Washington, DC: Brookings Institution, 1961), 348–49. There were over 100 rural health cooperatives, but the number fell to 54 by 1949 and continued to decline.

61. Committee on Cost of Medical Care, Medical care for the American people: Final report, 1932. Reprinted in U.S. Department of Health, Education, and Welfare, Public Health Service, Health Services and Mental Health Administration, Community Health Services (Washington, DC: Government Printing Office, 1970), 175–76.

62. AMA House of Delegates, Sickness insurance problems in the United States, *JAMA* 102, no. 26 (1934): 2200–2201.

63. For the French Medical Charter, see chapter 2, "Organized Medicine's Charter," pages 40–42. The AMA summarized the International Association of Physicians insurance principles: "The Medical services must remain autonomous as to all questions concerning the practice of Medicine." Insurance should be "applied only to those persons who are incapable of meeting the necessary cost of medical care in case of sickness from their own resources." The insurance should always share in the cost of medical care and drugs. There should be complete free choice of physician permitting all licenses who accept insurance regulations to share in the care of the sick. "Professional secrecy should be maintained." There should be no restriction of the right to prescribe although the medical organizations should always "seek to suppress all expensive and superfluous medication." Payments should not be by a fixed sum per person or by salary. AMA, Bureau of Economics, The insurance principle in the practice of medicine, *JAMA* 102, no. 19 (1934): 1616–17; Morris Fischbein, *Sickness insurance and sickness costs* (Chicago: AMA, 1934); AMA, Bureau of Medical Economics, *A critical analysis of sickness insurance* (AMA: Chicago, 1934).

64. The AMA presented these principles in this order: (1) Medical practice should be controlled by the medical profession. (2) No third party should come between the patient and physician. (3) Patients should have free choice of physicians. (4) The relationship between physician and patient is confidential. (5) All medical services should be under medical profession control. (6) Patients should pay physicians directly at the time of service. (7) Medical services should have no connection with cash benefits. (8) Insurance and medical benefits should allow all qualified physicians in the locality to participate. (9) Assistance should be limited to those below the

comfort level. (10) There should be no restrictions on treatment or prescribing not formulated by organized medicine.

65. See, e.g., *Weyrens v. Scotts Bluff County Med. Society*, 277 N.W. 378 (1938); Joseph Laufer, Ethical and legal restrictions on contract and corporate practice of medicine, *Law and Contemporary Problems* 6, no. 4 (1939): 517.

66. These decisions do not cite the AMA code. Although a few courts discussed corporate practice of medicine before the AMA's statements in 1932, 1933, and 1934, they all presented unusual situations. By 1932 the AMA had already opposed contract practice, and state medical societies had opposed employment of physicians. Some courts also held that public policy precluded corporations from employing physicians and drew on laws that prohibited corporations from employing lawyers to sell legal services to the public. A few state licensing laws prohibited corporations from employing physicians, but most of these were added through amendments after the AMA articulated its ethical stance. See Jerome L. Schwartz, Early history of prepaid medical care plans, *Bulletin of the History of Medicine* 39, no. 5 (1965): 450–75.

67. Albert W. Snoke, The future role of hospitals in medical care, *American Journal of Public Health* 48, no. 4 (1958): 468–72.

68. Mark A. Hall, Institutional control of physician behavior: Legal barriers to health care cost containment. *University of Pennsylvania Law Review* 137, no. 2 (1988): 431–536; Jeffrey F. Chase-Lubitz, The corporate practice of medicine doctrine: An anachronism in the modern health care industry, *Vanderbilt Law Review* 40, no. 2 (1987): 445–88.

69. *AMA v. United States*, 130 F. 2d 233 (D.C. Cir. 1942).

70. *Group Health Cooperative of Puget Sound v. King County Medical Society*, 29 Wash. 2d. 586, 237 P. 2nd 727 (1951).

71. *Washington Post*, 21 December 1938, quoted in Starr, *Social transformation of American medicine*, 305.

72. Horace R. Hansen, Group health plans: A twenty-year legal review. *Minnesota Law Review* 42, no. 4 (1958): 527–48.

73. Starr, *Social transformation of American medicine*, 331.

74. Robert Cunningham III and Robert Cunningham, Jr., *The Blues: A history of the Blue Cross and Blue Shield system* (DeKalb: Northern Illinois University Press. 1998).

75. Wing, *Law and American health care*, 8, 20.

76. Commission on Financing Hospital Care, Prepayment and community. In *Financing of hospital care in the United States*, vol. 2, ed. Harry Becker (New York: Blakiston, 1955), 11.

77. Odin W. Anderson, Patricia Collette, and Jacob J. Feldman, *Changes in family medical expenditures and voluntary health insurance: A five-year resurvey* (Cambridge, MA: Harvard University Press, 1963), 8–9.

78. AMA, Organization section. *JAMA* 119, no. 9 (1942): 727–28.

79. Leon Applebaum, The development of voluntary health insurance in the United States, *Journal of Risk and Insurance* 28, no. 3 (1961): 25–33; Special Ruling, 1943 T.C.M. (PH) P 66, 294 (Aug. 26, 1943); Special Ruling, 3 Stand. Federal Tax Reporter. (CCH) P 6587 (Oct. 26, 1943); 26 U.S.C. 106. Tax deductibility was extended to all employer-purchased medical insurance in 1954.

80. *Inland Steel v. National Labor Relations Board*, 170 F_2d_247 (7th Cir, 1948).

81. Rashi Fein, *Medical care, medical cost: The search for a national health insurance policy* (Cambridge, MA: Harvard University Press, 1986), 21.

CHAPTER 5

1. Peter Temin, *Taking your medicine: Drug regulation in the United States* (Cambridge, MA: Harvard University Press, 1980), 86.

2. AMA, *Proceedings of the House of Delegates* (hereafter *AMA Proceedings*) (December 1952): 97. Paul R. Hawley, American College of Surgeons restates principles of financial relations, *Bulletin of the American College of Surgeons* 37, no. 3 (1952): 233.

3. *AMA Proceedings* (June 1949): 39, Section 6; AMA, The trend in dispensing and prescribing, *Modern medicine topics, modern medicine medical market guide* 11 (November 1950): 1; *AMA Proceedings* (December 1953): 58; *AMA Proceedings* (June 1955): 52; Ownership of pharmacies, *AMA Proceedings* (December 1–4, 1959): 135–36.

4. U.S. Senate Subcommittee on Antitrust and Monopoly, Committee on the Judiciary, 1965, *Physician ownership in pharmacies and drug companies* 2nd Session August 4, 5, 6, 11, 12, and 14, Opening Statement of Senator Philip A. Hart, 1.

5. Dean Frye, Carrtone Labs, in which several thousand of MDs hold stock, had $237,297 loss on $340,421 sales; hope for comeback under new management, *Food-Drug-Cosmetic Reports* 25, no. 35 (1963): 8.

6. U.S. Senate Subcommittee on Antitrust and Monopoly, 1965, Testimony of George Woodhouse, 110.

7. U.S. Senate Subcommittee on Antitrust and Monopoly, Committee on Judiciary, 1967, *The medical restraint of trade act*. 1st Session (24, 25, 26, 30, and 31 January, 1, 6, 7, 9, and 23 February), 1.

8. George Hoffer, Physician-ownership in pharmacies and drug repackagers (Ph.D. diss., University of Virginia, 1972); George E. Hoffer, Physician-ownership in pharmacies and drug repackagers. *Inquiry* 12, no. 1 (1974): 26–36.

9. U.S. Department of Health and Human Services (DHHS), Office of the Inspector General, *Physician drug dispensing: An overview of state regulation* (Washington, DC: DHHS, 1988).

10. "Massachusetts, Montana, Texas, and Utah disallow physician dispensing except in emergencies, when pharmacy services are unavailable, or when the physician

is providing for the patient's immediate needs. Arizona either disallows physician dispensing altogether or allows it only in emergencies." U.S. DHHS, OIG, *Physician Drug Dispensing.*

11. *AMA Proceedings* (November–December 1948): 61, 71. Loyal Davis, *Fellowship of surgeons: A history of the American College of Surgeons* (Springfield, IL: Charles C. Thomas, 1960), 435.

12. Too much unnecessary surgery: Interview with Dr. Paul Hawley, *U.S. News and World Report,* 20 February 1953, 48–55; Resolution on Dr. Paul R. Hawley, resolution of Robert B. Homa, Jr., and resolution on public relations, *AMA Proceedings* (June 1–5, 1963): 36, 43, 34; Davis, *Fellowship of Surgeons,* 424–28.

13. *AMA Proceedings* (June 1954): 29–31.

14. *AMA Proceedings* (November 27–29, 1961): 201–3.

15. Frank G. Lydston, The surgical commission man and surgical canvassing, *Philadelphia Medical Journal* 4, no. 1 (1899): 837–40; W. L. Downing and Paul R. Hawley, Two physicians speak their minds on fee-splitting, *Bulletin of the American College of Surgeons* 37, no. 4 (1952): 393.

16. James C. McCann, Consideration of deduction and allocation of surgical fees by Blue Shield plans, *JAMA* 166, no. 6 (1958): 624–28; ACS, Position of American College of Surgeons on proration of insurance payments, *Bulletin of the American College of Surgeons* 44, no. 1 (1959): 5–8; John G. Bowman, General hospitals of 100 or more beds, *Bulletin of the American College of Surgeons* 5, no. 1 (1919): 6.

17. Greer Williams, The Columbus five-year cure for fee-splitting, *Modern Hospital* 78, no. 6 (1952): 67–69, 94–95.

18. Bernard D. Hirsh, *History of the Judicial Council of the American Medical Association* (Chicago: AMA, 1984), 110, citing the November 1965 meeting at Philadelphia; Physician ownership of expensive equipment, *AMA Proceedings* (19–23 June 1977): 176.

19. Senate investigations found that pharmaceutical industry net profits after taxes from 1958–1959 were 21 percent, U.S. Senate Subcommittee on Antitrust and Monopoly, 1965, 278. Peter Temin analyzed the data from the FTC, Securities Exchange Commission, and other studies and concluded that profits after taxes were between 17 percent and 19 percent from 1948 through 1973, Temin, *Taking your medicine,* 80–82. For spending on marketing, see U.S. Senate Subcommittee on Antitrust and Monopoly, 1961. *Administered prices drugs,* 1st Session, Washington, DC: U.S. GPO, 158.

20. Temin, *Taking your medicine,* 84–85.

21. Elihu Katz and George Menzel, Social relations and innovation in the medical profession: The epidemiology of a new drug, *Public Opinion Quarterly* 19, no. 4 (1955): 337–72; Norman G. Hawkins, The detailman and preference behavior, *Southwestern Social Science Quarterly* 40 (1959): 213–24; Robert R. Rehder, communication and opinion formation in a medical community: The significance of the detail man, *Journal of the Academy of Management* 8, no. 4 (1965): 282–91.

22. Temin, *Taking your medicine*, 115–16, 88–119.

23. U.S. Federal Trade Commission, *Economic report on antibiotics manufacturers* (Washington, DC: GPO, 1958), 128; Robert Ferber and Hugh G. Wales, The effectiveness of pharmaceutical promotion, *University of Illinois Bureau of Economic and Business Research Bulletin* No. 83 (Urbana: University of Illinois Press, 1958).

24. Jeremy A. Greene, Pharmaceutical marketing research and the prescribing physician, *Annals of Internal Medicine* 146, no. 10 (2007): 742–47.

25. Richard Steinbrook, For sale: Physicians' prescribing data, *NEJM* 354, no. 26 (2006): 2745–47.

26. Morris Fishbein, *A history of the American Medical Association: 1847 to 1947* (Philadelphia: W. B. Saunders, 1947), 872.

27. AMA, Council on Pharmacy and Chemistry, New program of operation for evaluation of drugs, *JAMA* 158, no. 13 (1955): 1171; Harry F. Dowling, *Medicines for man: The development, regulation and use of prescription drugs* (New York: Alfred A. Knopf, 1970), 164.

28. U.S. Senate Subcommittee on Antitrust and Monopoly, 1961–1962, *Drug industry antitrust act (S. 1551)*, 1st and 2nd Sessions, part 2, 1010. The hearings are recounted in Richard Harris, *The real voice* (New York: Macmillan, 1964). Previously, the AMA held that "the average physician has neither the time nor facilities to experiment with new drugs in order to determine their proper indications for use," Report of the Board of Trustees, *AMA Proceedings* (8–12 June 1942): 12.

29. The FDA regulations stated that "adequate and well controlled investigations" would constitute the "substantial evidence" necessary for drug approval, U.S. Food and Drug Administration, Hearing and regulations describing scientific content of adequate and well-controlled clinical investigations, *Federal Register* 35, no. 90 (1970): 7250.

30. Dowling, *Medicines for man*, 171.

31. For 1959 data, U.S. Senate, 1965, *Physician ownership in pharmacies*, 272, citing *JAMA* (29 April 1961): 310. For 1968 data, Milton Silverman and Philip R. Lee, *Pills, profits and politics* (Berkeley: University of California Press, 1974), 68.

32. Ben Gaffin, Report on a study of advertising and the American physician, part 1. Based on Ben Gaffin and Associates, *Fond du Lac study: An intensive study of the marketing of five new ethical pharmaceutical products in a single market, resulting in some theory of scientific marketing and service programs for action* (Chicago: AMA, 1956), reprinted in U.S. Senate Subcommittee on Antitrust and Monopoly, 1961–1962, *Drug industry antitrust act*, pt. 1, 490–529. The Gaffin report and AMA changes are summarized in Temin, *Taking your medicine*, 86–87.

33. U.S. Senate, Select Committee on Small Business, Subcommittee on Monopoly, 1968, *Present status of competition in the pharmaceutical industry* (Washington, DC: GPO, 1968), Testimony of Edward Pinkney, 14:5727.

34. Gaffin and Associates, Recommendations to the AMA, 3, reprinted in U.S. Senate Hearings 1961–1962, pt. 2, 524.

35. Scott H. Podolsky and Jeremy A. Greene, A historical perspective of pharmaceutical promotion and physician education, *JAMA* 300, no. 9 (2008): 1071–73, 832.

36. Ibid., 527; John G. Searle, L. D. Barney, Francis Boyer, et al., The pharmaceutical industry, *Journal of Medical Education* 36, no. 1 (1961): 24–25.

37. Gaffin and Associates, Recommendations to the AMA, 2, reprinted in U.S. Senate Hearings 1961–1962, 526.

38. Temin, *Taking your medicine*, 79 citing U.S. Senate Hearings 1961–1962, 749.

39. Gaffin Report, Part I, The advertisers' viewpoint, 3, reprinted in U.S. Senate Hearings 1961–1962, Exhibit 6, 492. Searle, Barney, Boyer, et al., Pharmaceutical industry.

40. Gaffin Report, reprinted in U.S. Senate Hearings 1961–1962, 505.

41. For Warner statement, U.S. Senate, Subcommittee on Antitrust and Monopoly, *Study of Administered Prices in the Drug Industry*, Report No. 448 (Washington, DC: GPO, 1961), Testimony of Charles May, 189, citing Tobias Warner, *Ethical pharmaceutical promotion: The workings and philosophies of the pharmaceuticals industry* (New York: National Pharmaceutical Council, Inc., 1959). For Smith statement, U.S. Senate Subcommittee on Antitrust and Monopoly, *Study of Administered Prices*, 210.

42. Searle, Barney, Boyer, et al., Pharmaceutical industry, 25.

43. Charles D. May, Selling drugs by educating physicians, *Journal of Medical Education* 36 (January 1961): 1; U.S. Senate Hearings, 1961–1962, Testimony of Dr. Charles D. May, 190, 177.

44. Ibid.

45. U.S. Senate Hearings, 1960, vol. 18, 10, 338, Testimony of William B. Bean.

46. U.S. Senate Hearings, 1961, 182. Other testimony revealed a practice called "seeding drugs," whereby drug companies initiated post-marketing trials at medical centers to get their new drug used, rather than conducting any significant research. Testimony of Dr. Frederick Meyers, professor of pharmacology at the University of California, 176–77.

47. Bernard D. Hirsh, statement before U.S. Senate, Committee on Ways and Means, 26 February 1969, quoted in Silverman and Lee, *Pills, profits and politics*, 53–54. At the time, tax-exempt organizations could obtain tax exemptions for commercial ventures related to their tax purpose.

48. Edwin Funk, Yesterday, today and tomorrow in drug advertising, *Drug Advertising, Pharmaceutical Marketing and Media* 2 (March 1968): 13–16; Pierre R. Garai, Advertising and promotion of drugs, in *Drugs in our society*, ed. Peter Talalay (Baltimore, MD: Johns Hopkins University Press, 1964), 195.

49. *Washington Post*, 7 December 1965, 12; *Washington Post*, 20 March 1969, 24.

50. Elmer Sevringhaus, Interdependence of the medical profession and the pharmaceutical industry, *JAMA* 152, no. 16 (1953): 1525.

51. U.S. Department of Health, Education, and Welfare (DHEW), Office of the Secretary, Task Force on Prescription Drugs, *The drug makers and the drug distributors* (Washington, DC: GPO, 1968), 6.

52. U.S. Senate, Committee on Small Business, Subcommittee on Monopoly, *Present status of competition* (Washington, DC: GPO, 1969), Testimony of James M. Faulkner, vol. 10, 4056; U.S. Senate, Committee on Small Business, Subcommittee on Monopoly, *Effect of promotion and advertising of over-the-counter drugs on competition, small business, and the health and welfare of the public* (Washington, DC: GPO, 1971), Testimony of Robert Seidenberg, vol. 2, 541.

53. Donald T. Rucker, Economic problems in drug distribution, *Inquiry* 9, no. 3 (1972): 43; U.S. DHEW, Office of the Secretary, *The drug makers and the drug distributors.*

54. Kenneth M. Ludmerer, *Time to heal: American medical education from the turn of the century to the era of managed care* (New York: Oxford University Press, 1999), 115–16. Industry leaders estimated that pharma then contributed over $15 million a year to medical education; Searle, Barney, Boyer, et al., Pharmaceutical industry.

55. Donald W. Petit, The physician recognition award, *JAMA* 213 no. 10 (1970): 1668–70; Norman S. Stearns, Marjorie E. Getchell, and Robert A. Gold, *Continuing medical education in community hospitals: A manual for program development* (Boston: Massachusetts Medical Society, 1971), 2. Jerome Kassirer, M.D., provided me extensive information on the history of continuing medical education.

56. Jose M. Ferrer, How are the costs of continuing medical education to be defrayed? *Bulletin of the New York Academy of Medicine* 51 (1975): 785–88.

57. Gaylord Nelson, U.S. Senate, Committee on Small Business, Subcommittee on Monopoly, *Present status of competition*, 13913–14.

58. Richard Crout, U.S. Senate, Committee on Small Business, Subcommittee on Monopoly, *Present status of competition*, 13919.

59. Jeremy A. Greene and Scott H. Podolsky, Keeping modern in medicine: Pharmaceutical promotion and physician education in postwar America, *Bulletin of the History of Medicine* 83, no. 2 (2009): 331–77, at 335.

60. Louis S. Reed, Private health insurance: Coverage and financial experience, 1940–66, *Social Security Bulletin* 30 (November 1967): 3–22.

61. David J. Rothman, A century of failure: Health care reform in America, *Journal of Health Politics, Policy and Law* 18, no. 2 (1993): 271–86.

62. Robert A. Caro, *Master of the senate: The years of Lyndon Johnson* (New York: Vintage Books, 1983). Theodore R. Marmor, *The politics of Medicare*, 2d ed. (Hawthorne: Aldine de Gruyter, 2000).

63. Harold B. Meyers, The medical industrial complex, *Fortune* 81 (January 1970): 1; Barbara Ehrenreich and Jon Ehrenreich, *The American health empire* (New York: Random House, 1970), 963–70; Bruce Steinwald and Duncan Neuhaurser, The role of the proprietary hospital, *Law and Contemporary Problems* 35, no. 4 (1970): 824.

64. Gordon K. MacLeod and M. Roy Schwartz, Faculty practice plans: Profile and critique, *JAMA* 256, no. 1 (1986):58–62. For teaching tracks, see Ludmerer, *Time to heal*, 328–29.

65. See Eli Ginzberg, ed. *Health service research: Key to health policy* (Cambridge, MA: Harvard University Press, 1991).

66. 42 United States Code Section 1320a-7a; David Hyman and Joel V. Williamson, Fraud and abuse: Regulatory alternatives in a competitive health care era, *Loyola University of Chicago Law Journal* 19, no. 4 (1988): 1131–96.

67. Bradford H. Gray and Marilyn J. Fields, eds., *Controlling costs and changing patient care: The role of utilization management* (Washington, DC: National Academy Press, 1989); Sharon McIllrath, AMA take on role as mediator between PROs and super-PRO, *American Medical News* 33, no. 44 (1990): 23.

68. P.L. 92–603 (1972); John McDonough, Tracking the demise of state hospital rate-setting, *Health Affairs* 16, no. 1 (1977): 142–49.

69. Milton I. Roemer and Max Shain, *Hospital utilization under insurance* (Ithaca, NY: Cornell University School of Business and Public Administration, 1959).

70. Victor G. Rodwin, *The health planning predicament: France, Québec, England, and the United States* (Berkeley: University of California Press, 1984); James A. Morone, *The democratic wish: Popular participation and the limits of the American government* (New York: Basic Books, 1990), 253–321.

71. Harold S. Luft, *Health maintenance organizations: Dimensions of performance* (New Brunswick, NJ: Transaction Books, 1987).

72. 42 U.S.C. Section 300e-10(a); Lawrence D. Brown, *Politics and health care organization: HMOs as federal policy* (Washington, DC: Brookings Institution, 1983).

73. Paul Starr, *The social transformation of American medicine* (New York: Basic Books, 1982), 415.

74. James C. Robinson, Theory and practice in the design of physician payment incentives, *Milbank Quarterly* 79, no. 2 (2002): 149–77.

75. Allan L. Hillman, W. Pete Welch, and Mark V. Pauly, Contractual arrangements between HMOs and primary care physicians: Three-tiered HMOs and risk pools, *Medical Care* 30, no. 2 (1992): 136–48.

76. Marc A. Rodwin, *Medicine, money, and morals: Physicians and conflicts of interest* (New York: Oxford University Press, 1993), 97–134.

77. *United States v. Oregon State Medical Society*, 343 U.S. 326 (1952); *Goldfarb v. Virginia State Bar*, 421 U.S. 773 (1975).

78. William M. Sage, David A. Hyman, and Warren Greenberg, Why competition law matters to health care quality, *Health Affairs* 22, no. 2 (2003): 31–43.

79. Carl F. Ameringer, *The health care revolution: From medical monopoly to market competition* (Berkeley: University of California Press, 2008); *In re American Medical*

Ass'n, 94 F.T.C., 701, (1979). For the FTC order, see [1979–1983 Transfer Binder] Trade Reg. Rep. (CCH) p. 21,955 at 22, 418–19.

80. *Michigan Optometric Association*, 106 F.T.C. 342 (1985); *American Academy of Ophthalmologists*, 108 F.T.C. 25 (1986); *FTC v. Indiana Federation of Dentists*, 476 U.S. 447 (1986); *Iowa Chapter of the American Physical Therapy Association*, No. 3242 (1988) (Consent Order); *Wilk v. AMA*, 895 F. 2d 352 (7th Cir. 1990).

81. *College of Physician-Surgeons of Puerto Rico*, Civ. No. 24–66-HL (D. Puerto Rico) (2 October 1997); *Arizona v. Maricopa County Medical Society*, 457 U.S. 332 (1982); Clayton Act, Section 6, 20, Norris LaGuardia Act, Section 4; National Labor Relations Act, Section 2 (3).

82. Donald H. Smith, Wishful thinking about unions, *Physician News Digest*, available at www.physiciansnews.com/discussion/smith.html (accessed 4 September 2007); Robert Carlson, Is there a physician union in your future? *Family Practice Management* 6, no. 1 (1999): 21–25.

CHAPTER 6

1. Thomas Rice, *The economics of health reconsidered*, 2nd ed. (Chicago: Health Administration Press, 2003); Stuart H. Altman and Marc A Rodwin, Halfway competitive markets and ineffective regulation: The American health care system, *Journal of Health Politics, Policy and Law* 13, no. 2 (1988): 323–39.

2. Arnold S. Relman, The new medical-industrial complex, *NEJM* 303, no. 17 (1980): 963–70; Arnold S. Relman, Dealing with conflicts of interest, *NEJM* 310, no. 18 (1984): 1182–83.

3. When borrowing money, firms pay interest instead of a share of all future profits. They can control the timing of their repayment to affect their interest payments, cash flow, and profit or loss, thereby reducing taxes.

4. Marc A. Rodwin, *Medicine, money and morals: Physicians' conflicts of interest* (New York: Oxford University Press, 1993).

5. *Walter Ford v. William Cabot*. Superior Court of Fulton County, Georgia. CA No. D-344. July 14, 1983. First Amendment to Complaint, and Exhibit A.

6. For a review of these studies, see Rodwin, *Medicine, money and morals*, 16–17, 67–79, 100–102.

7. Richard P. Kusserow, *Financial arrangements between physician and health care businesses: Report to Congress* (Washington, DC: OIG, DHHS, 1989); Jean M. Mitchell and Elton Scott, Evidence of complex structure of physician joint ventures, *Yale Journal on Regulation* 9, no. 2 (1992): 489–520; Jean M. Mitchell and Jonathan H. Sunshine, Consequences of physicians' ownership of health care facilities: Joint ventures in radiation therapy, *NEJM* 327, no. 21 (1992): 1497–501.

8. Author's analysis based on SEC, 10K Filing, filed on 8/27/97 Exhibit 21. Sometimes physicians invested as individuals, and at other times through physician-owned partnerships.

9. Margaret Jean Hall and Linda Lawrence, *Ambulatory surgery in the United States* (Vital and Health Statistics, National Center for Health Statistics, American Hospital Association, 1996); American Hospital Association, Trend watch chart book, 2009. Organization trends. Chart 2.6 Number of outpatient surgery centers, 2003–2008, available at http://www.aha.org/aha/trendwatch/chartbook/2009/chart 2–6.pdf (accessed 21 November 2009); Ambulatory surgery centers: A positive trend in health care, available at http://www.ascassociation.org/advocacy/Ambulatory SurgeryCentersPositive TrendHealthCare.pdf (accessed 13 November 2009).

10. *Specialty hospitals: Information on national market share, physician ownership and patients served* (Washington, DC: GAO, 2003); American Hospital Association, Trend watch: Physician ownership and self-referrals in hospitals, 2008, available at www. aha.org/aha/trendwatch/2008/twapr2008selfreferral.pdf (accessed 13 November 2009); Jean M. Mitchell, Utilization changes following market entry by physician owned specialty hospitals, *Medical Care Research and Review* 64, no. 4 (2007): 395–415.

11. AMA, Report of the Council on Ethical and Judicial Affairs, Report A (I-86): Conflicts of interest (1986); AMA, House of Delegates, Physicians' involvement in commercial ventures: Status report, *Proceedings* (December 1989): 131–32.

12. U.S. House of Representatives, Subcommittee on Health and the Environment, Committee on Energy and Commerce, *Medicare and Medicaid initiatives hearings*, 1st Session, 8 June 1989, Testimony of James Todd, 392; OBRA Act of 1989, P.L. 101–239, Title 6, § 620–4 Adding § 1877 to Title 18 of the Social Security Act.

13. AMA, Report of the CEJA, Report C (I-91), Conflicts of interest: Physician ownership of medical facilities.

14. AMA, House of Delegates, *Proceedings* (June 1992): 344; AMA, House of Delegates, *Proceedings* (December 1989): 108–11. Substitute resolution 4, adopted by the AMA House of Delegates, 8 December 1992.

15. U.S. House of Representatives, Committee on Ways and Means, Subcommittee on Health, *Physician ownership and referral arrangements*, 1st Session, vol. 2, 20 April 1993, testimony of Nancy Dicey, 200. I also testified at those hearings. The expanded law is OBRA, 1993, P.L. No. 103–66, § 13,500–664, codified as 42 U.S.C.A, 1395nn. Stark's 1989 bill would have banned physician self-referral to hospitals. However, the 1991 bill allowed self-referral to physician-owned hospitals. Representative James Pickle (D-TX) was on the committee with jurisdiction over the legislation, and his district was the home of a hospital chain that sought physician investors.

16. U.S. House of Representatives, Hearing before the Committee on Energy and Commerce, Subcommittee on Health and the Environment. 1987. *Physician dispensing of drugs: Hearings on H.R. 2093*, 1st Session, 22 April 1987, 1, quoting from Doctors shouldn't be pharmacists, *New York Times*, 28 March 1987.

17. U.S. House of Representatives, Committee on Energy and Commerce, *Physician dispensing of drugs*, Testimony of Nancy Dicey, 12, 15.

18. Carol Ukens, Long Island, R.I.'s picket physician-owned pharmacies, *Drug Topics* 136, no. 19 (1992): 110, 112; Richard L. Reece, Will dispensing make a comeback? *MD*

Options 2002, available at http://www.mdoptions.com/cgi-bin/article.cgi?article_id=1098 (accessed 10 January 2007).

19. Reed Ableson, Drug sales bring huge profits, and scrutiny, to cancer doctors, *New York Times*, 26 January 2003, 1; Alex Berenson and Andrew Pollack, Doctors reaping millions for use of anemia drugs, *New York Times*, 9 May 2007, 1.

20. Richard P. Kusserow, *Ensuring appropriate use of laboratory services: A monograph* (Washington, DC: OIG-DHHS, 1990).

21. Walt Bogdanich, Lax laboratories: The pap test misses much cervical cancer through labs' errors, *Wall Street Journal*, 2 November 1987, 1; U.S. House of Representatives, Committee on Energy and Commerce, Subcommittee on Oversight and Investigations, *Kickbacks in clinical laboratories*, 2nd Session, 5 March 1982 (Washington, DC: GPO, 1982). Laboratories were first regulated by the Clinical Laboratory Improvement Act of 1967, P.L. 90–174 (December 5, 1967) and later applied to doctors' offices by the Clinical Laboratory Improvement amendments of 1988, P.L. 100–578, codified as amended at 42 U.S.C § 263a (2006); Connie Laubenthal, Physician Office Laboratory (POL) adviser, Part 1, Physician office laboratories, history of government regulation on medical laboratories, *Medical Laboratory Observer* (November 1996), available at http://findarticles.com/p/articles/mi_m3230/is_n11_v28/ai_18899710/ (accessed 13 November 2009).

22. Dianne Miller Wolman, Andrea L Kalfoglou, and Lauren LeRoy, *Medicare laboratory payment policy: Now and in the future* (Washington, DC: National Academy Press, 2000), Table 2, at 5; John T. Benjamin, Effect of CLIA '88 and managed care on the medical lab market, *Medical Laboratory Observer* (November 1996), available at http://findarticles.com/p/articles/mi_m3230/is_n11_v28/ai/188999710 (accessed 13 November 2009).

23. Penny L. Havlicek, Ann Eiler, and Ondria T. Neblett, *Medical groups in the United States: A survey of practice characteristics* (Chicago: AMA, 1993); John D. Wassenaar and Sara L. Thran, *Physician socioeconomic statistics 2003* (Chicago: AMA, 2003). In addition, in 2001, 9 percent of employed physicians worked in group practices. David M. Frankford, Creating and dividing the fruits of collective economic activity: Referrals among health care providers, *Columbia Law Review* 89, no. 8 (1989): 1861–938.

24. Hospital corporation agrees to sell Los Angeles property to its physicians. *Hospital Business Week*, 10 October 2004.

25. Wassenaar and Thran, *Physician socioeconomic statistics 2003*.

26. Kenneth M. Ludmerer, *Time to heal: American medical education from the turn of the century to the era of managed care* (New York: Oxford University Press, 1999), 327–29.

27. Atul Gawande, The cost conundrum, *New Yorker*, 1 June 2009, 36–44.

28. American Hospital Association, *Hospital statistics 1980* (Chicago: American Hospital Association, 1981); Montague Brown, Michael Warner, Paul R. Luehrs, et al., Trends in multi-hospital systems: A multiyear comparison, *Health Care Management Review* 5, no. 4 (1980): 9–22; Kaiser State Health Facts, Hospitals by ownership

type, available at http://www.statehealthfacts.org/comparebar.jsp?ind=383&cat=8 (accessed 1 November 2010).

29. Health Care Advisory Board, *Physician bonding*, vol. 2, *Perfecting the physician network* (Advisory Board Company, 1989), Tactic #8, redoubled recruitment, conclusion #111, 138.

30. Robin Locke Nagele and Elizabeth B. Bradley, Physician-owned specialty hospital and hospital conflict-of-interest policies: Healthy competition or business opportunism? In A. G. Gosfield, *Health law handbook 2006* (St. Paul, MN: Thompson/West 2006), 691–725.

31. Health Care Advisory Board, *Physician bonding*, Tactic #3, massive contract management, 63.

32. Medicare program: Physicians' referrals to health care entities with which they have financial relationships: Exceptions for certain electronic prescribing and electronic health records arrangements, *Federal Register* 71, no.152 (8 August 2006): 45140–71.

33. John Blum, Evaluation of medical staff using fiscal factors: Economic credentialing, *Journal of Health and Hospital Law* 26, no. 3 (1993): 65–72, 82.

34. Paul Starr, *The Social transformation of American medicine* (New York: Basic Books, 1982) 436.

35. 42 USC 1395dd.

36. Lucette Lagnado, Twenty years and still paying, *Wall Street Journal*, 13 March 2003, A1; Lucette Lagnado, Medical seizures: Hospitals try extreme measures to collect their overdue debts, *Wall Street Journal*, 30 October 2003, A1; David U. Himmelstein, Elizabeth Warren, Deborah Thorne, and Steffie Woolhander, Illness and injury as contributors to bankruptcy, *Health Affairs*, W5 (2005): 63–73.

37. *Utah County v. Intermountain Health Care, Inc.* 709 P.2d 265 (Utah 1985).

38. Jack Needleman, Deborah J. Chollet, and JoAnn Lamphere, Hospital conversion trends, *Health Affairs* 6, no. 2 (1997): 187–95.

39. Jeff Goldsmith, *Can hospitals survive? The new competitive health care market* (Homewood, IL: Dow Jones-Irwin, 1981); Anthony R. Kovner and James R. Knickman, *Jonas and Kovner's health care delivery in the United States*, 9th ed. (New York: Springer, 2008).

40. Sylvia A. Law, *Blue Cross: What went wrong?* (New Haven, CT: Yale University Press, 1976); The Tax Reform Act of 1986, Internal Revenue Code, § 501(m).

41. Uwe E. Reinhardt, The economics of for-profit and not-for-profit hospitals, *Health Affairs* 19, no. 6 (2000): 178–86.

42. For the California conversion, see Consumers Union. *Blue Cross and Blue Shield: A historical compilation*, 17, available at http://yourhealthdollar.org/pdf/yourhealthdollar.org_blue-cross-history-compilation.pdf (accessed 12 September 2010); Blue Cross Blue Shield Association, *For-profit conversions and merger trends among Blue Cross Blue Shield health plans* (2004), 1–2.

43. Larry Kirsch, Report to the Pennsylvania insurance department concerning the applications of Blue Cross plans for the approval of reserves and surplus (2004), available at http://www.phlp.org/Website/Uninsured/The%20Kirsch%20Report.pdf (accessed 10 November 2009).

44. Center for Medicare and Medicaid Services. 2002. Trends and indicators in the changing health care marketplace, 2002—Chart book.

45. Uwe E. Reinhardt, A social contract for 21st century health care: Three-tier health care with bounty hunting, *Health Economics* 5, no. 6 (1996): 479–99. Statistics from Elizabeth Hoy, Richard E. Curtis, and Thomas D. Rice, Change and growth in managed care, *Health Affairs* 10, no. 4 (1991): 18–36.

46. Jerome P. Kassirer, The use and abuse of practice profiles, *NEJM* 330, no. 9 (1994): 634–36; Jon Gabel, Ten ways HMOs have changed during the 1990s, *Health Affairs* 16, no. 3 (1997): 134–45.

47. Marsha R. Gold and Ingrid Reeves, Preliminary results of the GHAA-BC/BS survey of physician incentives in health maintenance organizations (HMOs), *Research Briefs* 1 (November 1987): 1–15; Gloria J. Bazzoli, Stephen M. Shortell, Nicole Dubbs, et al., A taxonomy of health networks and systems: Bringing order out of chaos, *Health Services Research* 33, no. 3 (1999): 1683–717; Marsha Gold, Timothy Lake, and Robert Hurley, Provider organizations at risk: A profile of major risk bearing intermediaries, 1999, *Health Affairs* 20, no. 2 (2001): 175–85.

48. Health Maintenance Organizations, Competitive Medical Plans, and Health Care Prepayment Plans Subpart L, Medicare Contract Requirements, 42 C.F.R. §417.479.

49. Fred J. Hellinger, The impact of financial incentives on physician behavior in managed care plans: A review of the evidence, *Medical Care Research and Review* 53, no. 3 (1996): 294; Lawrence P. Casalino, Balancing incentives: How should physicians be reimbursed? *JAMA* 267, no. 3 (1992): 403; James C. Robinson, Blended payment methods in physician organizations under managed care, *JAMA* 282, no. 13 (1999): 1258–63.

50. Marc A. Rodwin and Estuji Okomoto, Physicians' conflict of interest in Japan and the United States: Lessons for the United States, *Journal of Health Politics, Policy and Law* 25, no. 2 (2000): 343–75; Mark Schlesinger, Countervailing agency: A strategy of principled regulation under managed competition, *Milbank Quarterly* 75, no. 1 (1997): 35–87.

51. James C. Robinson and Lawrence Casalino, Reevaluation of capitation contracting in New York and California, *Health Affairs* 20, no. 4 (2001): W3–W9.

52. Lawrence D. Brown and Elizabeth Eagan, The paradoxical politics of provider reempowerment, *Journal of Health Politics, Policy and Law* 29, no. 6 (2004): 1045–72; Marc A. Rodwin, Backlash: Prelude to managing managed care, *Journal of Health Politics, Policy and Law* 24, no. 5 (1999): 1115–26.

53. Leatrice Berman-Sandler, Independent medical review: Expanding legal remedies to achieve managed care accountability, *Annals of Health Law* 13, no. 1 (2004): 233–302.

54. James C. Robinson, The end of managed care, *JAMA* 285, no. 20 (2001): 2622–28; Medicaid managed care penetration rates, CMS, DHHS, available at http://www.cms.hhs.gov/MedicaidDataSourcesGenInfo/downloads/08Dec31f.pdf (accessed 28 November 2009); Center for Medicare and Medicaid Services (CMS), *Medicare advantage program facts and figures, January 2009*, available at http://www.ahip.org/content/default.aspx?docid=25733 (accessed 7 January 2009). See Marc A. Rodwin, The metamorphosis of managed care, *Journal of Law, Medicine & Ethics* 36, no. 2 (2010): 252–364.

55. For an overview, see David S. Shimm, Conflicts of interest in relations between physicians and the pharmaceutical industry. In *Conflicts of interest in clinical practice and research*, ed. R. Spece, D. S. Shimm, and A. E. Buchanan, 321–57 (New York: Oxford University Press, 1996).

56. The Patent and Trademark Amendments Act of 1980, P.L. 96–517. P. L. 97–34; Executive Order 12591 (19 April 1987); Robert Killoren and Susan Butts, Industry-university research in our times. White paper prepared for the Government-University-Industry Research Roundtable, National Academies, 26 June 2003, available at www7.nationalacademies.org/guirr/IP_background.html (accessed 10 November 2009); Douglas W. Jamison and Christina Jansen, Technology transfer and economic growth, *Journal of Association of University Technology Managers* 12 (2000): 24–35.

57. E. Ray Dorsey, Jason de Roulet, Joel P. Thompson, et al., Funding of US biomedical research, 2003–2008, *JAMA* 303, no. 2 (2010): 137–43.

58. Ludmerer, *Time to heal*, 341.

59. Anthony Flint, Stakes are high for BU in its response to AG: A fight seen as costly to reputation, *Boston Globe*, 17 March 1993, 1; David Barboza, Loving a stock, not wisely but too well, *New York Times*, 20 September 1998.

60. Thomas Bodenheimer, Uneasy alliance: Clinical investigators and the pharmaceutical industry, *NEJM* 342, no. 20 (2000): 1539–42; Marcia Angel, *The truth about drug companies: How they deceive us and what to do about it* (New York: Random House, 2004).

61. Nikolaos A. Patsopoulos, John P. A. Ioannidis, and Apostolos A. Analatos, Origin and funding of the most frequently cited papers in medicine: Database analysis, *British Medical Journal* 332, no. 7549 (2006): 1061–64; Bodil Als-Nielsen, Wendong Chen, Christian Glund, et al., Association of funding and conclusions in randomized drug trials: A reflection of treatment effect or adverse events? *JAMA* 290, no. 7 (2003): 921–28; Joel Lexchin, Lisa A. Bero, Benjamin Djulbegovic, et al., Pharmaceutical industry sponsorship and research outcome and quality: Systematic review, *British Medical Journal* 326, no. 7400 (2003): 1167–70.

62. Justin E. Bekelman, Yan Li, and Cary P. Gross, Scope and impact of financial conflicts of interest in biomedical research: A systematic review, *JAMA* 289, no. 4 (2003): 454–65; Helle Krogh Johansen and Peter C. Gotzche, Problems in the design and reporting of trials of antifungal agents encountered during meta-analysis, *JAMA* 282, no. 18 (1999): 1752–59; Lise L. Kjaergard and Bodil Als-Nielsen, Association between competing interests and authors' conclusions: Epidemiological study of

randomized clinical trials published in the *BMJ, British Medical Journal* 325, no. 7358 (2002): 249–52; S. Swaroop Vedula, Lisa Bero, Roberta W. Scherer, et al., Outcome reporting in industry-sponsored trials of Gabapentin for off-label use, *NEJM* 361, no. 20 (2009): 1963–71.

63. Shedon Krimsky, *Science in the private interest: Has the lure of profits corrupted biomedical research* (Lanham, MD: Rowman and Littlefield, 2003), 91–106; Robert Steinbrook, Financial conflicts of interest and the Food and Drug Administration's advisory committees, *NEJM* 353, no. 2 (2005): 116–18.

64. See John Lear, The unfinished story of Thalidomide, *Saturday Review of Literature* 45 (1 September 1962): 35–40; The Prescription Drug User Fee Amendments of 2007, Title I of the Food and Drug Administration Amendments Act of 2007.

65. Richard Smith, *The trouble with medical journals* (London: Royal Society of Medicine Press Ltd., 2006).

66. Sheldon Krimsky and L. S. Rothenberg, Conflict of interest policies in science and medical journals: Editorial practices and author disclosures, *Science and Engineering Ethics* 7, no. 2 (2001): 205–18; Marc A. Rodwin, Physicians' conflicts of interests: The limitations of disclosure, *NEJM* 321, no. 20 (1989): 1405–8.

67. John Abramson, *Overdo$ed America: The broken promise of American medicine* (New York: Harper, 2004), 13–22, 23–28.

68. On drug advertising, see Jerome Kassirer, *On the take: How America's complicity with big business can endanger your health* (New York: Oxford University Press, 2005), 90–91. Regarding dialysis, see Owen Dryer, Journal rejects article after objections from marketing department, *British Medical Journal* 328, no. 7434 (2004): 244.

69. Annette Flanagin, Lisa A. Carey, Phil B. Fontanarosa, et al., Prevalence of articles with honorary authors and ghost authors in peer-reviewed medical journal, *JAMA* 280, no. 3 (1998): 222–24; Troyen A. Brennan, Buying editorials, *NEJM* 331, no. 10 (1994): 673–75; Anna Matthews, Ghost story at medical journals: Writers paid by industry play big role, *Wall Street Journal*, 13 December 2005, A1; Joseph S. Ross, Kevin P. Hill, David S. Egilman, et al., Guest authorship and ghostwriting in publications related to Rofecoxib: A case study of industry documents from Rofecoxib litigation, *JAMA* 299, no. 15 (2008): 1800–12; Natasha Singer, Medical papers by ghostwriters pushed therapy, *New York Times*, 5 August 2009, 1. For ghostwriting in the 1950s, see chapter 5.

70. Niteesh K. Choudhry, Henry Thomas Stelfox, and Allan S. Detsky, Relationships between authors of clinical practice guidelines and the pharmaceutical industry, *JAMA* 287, no. 5 (2002): 612–17; Lisa Cosgrove, Sheldon Krimsky, Manisha Vijayaraghavan, et al., Financial ties between DSM-IV panel members and the pharmaceutical industry, *Psychotherapy and Psychosomatics* 75, no. 3 (2006): 154–60; Kassirer, *On the take*, 129.

71. Alice Dembner, A cure for fraud: Weston doctor saves taxpayers millions by blowing whistle, *Boston Globe*, 7 October 2001; Margaret M. Chren and C. Seth Landefeld, Physicians' behavior and their interactions with drug companies: A controlled

study of physicians who requested additions to a hospital drug formulary, *JAMA* 271, no. 9 (1994): 684–89.

72. Richard Steinbrook, Financial support of continuing education in the health professions. In *Continuing education in the health professions: Improving healthcare through lifelong learning*, ed. M. Hager, S. Russell and S. Fletcher, 110–11 (2007), available at www.joshiahmacyfoundation.org (accessed 10 November 2009).

73. Data supplied by ACCME for 2000 and 2006. Data for 1990 from interview with Murray Kopelow, president, ACCME.

74. AMA, *U.S. medical licensure statistics 1985 and licensure requirements* 1986 (Chicago: AMA1987), Table 14, p. 30; AMA, Continuing medical education for licensure reregistration. In *State medical licensure requirements and statistics 2009* (Chicago: AMA, 2008).

75. Arnold S. Relman, Separating continuing medical education from pharmaceutical marketing, *JAMA* 285, no. 15 (2001): 2009–12.

76. The ACCME distinguishes between commercial support (grants to CME providers) and income from advertising and exhibits at CME meetings. I included both under commercial support. Most funding comes from the grants. See ACCME, Annual Report Data 2004, available at http://www.accme.org/dir_docs/doc_upload/2130a818–1c9f-400b-9d54–56b3f8f9a2f6_uploaddocument.pdf (accessed 17 September 2006);

ACCME, Annual Report Data 1998, available at http://www.accme.org/dir_docs/doc_upload/dc316660–2a48–46d4–916f-60334f7527ba_uploaddocument.pdf (accessed 17 September 2006);

ACCME, Annual Report Data 2008, available at http://www.accme.org/dir_docs/doc_upload/1f8dc476–246a-4e8e-91d3-d24ff2f5bfec_uploaddocument.pdf (accessed 13 November 2009).

77. Eric Campbell et al., A national survey of physician-industry relationships.

78. U.S. Senate, Committee of Labor and Human Resources, *Advertising, marketing and promotion*, 11 and 12 December 1990, 19, 24–25.

79. Final Guidance on Industry-Supported Scientific and Educational Activities, *Federal Register* 62, no. 232 (December 3, 1997): 64074–64100.

80. David Armstrong, Drug firm's cash sways debate over test for pregnant women, *Wall Street Journal*, 13 December 2006, A1.

81. Anonymous interview with the author, fall 2007.

82. Interview with Mark Schaffer, October, 2007.

83. Marjorie A. Bowman, The impact of drug company funding on the content of continuing medical education, *Mobius* 6, no. 1 (1986): 66–69; Marjorie A. Bowman and David L. Pearle, Changes in drug prescribing patterns related to commercial company funding of continuing medical education, *Journal of Continuing Education in the Health Professions* 8, no. 1 (1988): 13–20; Roger W. Spingarn, Jesse A. Berlin, and Brian L. Strom, When pharmaceutical manufacturers' employees present

grand rounds, what do residents remember? *Academic Medicine* 71, no. 1 (1996): 86–88.

84. *Physicians World*, available at http://www.pwcg.com/whoweare/html (accessed 3 December 2001).

85. U.S. DHHS, OIG, Compliance program guidance for pharmaceutical manufacturers, *Federal Register* 68, no. 86 (May 5, 2003): 23731–43.

86. See Michael A. Steinman, Lisa A. Bero, Mary-Margaret Chren, et al., Narrative review: The promotion of Gabapentin: An analysis of internal industry documents, *Annals of Internal Medicine* 145, no. 4 (2006): 284–93. The documents are part of over 80,000 pages made available in *United States of America ex. Rel David Franklin vs. Pfizer, Inc, and Parke-Davis*, 1 September 2010, available at http://dida.library.ucsf.edu/.

87. Eric Campbell, Russell Gruen, James Mountford, et al., A national survey of physician-industry relationships, *NEJM* 356, no. 17 (2007): 1742–50.

88. Marc-André Gagnon and Joel Lexchin, The cost of pushing ills: A new estimate of pharmaceutical promotion expenditures in the United States, *PLoS Medicine* 5, no. 1 (2008), available at http://www.plosmedicine.org/article/info:doi/10.1371/journal.pmed.0050001 (accessed 10 November 2009). An extensive literature examines gifts and social exchange. See, e.g., Peter M. Blau, *Exchange and power in social life* (New York: John Wiley, 1964); Robert B. Cialdini, *Influence: Science and practice* (New York: HarperCollins, 1993); Jason Dana and George Loewenstein, A social science perspective on gifts to physicians from industry, *JAMA* 290, no. 2 (2002): 252–55. In medical practice, see Flora Haayer, Rational prescribing and sources of information, *Social Science and Medicine* 16, no. 23 (1982): 2017–23. Andrew Pollack, Secret rebates offered on costly eye drug, *New York Times*, 4 November 2010, B1, 6.

89. U.S. Senate, Committee on Labor and Human Resources, *Advertising, marketing and promotion* (December 1990), Testimony of Sidney Wolf, 4; John Graves, Frequent-flyer program for drug prescribing, *NEJM* 317, no. 4 (1987): 252.

90. Morten Andersen, Jakob Kragstrup, and Jens Sondergaard, How conducting a clinical trial affects physicians' guideline adherence and drug preferences, *JAMA* 295, no. 23 (2006): 2759–64.

CHAPTER 7

1. The AMA made some exceptions for medical society-owned insurance. AMA, House of Delegates, Sickness insurance problems in the United States, *JAMA* 102, no. 26 (1934): 2200–2201. It made some exceptions for medical society–owned insurance.

2. The AMA politics are discussed by George A. Woodhouse, past chairman of the AMA Judicial Council, in testimony before the U.S. House Committee on Energy and Commerce, Subcommittee on Health, *Physician dispensing of drugs: Hearings on H.R. 2093* (22 April 1987), 15, 105–24.

3. Mark Schlesinger, A loss of faith: The sources of reduced political legitimacy for the American medical profession, *Milbank Quarterly* 80, no. 2 (2002): 185–235.

4. Lawrence D. Brown, *Politics and health care organization: HMOs as federal policy* (Washington, DC: Brookings Institution, 1983); HMO Act of 1973, 42 U.S.C. Ch. 6a, Subchapter XI; *In re AMA*, 94 F.T.C., 701, 801 (1979); [1979–1983 Transfer Binder] Trade Reg. Rep. (CCH) p 21,955 at 22,418–19.

5. AMA, Report of the Council on Ethical and Judicial Affairs, A (I-86): Conflicts of interest (1986).

6. See Brown, *Politics and health care organization*; Harold S. Luft, *Health maintenance organizations: Dimensions of performance* (New Brunswick, NJ: Transaction Books, 1987).

7. Mark J. Schlesinger, Bradford H. Gray, and Krista M. Perreira, Medical professionalism under managed care: The pros and cons of utilization review, *Health Affairs* 16, no. 1 (1997): 106–24.

8. PriceWaterhouseCoopers, LLP, Study of pharmaceutical benefit management (2001), available at http://www.cms.hhs.gov/reports/downloads/cms_2001_4.pdf (accessed 17 November 2009).

9. Jerry Avorn and Stephen B. Soumerai, Improving drug-therapy decisions through educational outreach: A randomized controlled trial of academically based "detailing," *NEJM* 308, no. 24 (1983): 1457–63; Stephen B. Soumerai and Jerry Avorn, Principles of educational outreach ("academic detailing") to improve clinical decision making, *JAMA* 263, no. 4 (1990): 549–56; Stephen B. Soumerai and Jerry Avorn, Economic and policy analysis of university-based drug "detailing," *Medical Care* 24, no. 4 (1986): 313–31.

10. Elizabeth L. Mitchell, The potential for self-interested behavior by pharmaceutical manufacturers through vertical integration with pharmacy benefit managers: The need for a new regulatory approach, *Food & Drug Law Journal* 54, no. 1 (1999): 151; Barbara Martinez, Medco finds that old ties bind in contract with parent Merck after spinoff, it agrees to maintain market share for Merck medications, *Wall Street Journal*, 15 May 2002, 1; Stan Finkelstein and Peter Temin, *Reasonable Rx: Solving the drug price crisis* (Upper Saddle River, NJ: FT Press, 2008): 50–55.

11. U.S. Congressional Budget Office, *The effects of PSROs on health care costs: Current findings and future evaluations* (Washington, DC: CBO, 1979); Richard P. Kusserow, *State medical boards and medical discipline* (Washington, DC: OIG-DHHS, 1990).

12. Stephen F. Jencks and Gail Wilensky, The health care quality improvement initiative: A new approach to quality assurance in Medicare, *JAMA* 286, no. 7 (1992): 900–903; Institute of Medicine, *Medicare's quality improvement organization program: Maximizing potential* (Washington, DC: National Academy Press, 2006).

13. Medicare Payment Advisory Commission, *Medicare payment policy report to Congress*, Washington, D.C., 17 March 2009, 251–69.

14. 42 U.S.C. § 1320a-7a. Several states also have anti-kickback statutes that apply regardless of the insurer.

15. *United States* v. *Greber*, 760 F.2d 68 (3rd Cir.1985); Medicare Medicaid Patient and Program Protection Act of 1987, P. L. 100–93, § 14.

16. OBRA1993, P. L. No. 103–66, §§ 13,500–664, codified as 42 U.S.C.A, § 1395nn.

17. Final Decision Review of Administrative Law Judge Decision, *The Hansleter Network* et al., Doc. No. c-448; Doc. No. CR181. 42 C.F.R. § 1001.952(a), *Federal Register* 57 (29 January 1992): 3330, as amended at *Federal Register* 57 (5 November 1992): 52729; OIG Anti-Kickback Regulations, *Federal Register* 56 (29 July 1991): 35952.01. In addition, business cannot require that physicians make referrals, be in a position to make referrals, or promote business to be investors; they cannot lend funds or guarantee loans to individuals to finance their investment.

18. The Health Insurance Portability and Accountably Act (HIPAA) of 1996, 5 U.S.C.A. §§ 601 et seq. The Balanced Budget Act of 1997. False Claims Act, 47 U.S.C.A§ 337 et seq. 42 U.S.C.A. § 1320 a-7b(a); 18 U.S.C.A. § 286; 31 U.S.C A. § 3730(b). Federal Qui Tam Statute, 31 U.S.C.A., § 3730.

19. OBRA 1986, § 9313 (c), 42 U.S.C. 1320a-7(b). OBRA 1990, 2 U.S.C. §1395 mm(I)(8)(1996); § 4204, Health Maintenance Organization. (a) Regulation of Incentive Payments to Physicians. 42 CFR. Parts 417, 434, 1003. Beth Schermer and Lawrence Foust, Assumption of risk: Federal regulation of physician incentive plans, *Journal of Health and Hospital Law* 30, no. 1 (1997): 1–10.

20. OIG, Gain sharing arrangements and CMPs for hospital payments to physicians to reduce or limit services to beneficiaries, 1999; OIG Advisory Opinion No.01 18 January 2001; Gail R. Wilensky, Nicholas Wolter, and Michelle M. Fischer, Gain sharing: A good concept getting a bad name, *Health Affairs* 26, no. 1 (2007): 58–67.

21. Marc A. Rodwin, Backlash: Prelude to managing managed care, *Journal of Health Politics, Policy and Law* 24, no. 5 (1999): 1115–26; Marc A. Rodwin, Consumer protection and managed care: Issues, reform proposals, and trade-offs, *Houston Law Review* 32, no. 5 (1996): 1319–81; Barry R. Furrow, Thomas L. Greaney, Sandra H. Johnson, et al., *Health law*, 2nd ed. (Saint Paul, MN: West, 2000), 501–8. In 2010, the Patient Protection and Affordable Care Act mandated external review for all states and regulations adopted the National Association of Insurance Commissions model guidelines as initial standards.

22. Personal communication from David A. Richardson, Center for Health Care Dispute Resolution, 4 March 1999.

23. Peter Jacobson, Legal challenges to managed care cost containment programs: An initial assessment, *Health Affairs* 18, no. 4 (1999): 69–85; Peter Jacobson, *Strangers in the night: Law and medicine in the managed care era* (New York: Oxford University Press, 2002).

24. *Pegram v. Herdrich*, 530 U.S. 211 (2000).

25. Barry Furrow, Managed care organizations and patient injury: Rethinking liability, *Georgia Law Review* 31, no. 2 (1997): 443–73; *Bush v. Dake*, C.A. No. 86–25767 Circuit Court, Saginaw County, Michigan.

26. Paul C. Weiler, Howard H. Hiatt, Joseph P. Newhouse, et al., *A measure of malpractice: Medical injury, malpractice litigation, and patient compensation* (Cambridge, MA: Harvard University Press, 1993).

27. For a RICO cases, see *Tetti v. U.S. Healthcare* U.S. Ct. of App, 3rd Cir., Judge Sloviter Order Nos. 89–2091/89–2092 (23 May 1990). For bad faith case, see *Morris v. HealthNet of California, Inc.* 988 P.2d 940 (Utah 1999). See also *Pulvers v. Kaiser Foundation Health Plans*, 99 Cal. App. 3d 560 (1980).

28. *Pilot Life Insurance Company v. Dedeaux*, 107 S.Ct. 1549 (1987); *Aetna v. Davilla*, 542 U.S. 200 (2004).

29. ERISA imposes no duty to disclose, *Shea v. Esensten*, 107 F.3d 625 (34d Cir.1997). ERISA imposes a duty to disclose, *Ehlmann v. Kaiser Health Plan of Texas*, 198 F.3d 552 (5th Cir. 2000); *Horvath v. Keystone Health Plan*, 333 F.3d 450 (3d Cir.2003); Marc A. Rodwin, Physicians' conflicts of interests: The limitations of disclosure, *NEJM* 321, no. 20 (1989): 1405–8; Tracy E. Miller and William M. Sage, Disclosing physician financial incentives, *JAMA* 281, no. 15 (1999): 1424–30.

30. Bradford H. Gray and Marilyn J. Fields, eds., *Controlling costs and changing patient care: The role of utilization management* (Washington, DC: National Academy Press, 1989), Appendix E, Summaries of Committee Site Visits to Utilization Management Organizations, 10, 270.

31. Howard Wolinsky and Tom Brune, *The serpent on the staff: The unhealthy politics of the American Medical Association* (New York: G. P. Putnam, 1994), 94–120.

32. U.S. Senate, Subcommittee on Health and Committee on Labor and Public Welfare, *Examination of the pharmaceutical industry: Hearings on Section 3441 and Section 966*, Part 3, March 8, 1974, 12, 13, 1974, Testimony of Gerald D. Laubach, President Pfizer, 793–866; excerpts from gift catalogues, 1014–37.

33. Ibid., 1348.

34. Ibid., 1348, 1353–54, 1361.

35. Telephone interview by author with David Orentlicher, former counsel, AMA CEJA, 12 December 2006.

36. AMA CEJA, Opinion 8.061, Gifts to physicians from industry, 1990; Gifts to physicians, *JAMA* 265, no. 4 (1991): 501.

37. U.S. Senate, Committee on Labor and Human Resources, Hearings on *Advertising, Marketing and Promotional Practices of the Pharmaceutical Industry*, 101st Cong., 2nd Session, 11 and 12 December 1990, 174–75.

38. Ibid., 173, 176.

39. Charles Bosk and Eliot Freidson make a similar distinction. They call errors that are technical and any physician can make *normal errors*; *abnormal errors* have a moral component that call the physician's character and judgment into question. Charles Bosk, *Forgive and remember: Managing medical failure* (Chicago: University of Chicago Press, 1979); Eliot Freidson, *Doctoring together: A study of professional social control* (Chicago: University of Chicago Press, 1984), 127–37.

40. AMA Council on Ethical and Judicial Affairs, Opinion 8.061, Gifts to physicians.

41. Richard P. Kusserow, *Promotion of prescription drugs through payment and gifts: Physicians' perspectives* (Washington, DC: OIG-DHHS, 1992); Adam O. Goldstein, Gifts to physicians from industry, *JAMA* 266, no. 1 (1991): 61; Leigh Page, Are goody grab bag days over? Dermatologists eye new ethics, *American Medical News* 35, no. 5 (1992): 30–31.

42. Susan Okie, AMA blasted for letting drug firms pay for ethics campaign, *Washington Post*, 30 August 2001, A3.

43. U.S. DHHS, OIG, 2002, Draft OIG compliance program guidance for pharmaceutical manufacturers, *Federal Register* 67, no. 192 (5 May 2003): 62057–67; PhRMA's comments on the draft, submitted by Sidley Austin Brown and Wood LLP, Comment No. 119, Comments from nineteen pharmaceutical companies on the draft, submitted by Arnold & Porter and PriceWaterhouseCoopers LLP.

44. U.S. DHHS, OIG, Compliance program guidance for pharmaceutical manufacturers, *Federal Register* 68, no. 86 (2003): 23731–43, at 23737–2378.

45. Melody Petersen, Vermont to require drug makers to disclose payments to doctors, *New York Times*, 13 June 2002, 1. States with such laws include California, Washington, D.C., Maine, Minnesota, and Vermont. A table of state legislation is available at http://www.ncsl.org/IssuesResearch/Health/2007PrescriptionDrugStat eLegislationNCSL/tabid/14423/Default.aspx (accessed 21 November 2009). Physician Payment Sunshine Act S.2029, introduced by Senator Charles Grassley (R-IA); Gardiner Harris, Senator Grassley seeks financial details from medical groups, *New York Times*, 7 December 2009.

46. Patient Protection and Affordable Care Act, Section 1128 G (a) Physician Payment Sunshine Act Transparency Reports.

47. U.S. Senate, Select Committee on Small Business, Subcommittee on Monopoly, *Present status of competition in the pharmaceutical industry* (Washington, DC: GPO, 1976).

48. A. Witt, for FDA, Drug company supported activities in scientific or education contexts: Draft concept paper (1991). The draft was announced in the *Federal Register* and publicly available. AMA guidelines, "We'll stay the course. Here's why," *Medical Marketing & Media* 26 (1991): 82–88.

49. The FDA said a CME program is unlikely to be independent if it focuses on a single product; a commercial firm owns the CME provider or employs it for marketing or sales, or recommends individuals who promote its products as faculty, or arranges program invitations or disseminates program materials through its marketing department; a provider is not financially viable without a single commercial firm's support, has significant contacts with FDA-regulated firms, or previously organized programs that did not meet standards for independence.

50. FDA, Citizen petition regarding the FDA's policy promotion of unapproved uses of approved drugs and devices; requests for comments, *Federal Register* 59, no. 222 (1994): 59820.

51. FDA, Final guidance on industry-supported scientific and educational activities, *Federal Register* 62, no. 232 (1997): 64074–100, 64074–79. See the FDA

guidelines, Guidance for industry good reprint practices for the distribution of medical journal articles and medical or scientific reference publications on unapproved new uses of approved drugs and approved or cleared medical devices, *Federal Register* 74, no. 8 (13 January 2009): 1694–95. For a summary of the WLF challenge and current law, see FDA, Decision in *Washington Legal Foundation v. Henney, Federal Register* 65, no. 52 (2000): 14286–88, FDA Docket No. 98N–0222.

52. ACCME, *Standards for commercial support,* 1992, available at www.accme.org; Arnold S. Relman, Separating continuing medical education from pharmaceutical marketing, *JAMA* 28, no. 15 (2001): 2009–12; Arnold S. Relman, Defending professional independence: ACCME's proposed new guidelines for commercial support of CME, *JAMA* 289, no. 18 (2003): 2418–20.

53. U.S. DHHS, OIG. 2002. Draft OIG compliance program, 62057–67; Susan Chimonas and David J. Rothman, New federal guidelines for physician-pharmaceutical industry relations: The politics of policy formation, *Health Affairs* 24, no. 4 (2005): 949–60; AMA comments on the draft, submitted by Michael Maves, executive vice president, obtained via FOIA.

54. See, for example, American Association of Electro-diagnostic Medicine, Comment No. 55, American College of Rheumatology, American College of Chest Physicians, Comment No. 87, The Endocrine Society, comment No. 106.

55. U.S. DHHS, OIG, Compliance program guidance, Federal Register 68, no. 86 (5 May 2003): 23731–43, at 23738.

56. ACCME, *Updated standards for commercial support: With back-ground rationale and answers to questions about compliance* (Chicago: ACCME, 2004); Robert Steinbrook, Commercial support and continuing medical education, *NEJM* 352 no. 6 (2005): 534–35.

57. ACCME Standard for Commercial Support, 3.2.

58. Letter from Max Baucus, Chair, Senate Finance Committee, to Murray Kopelow, ACCME, 27 April 2007, Committee on Finance, United States Senate, 2007, *Use of educational grants by pharmaceutical manufacturer,* Prt. 110–21, 110th Cong., 1st Session (April). Available at http://www.arbo.org/cope/SCF%20report%20 june%202005.pdf (accessed 12 September 2010).

59. Letter from Murray Kopelow, Chief Executive of ACCME, to Max Bucus and Charles Grassley, Senate Committee on Finance (3 August 2007), http://www.accme.org/dir_docs/doc_upload/ff745720–2080–496a-bece-2c50b09d4c7c_uploaddocument.pdf (accessed 16 August 2010); see also ACCME 24 August 2007 Announcements, http://accme.org/index.cfm/fa/news.detail/news_id/3605f21a-302a-40d1-ab4d-3ceb88087b1a.cfm (accessed 16 August 2010).

60. The ACCME statement was in its response to frequently asked questions; see ACCME response to frequently asked questions regarding commercial support and independence, http://www.accme.org/index.cfm/fa/faq.detail/category_id/667b72cf-6277–4317–99f9–1e476b621e76.cfm> (accessed 18 August 2010). Yet, the ACCME kept its standards for commercial support, which states only that providers "cannot be required by a commercial interest to accept advice."

61. Testimony of Murray Kopelow, chief executive, Accreditation Council for Continuing Medical Education (ACCME) Before the Special Committee on Aging, U.S. Senate, 29 July 2009, http://www.accme.org/dir_docs/doc_upload/0e7fba7d-9d68–4414–901b-aebb44c60dda_uploaddocument.pdf (accessed 9 September 2010).

62. AMA, CEJA, 2009, Report–A-09 *Financial relationships with industry in continuing medical education*, available at http://www.ama-assn.org/ama1/pub/upload/mm/475/ceja0109.pdf (accessed 7 August 2009).

63. Lewis Morris and Julie K. Taitsman, The agenda for continuing medical education—Limiting industry's influence, *NEJM* 361, no. 25 (2009): 2478–82.

64. DHHS, Public Health Service, Objectivity in research, *Federal Register* 60, no. 132 (1995): 35810–19; DHHS, National Institutes of Health, Scientific peer review of research grant applications and research and development contract projects, *Federal Register* 69, no. 2 (2004): 272–78, sets criteria for conflicts of interest in the application or proposal process; DHHS, FDA, Financial disclosure by clinical investigators; proposed rule, *Federal Register* 59, no. 183 (1994): 46708–19; *FDA guidance on conflicts of interest for advisory board members, February 2000*; available at http://www.fda.gov/oc/advisory/conflictofinterest/guidance.html (accessed 1 September 2010); DHHS, Financial relationships and interests in research involving human subjects: Guidance for human subject protection, *Federal Register* 69, no. 92 (2004): 26393–97, final guidance document on points to consider in determining whether specific financial interests in research affect the rights and welfare of human subjects. U.S. General Accounting Office, *University research: Most federal agencies need to better protect against financial conflicts of interest* (Washington, DC: GPO, 2003).

65. Mark Barnes and Patrik S. Florencio, Financial conflicts of interest in human subjects research: The problem of institutional conflicts, *Journal of Law, Medicine & Ethics* 30, no. 3 (2002): 390; Ezekiel J. Emanuel and Daniel Steiner, Institutional conflict of interest, *NEJM* 332, no. 4 (1995): 262–68.

66. Sheldon Krimsky, *Science in the private interest: Has the lure of profits corrupted biomedical research?* (Lanham, MD: Rowman and Littlefield, 2003).

67. Elaine Gibson, Françoise Baylis, and Stevan Lewis, Dances with the pharmaceutical industry, *Canadian Medical Association Journal* 166, no. 4 (2000): 448–50.

68. Kevin A. Schulman, Damon M. Seils, Justin W. Timbie, et al., A national survey of provisions in clinical-trial agreements between medical schools and industry sponsors, *NEJM* 347, no. 17 (2002): 1335–41.

69. GAO, *Biomedical research*, 11, 16.

70. Office of Inspector General, *How grantees manage financial conflicts of interest in research funded by the National Institutes of Health* (Washington, DC: OIG, 2009).

71. DHHS, Responsibility of applicants for protecting objectivity in research for which public health service funding is sought and responsible prospective contractors, *Federal Register* 75, no. 98 (May 21, 2010): 28688–28712.

CHAPTER 8

1. Kenpōren, *Health insurance, long-term care insurance and health insurance societies in Japan 2007* (Tokyo: Kenpōren, 2007). The social insurance agency provides an overview of employment-based insurance at http://www.sia.go.jp/e/ehi.html (accessed 13 November 2009). For an overview, see Kōzō Tatara and Estuji Okamoto, Japan: Health system review, *Health Systems in Transition* 11, no. 5 (2009), available from *European Observatory on Health Systems and Policies* at http://www.euro.who.int/Document/E92927.pdf (accessed 10 November 2009). John K. Iglehardt, Japan's medical system, Part I, *NEJM* 319, no. 12 (1988): 807–12. John K. Iglehardt, Japan's medical system, Part II, *NEJM* 319, no. 17 (1988): 1166–72.

2. Health and Medical Services for the Aged Act, 1982; Elderly Health Act reformed, 1983.

3. MHLW, 2007 Survey of Medical Institutions. Available at http://www.mhlw.go.jp/english/database/db-hss/mi.html (accessed 16 December 2009). Public authorities that owned hospitals included prefectures, municipalities, the national government, and public organizations such as the Red Cross or agricultural cooperatives. Public service organizations included public welfare corporations, private schools, social insurance organizations, and health cooperatives. For long-term care facilities, see Yuko Suda, Devolution and privatization proceed and centralized system maintained: A twisted reality faced by Japanese nonprofit organizations, *Nonprofit and Voluntary Sector Quarterly* 35, no. 3 (2006): 430–52, at 449–50.

4. This social stratum lacked authority and productive landholdings but included groups that later became the middle class. Merchants were not producers and so ranked below physicians and craftsmen.

5. Natito Museum of Pharmaceutical Science and Industry. *Medicine case* (Gifu-ken Hashima-gun Kawashima-chō: Naitō Kinen Kusuri Hakubutsukan, 1998), 98.

6. Margaret M. Lock, *East Asian medicine in urban Japan* (Berkeley: University of California Press, 1980); Naoki Ikegami and John Creighton Campbell, Medical care in Japan, *NEJM* 333, no. 19 (1995): 1295–99.

7. Naoki Ikegami, Economic aspects of the doctor-patient relationship in Japan from eighteenth century until the emergence of social insurance. In *History of the doctor-patient relationship: Proceedings of the 14th international symposium on the comparative history of medicine—East and West*, ed. Y. Kawakita, S. Sakai, and Y. Otsuka, 131–46 (Tokyo: Ishiyaku EuroAmerica, 1989); Shouichi Fuse, *Ishi no rekisi* [*History of doctors—its Japanese characteristics*] (Tokyo: Chūō Kōronsha, 1979).

8. In the twentieth century, Christian missionaries, including the Salvation Army, established a few charitable hospitals; the Emperor also established one. Wilhelm Röhl, *A history of law in Japan since 1868* (Leiden: Brill, 2005), 570–72.

9. Kodansha Encyclopedia of Japan (Tokyo: G. Itasaka/Kodansha America, 1983).

10. Fujia Ohtani, *One hundred years of health progress in Japan* (Tokyo: International Medical Foundation of Japan, 1971); Ikegami, Economic aspects of the doctor-patient relationship in Japan, 135.

11. Susan Orpett Long, Health care providers: Technology, policy, and professional dominance. In *Health, illness, and medical care in Japan: Cultural and social dimensions*, ed. E. Norbeck and M. Lock, 66–88 (Honolulu: University of Hawaii, 1987).

12. See Frank J. Schwartz and Susan. J. Pharr, eds., *The state of civil society in Japan* (Cambridge: Cambridge University Press, 2003), particularly Robert Pekkanen, Molding Japanese civil society: State-structured incentives and the patterning of civil society, 117–34, at 130–31, and Margarita Stevez-Abe, State-society partnership in the Japanese welfare state, 154–72, at 162.

13. The Civil Code of Japan, chapter 2, Article 34, defines a public interest juristic person as "An association or foundation related to worship, religion, charity, science, article or other related to public interest and not having for its object the acquisition of gain."

14. *Jyorei* means giving affordable compensation in a regular manner. Sumiko Ogawa, Toshihiko Segawa, Guy Carrin, et al., Scaling up community health insurance: Japan's experience with 19th century Jorei scheme, *Health Policy and Planning* 18, no. 3 (2003): 270–78; I. Aoki, *Shōki iryō-riyō kumiai no shōsō* [Evolution of early state of medical co-operatives society], *Han-Nan Rōnshū* [Social Science] 24 (1988): 1–18, 41–55 (in Japanese).

15. Seikyō Iryōbukai, *Iryō seikyō no rekishi to tokuchō* [The history and characteristics of health care cooperatives] (Tokyo: Iryō Seikyō, 1982).

16. Tarō Takemi, A history of the Japan Medical Association. In Takemi, *Socialized medicine in Japan: Essays, papers and addresses* (Tokyo: JMA, 1982), 5.

17. Kenpōren, *History of Japanese NHI* (Tokyo: Kenpōren, 1990), 9.

18. Ikegami, Economic aspects of the doctor-patient relationship in Japan, 135.

19. Andrew Gordon, *The evolution of labor relation in Japan: Heavy industry 1853–1955* (Cambridge, MA: Council on East Asian Studies, Harvard University, 1985); Mutsuko Takahashi, *The emergence of welfare society in Japan* (Brookfield: Ashgate, 1997); George Oakley Totten, *The social democratic movement in prewar Japan* (New Haven, CT: Yale University Press, 1966); Takeshi Takahashi, Social security for workers. In *Workers and employers in Japan: The Japanese employment relations system*, ed. K. Okochi, B. Karsh, and S. B. Levine, 442–43 (Princeton, NJ: Princeton University Press, 1974).

20. Takemi, History of the Japan Medical Association, 4.

21. Supreme Commander of the Allied Powers (SCAP), General Headquarters, Social Security Mission, *Report of the social security mission* (1947), Papers of George Fr. Rohlick, Library, Special Collections Dept., SUNY Albany.

22. Gregory J. Kasza, War and welfare policy in Japan, *Journal of Asian Studies* 61, no. 2 (2002): 417–27. See also Gregory J. Kasza, *One world of welfare: Japan in comparative perspective* (Ithaca, NY: Cornell University Press, 2006).

23. Sumiko Ogawa et al., Scaling up community health insurance, 274.

24. "Military industry was prioritized in allocation of funds and imported materials. Starting in 1939, citizens were mobilized to work for military industry pursuant

to the National Draft Ordinance" (translated by Estuji Okomoto). Mitsusada Inoue, Kazuo Kasahara, and Kota Kodama, *Japan's history* (Tokyo: Yamakawa, 1975), 313. This high school text is government approved.

25. Nishimura Yumiko and Aki Yosikawa, A brief history of Japan: Passage to the universal health insurance system. In *Japan's health system: Efficiency and effectiveness in universal care*, ed. D. I. Okimoto and A. Yoshikawa (Washington, DC: Falkner and Gray, 1993), 14–15; Margaret Powell and Masahira Anesaki, *Health care in Japan* (London: Routledge, 1990).

26. SCAP, Report of the social security mission, 88–89; L. E. Henderson, R. L. Sensenich, and Ernest E. Irons, Medicine in Japan: A report to General Douglas MacArthur, SCAP, *JAMA* 139, no. 18 (1949): 1280.

27. For the medical history, see Supreme Commander for the Allied Powers, *Public health and welfare in Japan, with annex and charts* ([Tokyo]: Supreme Commander for the Allied Powers, Public Health and Welfare Section, 1948). Yoneyuki Sugita, Universal health insurance: The unfinished reform of Japan's health care system. In *Democracy in occupied Japan: The U.S. occupation and Japanese politics and Society*, ed. M. E. Caprio and Y. Sugita (London: Routledge, 2007). For postwar medical politics, see Paul David Talcott, Why the weak can win: Healthcare policies in postwar Japan (Ph.D. diss., Harvard University, 1999).

28. Talcott, Why the weak can win, 90–99.

29. Medical Services Law, Article 7, 5, allows physician-owned medical corporations. The requirement that medical corporations be directed by physicians was dropped in 1999. Although investor-owned firms cannot own and direct medical corporations, they can invest in them. The restrictions on ownership by investor-owned firms do not apply to long-term care facilities or to pharmacies. An MHLW history describes the legislation as follows. The 1948 Medical Services Law prohibited for-profit organizations from operating medical service facilities (hospitals, clinics, childbirth facilities). The law was revised in 1950 to allow new medical corporation status for certain hospitals operating as privately owned corporations in the public interest under strict regulation, which in order to qualify for not-for-profit status could not be operated as publicly listed companies but needed some form of organization larger than a single individual. The legislation prohibited the distribution of surplus revenues as part of the definition of medical corporations as inherently not-for-profit. Health Policy Bureau, Guidance Section, *Iryō hōjin seidō no kaisetsu* [Understanding the medical corporation system] (Tokyo: Nihon Horei, 1996), 10, 11, based on translation provided to the author by Paul Talcott.

30. Robert Pekkanen and Karla Simon, Taxation of not-for-profit organizations and their donors in Japan: Is this tax reform or not? *International Journal of Not-for-Profit Law* 4, no. 2/3 (2002): 1–5.

31. I have found no texts that explain the reasons for this legislation.

32. SCAP, *Report of the social security mission*, 60.

33. SCAP, *Report of the social security mission*, 133, 12, 16.

34. Major Crawford Sams wrote in his memoir: "A certain American congressman thought that he had discovered a deep dark plot . . . [to] impose state medicine and compulsory national health insurance in Japan. . . . As a result, we invited a mission of the American Medical Association to come to Japan and review the situation. . . . It must be recalled that during the years from 1946 through 1949, a great controversy in our county was underway between the medical profession and those who would impose socialized state medicine. . . . We were able to show to the various groups concerned what we were doing and why we doing these things. We received . . . the support of the American medical profession in carryout our program." Crawford F. Sams, *"Medic": The mission of an American military doctor in occupied Japan and war-torn Korea* (Armonk, NY: M. E. Sharp, Controversies of State Medicine, 1998), 171.

35. Henderson, Sensenich, and Irons, Medicine in Japan, 1281.

36. JMA, *Physician's ethics code* (Tokyo: JMA, 1951); see Remuneration of doctors, ethical codes for doctors, ch. 3, clause 3. The current summary is JMA, *Principles of medical ethics*, available at http://www.med.or.jp/english/02_princ.html (accessed 9 June 2009).

37. Talcott, Why the weak can win, 40; Naoki Ikegami, Japanese health care: Low cost through regulated fees, *Health Affairs* 10, no. 3 (1991): 87–109; Etsuji Okamoto, *Public health of Japan, 2004* (Tokyo: Japan Public Health Association, 2004), 41.

38. Satoru Sugita, A historical study of *Iyaku-Bungyō* (the separation of the dispensary from medical practice) in Japan. In *History of the doctor-patient relationship*, ed. Kawakita, Sakai, and Otsuka, 147–64; Talcott, Why the weak can win, 40–48.

39. Exceptions allowed doctors to dispense drugs if in the doctor's judgment the patient might become "anxious" upon receiving a prescription, interfering with treatment. Medical Practitioners' Law, Art. 22(2). See Robert B. Leflar, Informed consent and patients' rights in Japan, *Houston Law Review* 33, no. 1 (1996): 40–43.

40. William E. Steslicke, *Doctors in politics: The political life of the Japan Medical Association* (New York: Praeger, 1973), 49.

41. William E. Steslicke, Development of health insurance policy in Japan, *Journal of Health Politics, Policy and Law* 7, no. 1 (1982): 210.

42. SCAP, *Report of the social security mission*, 88. Quotation from Talcott, Why the weak can win, 87.

43. Steslicke, *Doctors in politics*, 95–101.

44. Talcott, Why the weak can win, 44–66; Henderson, Sensenich, and Irons, Medicine in Japan, 1281.

45. Steslicke, *Doctors in politics*, 80–81, 207.

46. Takemi, History of the Japan Medical Association, 16–17.

47. Arahira Shoji and Onishi Hironari, Reform of the Japanese health insurance system, *International Social Security Review* 52, no. 2 (1999): 101–8. Copayments are

typically 30 percent until age 70 and 10 percent thereafter. Individuals with higher incomes pay 30 percent.

48. In most hospitals, nearly half of rooms are private, the maximum amount allowed. Typically, they are ¥30,000 ($336) a day. Luxury rooms can be ¥40,000 ($448). In Tokyo, VIP suites cost up to ¥100,000 ($1,120). One industry observer reports that fees from private rooms make the difference between a hospital's loss and profit. Interview with John Wocher, 21 November 2002.

49. For fee schedule and its politics, see John Creighton Campbell and Naoki Ike-gami, *The art of balance in health policy: Maintaining Japan's low-cost, egalitarian system* (New York: Cambridge University Press, 1998), 116–44; Naoki Ikegami and John Creighton Campbell, Health care reform: The virtues of muddling through, *Health Affairs* 18, no. 3 (1999): 56–75, at 63–65. The similarity to governmental budget ne-gotiations is discussed in Mikitaka Masuyama and John Creighton Campbell, The evolution of fee-schedule politics in Japan. In *Containing health care costs in Japan*, ed. N. Ikegami and J. C. Campbell, 265–77 (Ann Arbor: University of Michigan Press, 1996).

50. Japan had the lowest staff-to-bed ratio in OECD nations; see OECD Health Data, 1993.

51. Ryu Niki, Integrated delivery systems in Japan: Brief summary of a national survey and future predictions, paper presented at Pacific Research Center, Stanford University, 2 September 1999; Ryu Niki, Rapid increase in private multi-hospital systems in Japan, paper presented at the Comparative Health Care Research Series, Stanford University, 1993; Ryu Niki, *Hoken iryō fukushi fukugotai* [Integrated delivery systems] (Tokyo: Igaku Shoin, 1998).

52. Aki Yoshikawa, Doctors and hospitals in Japan. In *Japan's health system: effi-ciency and effectiveness in universal care*, ed. D. I. Okimoto and A Yoshikawa, 63–89, at 65 (Washington, DC: Faulkner and Gray, 1993). The data are from MHW, *Survey of doctors, dentists, and pharmacists*, 1990. Yoshikawa reports that although more than half of hospital beds were physician-owned, less than 1.5 percent of physicians owned hospitals. However, 27.5 percent of physicians owned clinics, either with no beds or under twenty beds. About one-third of clinics had beds, so he estimated that 9 percent of physicians owned clinics with beds.

53. William C. Ouchi, *Theory Z: How American business can meet the Japanese chal-lenge* (Reading, MA: Addison-Wesley, 1981); James R. Lincoln and Arne L. Kalleberg, Work organization and workforce commitment: A study of plants and employees in the U.S. and Japan, *American Sociological Review* 50, no. 6 (1985): 738–60.

54. A 1992 survey indicated that nearly 8 percent of hospitals linked salary to utili-zation of services and 41 percent said they might do so. *Nikkei Health Care*, Septem-ber 1992, 59.

55. Long, Health care providers, 81.

56. Patients' gifts to physicians are part of a broader gift-giving practice. It is cus-tomary to give gifts in July and at the end of the year. Gifts are given among colleagues,

to teachers, to social superiors with whom one has a relationship, to professionals, and to those who have shown benevolence. Anthropologist Margaret Lock reported that families which gave their physicians gifts prior to World War II often did not following the war, presumably because the NHI changed the relationship: Lock, *East Asian medicine in urban Japan*, 241–43. However, more recently another anthropologist found that the practice thrives: Katherine Rupp, *Gift-giving in Japan: Cash, connections, cosmologies* (Stanford, CA: Stanford University Press, 2003). Hospital visits have traditionally been an occasion for making gifts to patients by family and colleagues, and patients have made return gifts later. Emiko Ohnuki-Tierney, *Illness and culture in contemporary Japan: An anthropological view* (Cambridge: Cambridge University Press, 1984), 203–6.

57. Rupp, *Gift-giving in Japan*, 75–76, 163–65, 169–74.

58. Ikegami, Japanese health care, 104; interview with Yoshi Nomi, fall 2002.

59. Hospitals might also make it clear to patients who want access to other supplemental services that they need to be treated in private rooms. Mark A. Colby, *The Japan healthcare debate: Diverse perspectives* (Folkestone: Global Oriental, 2004), 110.

60. OECD Statistics, 2003.

61. Administrative Procedure Act (Act No. 88 of 1993); OECD Reviews of Regulatory Reform. Japan progress in implementing regulatory reform executive summary, available at http://www.oecd.org/dataoecd/56/2/32983995.pdf (accessed 17 November 2009).

62. Office of the U.S. Trade Representative, Third report to the leader on the U.S.-Japan regulatory reform and competition policy initiative, 8 June 2004, 25. For discussion of American firm influence of U.S. trade policy, see Michael Watkins, *The medical technology industry and Japan* (Cambridge, MA: Harvard Business School, 2004), Case No. 9–904–018; Nathan Corteze, International health care convergence: The benefits and burdens of market-driven standardization, *Wisconsin International Law Journal* 26, no. 3 (2008): 646–704.

63. Okamoto, *Public health of Japan*, 41.

64. This followed the government's prosecution of the CSIMC representatives from organized labor and the Kenpōren for corruption.

65. Health Care Reform Act of 2006.

66. Each case is assigned to one of sixteen categories based on primary and secondary diagnoses, then to subcategories for medical or surgical care, and classified using the ICD-10 codes for primary diagnoses. Then each case is assigned reimbursement points for three stages of hospitalization. Kazuhiro Ishikawa, Masato Yamamoto, Donald T. Kishi, et al., New prospective payment system in Japan, *American Journal of Health-System Pharmacy* 62, no. 15 (2005): 617–19.

67. Tetsurō Chino, An economic analysis of institutions and regulations in the Japanese healthcare system, *Government Auditing Review* 14 (2007): 13–25; Council for the Promotion of Regulatory Reform (CPRR), First report on the promotion

of regulatory reform and the opening up of government-driven markets for entry into the private sector (24 December 2004), available at http://www8.cao.go.jp/kisei-kaikaku/old/publication/2004/1224/item041224_02e.pdf (accessed 1 September 2010).

68. These were part of the Special Zones for Structural Reform. There are other deregulation zones for other activities. In 2008, the government designated zones for development of advanced medicine to encourage university hospital and research facilities to develop projects in regenerative medicine, medical devices, biotechnology-based drugs, and joint international research on cancer and other diseases. See Reform zones to be set up for medicine development, *Daily Yomiuri*, 26 April 2008.

69. CPRR, First report, 11, 62–68.

70. U.S.-Japan Economic Partnership for Growth, U.S.-Japan Investment Initiative 2005 Report, 7 July 2005.

71. Tokyo district court, 23 January 1989.

72. Naoki Ikegami, Should providers be allowed to extra-bill for uncovered services? Debate, resolution and the sequel in Japan, *Journal of Health Politics, Policy and Law* 31, no. 6 (2006): 1129–49.

73. Lifting of ban on mixed use of health plans to be postponed, *Daily Yomiuri*, 16 December 2004.

74. Editorial, Mixed-treatment conundrum, *Japan Times*, 8 October 2009, available at http://search.japantimes.co.jp/cgi-bin/ed20091008a1.html (accessed 16 December 2009).

75. Ikegami, Should providers be allowed to extra-bill for uncovered services?

76. Bureaucrats give reform panel the runaround, *Daily Yomiuri*, 30 December 2005. Tokyo University hospital offers cancer exam for 6 million yen, *Daily Yomiuri*, 26 April 2008.

CHAPTER 9

1. This work grows out of research conducted with Estuji Okmoto: Marc A. Rodwin and Estuji Okamoto, Physicians' conflict of interest in Japan and the United States: Lessons for the United States, *Journal of Health Politics, Policy and Law* 25, no. 2 (2000): 343–75.

2. The Ministry of Health and Welfare (MHW) was renamed the Ministry of Health, Labor and Welfare (MHLW) in 2001. I refer to it as the MHW for decisions before 2001 and as the MHLW for policies initiated thereafter or that span both periods.

3. John Creighton Campbell and Naoki Ikegami, *The art of balance in health policy: Maintaining Japan's low-cost, egalitarian system* (New York: Cambridge University Press, 1988), 159.

4. Michio Kodaka, Present status of hemodialysis in Japan, *Journal of the Japanese Society for Dialysis Therapy* 19 (1986): 1–21; K. Sawanishi, Follow up on dialysis patients initiated below serum creatinine level 8.0 mg/dl, *Journal of Japanese Society of Dialysis Therapy* 23 (1990): 1–10; M. Yamagami and Y. Seoka, Health economics analysis on dialysis treatment, *Banboo* 163 (January 1995): 64–68.

5. MHW, 5 National trends of health [*Kokumin eisei no dōkō*] (Tokyo: Health and Welfare Statistics Association, 1996), 180. Statistic for 25 percent of the world's dialysis patients from Yamagami and Seoka, Health economic analysis. The mean number of dialysis patients for OEDC nations in 1994 was 501 per million, while Japan has 1,149 per million. Eric A. Feldman, Legal transplants, organ transplants: The Japanese experience, *Social and Legal Studies: An International Journal* 3, no. 1 (1994): 71–91; G. Ohi, T. Hasegawa, H. Kumano, I. Kai, et al., Why are cadaveric renal transplants so hard to find in Japan? An analysis of economic and attitudinal aspects, *Health Policy* 6, no. 3 (1986): 269–78.

6. Japan Government Auditing Office, *Audit report for the fiscal year 1993* (Tokyo: Ministry of Finance Printing Bureau, 1994), 76.

7. *Yomiuri Newspaper*, 9 October 1994; Oshamu Kozeki, Consequences of fixed-payment for dialysis, *Banboo* 164 (February 1995): 68–72; *Kyodo News*, 30 March 1995.

8. Shunichi Fukuhara, Chikao Yamazaki, Yasuaki Hayashino, et al., The organization and financing of end-stage renal disease, *International Journal of Health Care Finance and Economics* 7, no. 2 (2007): 219.

9. Report by MHW, quoted in Yukata Nakano and Hiroshi Ohama, *Fee schedule made easy '98* (Tokyo: UtoBrain, 1998), 92; MHW, *A survey result on per-diem payment hospitals*, May 1991; Yasuo Takagi, Effects of per-diem payment method in geriatric care: Changes in pharmaceutical and laboratory costs and ADL of the inpatients, *Medicine and Society* 2, no. 1 (1992): 43–62.

10. Naoki Ikegami, Games policy makers and providers play: Introducing case-mix-based payment to hospital chronic care units in Japan. *Journal of Health Politics Policy and Law* 34, 3 (2009): 361–80.

11. Naoko Muramatsu and Jersey Liang, Hospital length of stay in the United States and Japan: A case study of myocardial infarction patients, *International Journal of Health Services* 29, no. 1 (1999): 189–209. The statistic for France is from OECD, *Health data at a glance: OCCD indicators, 2003.*

12. Fukuhara, Yamazaki, Hayashino, et al., The organization and financing of end-stage renal disease.

13. Interview with Estuji Okamoto, 10 September 2002. The television program was titled *How a broken hospital is revived*. MHW: Health Insurance Bureau, Administrative directive 32, 16 March 1998.

14. Robert B. Leflar, Informed consent and patients' rights in Japan, *Houston Law Review* 33, no. 1 (1996): 1–112. But cf. Eric Feldman, Suing doctors in Japan: Structure, culture, and the rise of malpractice litigation. In *Fault lines: Tort law as cultural*

practice, ed. M. McCann and D. Engel, 211–32 (Stanford, CA: Stanford University Press, 2009).

15. Uwe Reinhardt, Is the target-income hypothesis an economic heresy? *Medical Care Research and Review* 53, no. 3 (1996): 274–87.

16. Naoki Ikegami, Efficiency and effectiveness in health care, *Daedalus* 123, no. 4 (1994): 119.

17. The agreement between the MHLW and JMA that claims would not be electronically reviewed was informal, not a regulation or official document, but it is widely acknowledged.

18. Naoki Ikegami, Japanese health care: Low cost through regulated fees, *Health Affairs* 10, no. 3 (1991): 107.

19. Ikegami, Japanese health care, 97. Less than half of insurance carriers check the content of claims for appropriateness. Institutions can be audited if suspected of engaging in egregious violations of law, such as billing for services not provided. Providers can be suspended or removed from the list that insurers pay. None of these procedures enable evaluation of the appropriateness or quality of treatment.

20. Social Insurance Payment Fund, http://www.ssk.or.jp/rezept/pdf/hukyu02.pdf.

21. Kenzō Kikuni, Quality assurance programs in Japan, *Japan Hospitals* 3 (July 1984): 29–31; John Wocher, TQM/CQI efforts in Japanese hospitals—Why not? In *The effectiveness of CQI in health care: Stories from a global perspective,* ed. V. A. Kazandjian (Milwaukee, WI: ASQ Quality Press, 1997), 56; John C. Wocher, The Japanese health care system: Planning the extinction of the private hospitals, *Japan Hospitals* 13 (July 1994), 39.

22. Wocher, TQM/CQI efforts in Japanese hospitals, 61

23. Personal correspondence, 4 January 2009. Kameda became the first Joint Commission International (JCI) accredited hospital in Japan in 2009, and such quality reporting is a JCI requirement. Developments in criminal and civil law, however, are beginning to promote quality assurance. See Robert B. Leflar, Unnatural deaths, criminal sanctions, and medical quality improvement in Japan, *Yale Journal of Health Policy, Law and Ethics* 9, no. 1 (2009): 11; Robert B. Leflar, Law and patient safety in the United States and Japan. In *Readings in comparative health law and bioethics,* ed. T. S. Jost, 124–26 (Durham, NC: Carolina Academic Press, 2007); Robert B. Leflar and Futoshi Iwata, Medical error as reportable event, as tort, as crime: A transpacific comparison, *Widener Law Review* 12, no. 1 (2005): 189–225.

24. MHW, Statistics and Information Bureau, *Social insurance claims survey 1994—Pharmaceutical utilization* (Tokyo: Health and Welfare Statistics Association, 1994), 14. The average number of medications prescribed per patient visit that are specified on insurance claims was 3.25. However, claimants are permitted to omit the names of drugs if they are priced less than ¥ 205 ($1.70) per daily dose. Approximately 36.5 percent of outpatient drug cost is unaccounted for. Margaret M. Lock, *East Asian medicine in urban Japan* (Berkeley: University of California Press, 1980), 242–43.

25. Drug spending statistics from Arahira Shoji and Onishi Hironari, Reform of the Japanese health insurance system, *International Social Security Review* 52, no. 2 (1999): 105. Generic drug statistics are from 2004 from Japan Fair Trade Commission, *Report on distribution of pharmaceuticals* (*Overview*), 2006, 2.

26. Interview with John Wocher, 21 November 2002. However, in personal correspondence, Read Mauer notes that differences in culture and population explain some differences in drug use. In Japan, daily doses are typically lower, and if the lower dose is not effective, another drug is added to the daily regimen. Two drugs may be used in Japan where one would be in the United States. Drug use also varies among therapeutic areas; Japan uses more antibiotics than the United States but less often uses central nervous system drugs to treat psychiatric and neurological problems.

27. John K. Iglehart, Japan's medical system, Part II, *NEJM* 319, no. 17 (1988): 1166–72; Campbell and Ikegami, *Art of balance in health policy*, 166.

28. The permitted profit margins were 15 percent in 1992, 13 percent in 1994, 11 percent in 1996, 10 percent in 1997, and 5 percent in 1998. English Regulatory Information Task Force, Japan Pharmaceutical Manufacturers Association, *Pharmaceutical administration and regulations in Japan* (2008), 166–67, available at http://www.jpma.or.jp/english/parj/pdf/2008.pdf (accessed 17 November 2009)

29. The MHW increased the fee for prescribing without dispensing from ¥60 to ¥500 in 1974 and to ¥810 (about $6) in 1998. The prescribing fee for dispensing physicians was then ¥370 (about $2.50). Data from Jeong Hyoung-Sun and Jeremy Hurst, 2001, An assessment of the performance of the Japanese health care system, *OECD Labor Market and Social Policy Occasional Papers*, no. 56 (2001), OECD Publishing. http://www.oecd.org/dataoecd/35/28/34687614.pdf (accessed 17 November 2009).

30. Interview with John Wocher, 21 November 2002.

31. Health Insurance Providers' Practicing Rules, § 19–3.

32. Incentive payment may backfire. Since patients pay a 10 percent to 30 percent copayment on the dispensing fee, it is less expensive for patients to use a pharmacy that receives most of its prescriptions from one hospital.

33. The 2008 statistic comes from a survey by Japan Pharmacist Association. source: *Kokumin eisei no dōkō* 2010, 248. The 1997 statistic comes from MHW, Statistics and Information Bureau, Social Insurance Claims Survey 1996 (Health and Welfare Statistics Association), 38.

34. MHLW Central Social Insurance Medical Care Committee, Subcommittee on Price Setting, *Report on pharmaceutical evaluation and price setting in foreign countries*. March 1995.

35. Jeong and Hurst, Assessment of the performance of the Japanese health care system, 30–31.

36. Interview with John Wocher, 21 November 2002.

37. Norio Sasamori, The present condition of the human dry dock in Japan and its outlook for the future, *Japan Hospitals* 1 (1978): 49–55; Mark A. Colby, *The Japan healthcare debate: Diverse perspectives* (Folkestone: Global Oriental, 2004), 90–94. However, Japan performs more diagnostic testing generally. Most schools provide electrocardiogram screening of children twice during their school years. Naoki Ikegami, Health technology development in Japan, *International Journal of Technology Assessment in Health Care* 4, no. 2 (1988): 248–49.

38. Maratoshi Abe, Japan's clinic physicians and their behavior, *Social Science and Medicine* 20, no. 4 (1985): 333–40.

39. Article 67, Section 2 of the Special Tax Regulations (*sozei tokubetsu sochiho*).

40. Hospital reform plan in works: Government aims to promote increased involvement of local residents, *Daily Yomiuri*, 4 December 2004.

41. Medical Services Act, Section 44, paragraph 4.

42. Nikkei Health Care, *Survey of hospitals on measures for taxation*, February 1991, 35.

43. Colby, *Japan healthcare debate*, 30–37, 99–100.

44. Okamoto and Kōzō Tatara, *Public health of Japan, 2007*, 46. The Japan Council for Quality in Health Care (JCQHC) has overseen voluntary hospital accreditation since 1997. International accreditation standard organizations also accredit hospitals and clinical laboratories. American firms spearheaded voluntary clinical laboratory accreditation and ran consulting companies that helped hospitals comply. In the 1990s, the American Joint Commission on Accreditation of Healthcare Organizations (JCAHO) developed accrediting standards for foreign hospitals through its affiliate, Joint Commission International. See http://www.colbygroup.com/en/president.html; http://www.jointcommissioninternational.org/.

45. Okamoto and Tatara, *Public health of Japan, 2007*, 43; Ikegami and Campbell, *Art of balance*, 34. However, some physicians say relaxing such networks makes it difficult for rural hospitals to find staff and causes dislocation.

46. See *Mainichi Newspaper*, 22 September 1992; *Yomiuri Newspaper*, 19 November 1992; *Kyodo News*, 28 January 1993; *Asahi Newspaper*, 23 February 1993; MHW, Medical Economics Division, On the pacemaker problem, 20 April 1993.

47. See Rodwin and Okamoto, Physicians' conflict of interest in Japan and the United States.

48. Good Clinical Practice Guidelines, Notice from Chief of Pharmaceutical Affairs Bureau, 2 October 1989.

49. See the textbook for medical representatives: *Iyaku jōhōtantōsha no jōshiki to rinri [Knowledge and ethics for MR/ textbook for medical representatives]* (Tokyo: MIX Publishing, 1995).

50. Katherine Rupp, *Gift-giving in Japan: Cash, connections, cosmologies* (Stanford, CA: Stanford University Press, 2003).

51. In 2009, JFTC guidelines restricted these loans.

52. Anonymous interview 1, fall 2002.

53. Anonymous interview 2, fall 2002.

54. Anonymous interview 3, fall 2002.

55. The Premiums and Representations Act was amended and since 1 September 2009, the Consumer Affairs Agency has enforced it, not the JFTC.

56. Act against Unjustifiable Premiums and Misleading Representations, Act no. 134 of 15 May 1962, as amended by Act No. 44 of 30 May 1977. The act authorizes the JFTC to certify industry associations to develop codes to promote industry compliance. The Fair Trade Council of the Ethical Pharmaceutical Drugs Manufacturing Industry (FTCEPM) developed a Fair Competition Code. However, the code's definition of premiums is not clear. It allows payments that are "economic benefits which are found as discounts or after-sales services as part of normal business practices." It also allows firms to pay for business entertainment, labor, and other services, which might facilitate surreptitious payments.

57. Drug firms engaged in similar manipulation of average wholesale prices in the United States, with the result that Medicaid paid inflated prices for drugs. Around 2001, private firms and federal and state governments sued drug companies for fraud. Alex Sugerman-Brozan and James Woolman, Drug spending and the average wholesale price: Removing the AWP albatross from Medicaid's neck, *Pharmaceutical Law & Industry Report* 3, no. 35 (9 September 2005): 1–8.The problem persists. See Robert Pear, Drug makers accused of ignoring price law, *New York Times*, 3 October 2010, 22.

58. The Japan Fair Trade Commission Public Notice No. 31 of 1991. Restriction on Premium Offers in the Ethical Pharmaceutical Drugs Industry, the Medical Devices Industry and the Hygienic Inspection Laboratory Industry (The Japan Fair Trade Commission Public Notice No. 54 of 11 August 1997; Secretary General JFTC, *Guidelines concerning distribution systems and business practices under the anti-monopoly act*, 1991, Japan Fair Trade Commission, available at http://www.jftc.go.jp/e-page/legislation/ama/distribution.pdf (accessed 9 February 2010).

59. Resale price maintenance is prohibited by the Act on Prohibition of Private Monopolization and Maintenance of Fair Trade (1947, revised 2005) and implemented by the JFTC Unfair Trade Code issued 18 June 1982.

60. Japan Fair Trade Commission, *Fair competition code concerning restriction on premium offers in ethical pharmaceutical drugs marketing industry*, issued 10 March 1984, revised 11 August 1997 and 1 October 2007; Japan Fair Trade Commission, Public notice no. 31 of 1991; Japan Fair Trade Commission, Public notice no. 54 of 11 August 1997.

61. Fair Trade Council of the Ethical Pharmaceutical Drugs Marketing Industry, *Fair competition code concerning restrictions on premium offers in ethical pharmaceutical drugs marketing industry* 1984, as revised in 1997 and 2007; Fair Trade Council of the Ethical Pharmaceutical Drugs Marketing Industry, *Enforcement rules of the fair competition code concerning restrictions on premiums officers in the ethical pharmaceutical drugs marketing industry*, 1984 as revised in 1997 and 2005.

62. In 1993, the JPMA developed three sets of guidelines: (1) *Promotional code of pharmaceuticals* (March 1993), a revision of the 1976 Federation of Pharmaceutical Manufacturer Associations of Japan's *Code of practices for the promotion of ethical drugs*; (2) *Guidelines on gift-giving to health care providers permissible under JFTC rules*; (3) *Guidelines on remuneration for case reporting allowable under JFTC rules* (1993), revised as *Promotion code for prescription drugs* (23 May 2008), available at http://www.jpma.or.jp/english/isuues/pdf/2007code_e.pdf (accessed 17 November 2009). The JPMA modified its code of conduct again in 2008.

63. *Gekkan detēruman. Shin rūru no jisshi to māketingu no henka. [Monthly Detail-man*, Behavioral change under new rules] 21, no. 8 (1993): 48–51.

64. PMAT, *Organization correspondence contribution scheme for academic society which used the associations as a focal point* (typescript); interview with Osamu Nagayama, president and chief executive officer of Chugai Pharmaceutical Co. and president of the JPMA, 12 November 2002; correspondence with Takashi Sakabe, executive secretary to Osamu Nagayama, 18 November 2002. The 2007 data are from correspondence with Shigeo Morioka, 25 June 2008.

65. Interview with Ouchi Yasuyush, Tokyo University Medical School, 14 October 2002.

66. Japan Medical Association, *Physician's ethics code* (Tokyo: JMA, 1951); JMA Principles of medical ethics (Tokyo: JMA 2002). English summary of twenty-five-page text available at http://www.med.or.jp/english/about_JMA/principles.html (accessed 15 November 2009). The JMA guidelines for physician's professional ethics 2008, *Japan Medical Association Journal* 52, no. 2 (2009): 75–91.

67. Japan Medical Association, *Physician's ethics code* (1951), Principle 6; JMA, *Remuneration of doctors* (1951), ch. 3, clause 3.

68. This report is a revision of Japan Medical Association, Committee on Bioethics, Social responsibility expected of doctors: In search of good professionalism, *Journal of the Japan Medical Association* 116, no. 3 (1996): 243–50.

69. Physicians' Act, Sec. 7 (1) (2).

70. There are set terms for suspension: one month, two months, three months, one year, two years, three years, or five years, depending on the severity of the offense.

71. Nikkei.net Interactive, reporting on Nihon Keizai Shimbun, 9 February 2004.

72. Analysis by Estuji Okomoto using MHLW data.

73. The mix of incentives resembles an American proposal to pay hospitals a combination of prospective payment and fees for services actually used. See R. P. Ellis and Thomas G. McGuire, Provider behavior under prospective payment, *Journal of Health Economics* 5 no. 2 (1986): 129–51.

74. There are a few exceptions, however. See Eric Feldman, Blood justice: Courts, conflict, and compensation in Japan, France, and the United States, *Law and Society Review* 34, no. 3 (2000): 651–702; Eric Feldman, *The ritual of rights in Japan: Law, society, and health policy* (New York: Cambridge University Press, 2000).

CHAPTER 10

1. This typology is a revision of one that appeared in Marc A. Rodwin, *Medicine, money and morals: Physicians' conflicts of interest* (New York: Oxford University Press, 1993), 209.

2. *Shea v. Esensten*, 107 F.3d 625 (1997).

3. Arnold S. Relman and Uwe E. Reinhardt, An exchange on for-profit health care. In *For-profit enterprise in health care*, ed. B. H. Gray, 209–23 (Washington, DC: National Academy Press, 1986).

4. Maratoshi Abe, Japan's clinic physicians and their behavior, *Social Science and Medicine* 20, no. 4 (1985): 333–40.

5. 1928 Income Tax Unit Ruling 2421, I.T. 2421, VII-2 C.B. 150 (1928); IRS Revenue Ruling 69–545 (1969).

6. Carl F. Ameringer, *State medical boards and the politics of public protection* (Baltimore MD: Johns Hopkins University Press, 1999).

7. E. Haavi Morreim, Physician investment and self-referral: A philosophical analysis of a contentious debate, *Journal of Medicine and Philosophy* 15, no. 4 (1990): 425–48.

8. Tom Baker, *The medical malpractice myth* (Chicago: University of Chicago Press, 2005); Marc A. Rodwin, Hak J. Chang, Melissa M. Ozaeta, et al., Malpractice premiums in Massachusetts, a high-risk state: 1975 to 2005, *Health Affairs* 27, no. 3 (2008): 835–44.

9. See the articles by Robert Leflar cited in chapter 9, note 23.

10. This section draws on Marc A. Rodwin, Conflicts of interest: The limitations of disclosure, *NEJM* 321, no. 20 (1989): 1405–8; Don A. Moore and George Loewenstein, Self-interest, automaticity, and the psychology of conflict of interest, *Social Justice Research* 17, no. 2 (2004): 189–202; Don A. Moore, Daylian M. Cain, George Loewenstein, et al., *Conflicts of interest: Challenges and solutions from law, medicine and organization settings* (Cambridge: Cambridge University Press, 2004); Daylian M. Cain, George Loewenstein, and Don A. Moore, The dirt on coming clean: Perverse effects of disclosing conflicts of interest, *Journal of Legal Studies* 34, no. 1 (2005): 1–23.

11. Ruth R. Faden and Thomas L. Beauchamp, *A theory and history of informed consent* (New York: Oxford University Press, 1986), 298–336; Paul S. Appelbaum, Charles W. Lidz, and Alan Meisel, *Informed consent: Legal theory and clinical practice* (New York: Oxford University Press, 1987); T. M. Graunder, On the readability of surgical consent forms, *NEJM* 302, no. 16 (1980): 900–902.

12. Wim B. Liebrand, David M. Messick, and Fred J. Wolters, Why we are fairer than others? A cross-cultural replication and extension, *Journal of Experimental Social Psychology* 22, no. 6 (1986): 590–604.

13. Stanley Milgram, *Obedience to authority* (New York: Harper and Row, 1974); Leonard Bickman, The social power of a uniform, *Journal of Applied Social Psychology* 4, no. 1 (1974): 47–61.

14. Robert B. Cialdini, *Influence: Science and practice* (New York: HarperCollins, 1993).

15. Jay Katz, *The silent world of doctor and patient* (Baltimore, MD: Johns Hopkins University Press, 1984).

16. Robert Gibbons, Frank J. Landry, Denise Blouch, et al., A comparison of physicians and patients' attitudes toward pharmaceutical industry gifts, *Journal of General Internal Medicine* 13, no. 3 (1998): 151–54.

17. Timothy D. Wilson and Nancy Brekke, Mental contamination and mental correction: Unwanted influences on judgments and evaluations, *Psychological Bulletin* 116, no. 1 (1994): 117–42.

18. Judith H. Hibbard, Paul Slovic, and Jacquelyn J. Jewett, Informing consumer decisions in health care: Implications from decision-making research, *Milbank Quarterly* 75, no. 3 (1997): 395.

19. Leon Festinger, Informal social communication, *Psychology Review* 57, no. 5 (1950): 271–82; Jennifer Campbell Abraham and Susan Mickler, The role of social pressure, attention to the stimulus and self-doubt in conformity, *European Journal of Social Psychology* 13, no. 3 (1983): 217–33.

20. *Cipollone v. Liggette Group, Inc.*, 789 F. 2d 181 (3rd Cir. 1986).

21. *Riegel v. Medtronic, Inc.*, 552 U.S. 312 (2008).

22. Ashish K. Jha, Jonathan B. Perlin, Kenneth W. Kizer, et al., Effect of the transformation of the veterans affairs health care system on the quality of care, *NEJM* 348, no. 22 (2003): 2218–27.

23. Arnold S. Relman, The reform we need. In A. S. Relman, *A second opinion: Rescuing America's health care* (New York: Public Affairs, 2007), 111–30; Atul Gawande, The cost conundrum, *New Yorker*, 1 June 2009, 36–44.

24. There is also the risk that when these hospitals depend on the revenue they generate they will pay physicians in ways that create conflicts of interest.

25. For a discussion of various kinds of post-marketing clinical trials, see Stephen Glasser, Maribel Salas, and Elizabeth Delzell, Importance and challenges of studying marketed drugs: What is a phase IV study? Common clinical research designs, registries, and self-reporting system, *Journal of Clinical Pharmacology* 47, no. 9 (2007): 1074–86.

26. Some writers propose that medical societies cut the financial link but do not advocate legal prohibition. David J. Rothman, Walter J. McDonald, Carol D. Berkowitz, et al., Professional medical associations and their relationships with industry: A proposal for controlling conflicts of interest, *JAMA* 301, no. 13 (2009): 1367–72.

27. National health spending for 2008 was estimated at $2.4 billion, or about $7,900 per person, based on a July 2008 U.S. population estimate of 303,824,640. Sean Keehan, Andrea Sisko, Christopher Truffer, et al., Health spending projections through 2017: The baby-boom generation is coming to Medicare, *Health Affairs* 27 (2008): W145–55.

28. Benjamin Falit, Curbing industry sponsors' incentive to design post-approval trials that are suboptimal for informing prescribers but more likely than optimal designs to yield favorable results, *Seton Hall Law Review* 37, no. 4 (2007): 969–1049.

29. For similar proposals, see Marcia Angell, *The truth about drug companies: How they deceive us and what to do about it* (New York: Random House, 2004), 244–45; John Abramson, *Overdo$ed America: The broken promise of American medicine* (New York: Harper, 2004), 251.

30. Pascale Santi, Recours devant le conseil d'état contre les liens entre médecin et laboratoires, *Le Monde* 9 December 2009.

31. Marc A. Rodwin, Patient appeals as policy disputes: Individual and collective action in managed care. In *Impatient voices: Patients as policy actors*, ed. B. Hoffman, N. Tomes, R. Grob, et al. (New Brunswick, NJ: Rutgers University Press, in press). Marc A. Rodwin, Health reform, independent medical review, and the neglected complaint data (under review).

32. *Abdullahi v. Pfizer*, 562 F.3d 163 (2009); George J Annas, Globalized clinical trials and informed consent, *NEJM* 360, no. 20 (2009): 2050–53.

33. Deborah Cohen and Philip Carter, WHO and the pandemic flu "conspiracies," *British Medical Journal* 340, no. 7759 (2010): 1274–79.

CHAPTER 11

1. Eliot Freidson, States and associations. In Friedson, *Professionalism: The third logic* (Chicago: University of Chicago Press, 2001), 215.

2. There are few books that focus on comparative cross-national analysis of professions, particularly the medical profession. But see Elliot A. Krause, *Death of the guilds: Professions, states, and the advance of capitalism, 1930 to the present* (New Haven, CT: Yale University Press, 1996); Frederick Hafferty and John McKinlay, eds., *The changing medical profession: An international perspective* (New York: Oxford University Press, 1993); Patrick Hassenteufel, *Les médecins face à l'état* (Paris: Presses De Sciences Po, 1997); David Wilsford, *Doctors and the state: The politics of health care in France and the United States* (Durham, NC: Duke University Press, 1991).

3. I have edited and slightly revised his formulation: Eliot Freidson, *Professionalism: The third logic*, ch. 6, 127–51.

4. Sydney Webb and Beatrice Webb, Special supplement on professional associations, parts 1 and 2, *New Statesmen* 9, no. 211 (21 April 1917): 1–24; R. H. Tawney, *The acquisitive society* (New York: Harcourt Brace, 1920); Alexander Morris Carr-Saunders and P. A. Wilson, *The professions* (Oxford: Clarendon Press, 1933); T. H. Marshal, The recent history of professionalism in relation to social structure and social policy, *Canadian Journal of Economics and Political Science* 5, no. 3 (1939): 325–40. After World War II, American scholars recognized that professions could promote their self-interest, but they distinguished professions from other occupations because of their ethical values. Ernest Greenwood, Attributes of a profession, *Social Work* 2, no. 3 (1957): 45–55; Bernard Barber, Some problems in the sociology

of the professions, *Daedalus* 92, no. 43 (1963): 669–88; Harold L. Wilensky, The professionalization of everyone? *American Journal of Sociology* 70, no. 2 (1964): 137–58; Talcott Parsons, Professions. In *International encyclopedia of the social sciences*, ed. D. Sills, 536–47 (New York: Macmillan, 1968); William J. Goode, The theoretical limits of professionalization. In *The semi-professions and their organizations*, ed. A. Etzioni, 266–313 (New York: Free Press, 1969); Wilbert E. Moore, *The professions: Roles and rules* (New York: Russell Sage Foundation, 1971); Everett C. Hughes, *The sociological eye* (Chicago: Aldine, 1971).

5. For discussion of the relation of medieval corporations and guilds on modern French professions, see William H. Sewell, Jr., *Work and revolution in France: The language of labor from the old regime to 1848* (Cambridge: Cambridge University Press, 1980); Jacques Le Goff, Les métiers et l'organisation du travail dans la France médiéval. In *La France et les français*, ed. M. François, 310–33 (Paris: Gallimard, 1980). For the relation of the state to the creation of professions and social groupings in France, see Pierre Rosanvallon, *L'État en France de 1789 a nos jours* (Paris: Seuil, 1990); François Edwald, *L'État-providence* (Paris: Fayard, 1986); Jean-Daniel Reynaud, *Les règles du jeu: L'action collective et la régulation sociale* (Paris: Armand Colin, 1989). Occupational and religion are explored by the great French sociologist Émile Durkheim, in *The division of labor in society*, trans. George Simpson ([1893] New York: Free Press, 2008) and *The elementary forms of religious life*, trans. Joseph Ward Swain ([1912] Mineola, NY: Dover 2008). For contemporary French sociology on professions, see Claude Dubar et Pierre Tripier, *Sociologie des professions* (Paris: Armand Colin, 1998). For discussion of professions in France, see particularly ch. 1, La profession-corps, Le modèle "catholique" des corps d'état, 21–35, and ch. 7–13, 141–245. See also Florent Champy, *La sociologie des professions* (Paris: Presses Universitaires de France, 2009).

6. George Bernard Shaw, Preface to *The doctor's dilemma* ([1913]; Baltimore: Penguin, 1988); Adam Smith, *The wealth of nations* ([1776]; Baltimore: Penguin, 1970).

7. Robert M. Veatch, *Patient-physician relationship. The patient as partner*, part II (Bloomington: Indiana University Press, 1991); James I. Charlton, *Nothing about us without us: Disability, oppression, empowerment* (Berkeley: University of California Press, 1998).

8. Irving Kenneth Zola, Medicine as an institution of social control, *Social Review* 20, no. 487 (1972): 487–504; Sandra Morgen, *Into our own hands: The women's health movement in the United States, 1969–1990* (Rutgers: Rutgers University Press, 2002); Marc A. Rodwin, Patient accountability and quality of care: Lessons from medical consumerism and the patients' rights, women's health and disability rights movements, *American Journal of Law and Medicine* 20, no. 1 and 2 (1994): 147–67.

9. Ivan Illich, *Medical nemesis: The expropriation of health* (New York: Pantheon Books, 1976); Deborah Stone, *The limits of professional power: National health care in the Federal Republic of Germany* (Chicago: University of Chicago Press, 1980).

10. Julius A. Roth, Professionalism: The sociologists' decoy, *Work and Occupations* 1, no. 1 (1974): 6; Corinne Lathrop Gilb, *Hidden hierarchies: The professions and*

government (Westport, CT: Greenwood Press, 1976); Caroline Barth et Richard Vargas, *Quand l'ordre règne: L'ordre des médecins en question* (Paris: Mango Document, 2001); Claude Béraud, Le rapport Béraud, *Le Concours Médical* 114, no. 30 (3 October 1992): 2616–2724; Y. Audere et G. Delteil, *La médecine malade de l'argent* (Paris: Edition de l'Atelier, 1994).

11. Milton Friedman and Simon Kuznets, *Income from independent professional practice* (New York: National Bureau of Economic Research, 1945); Milton Friedman and Rose D. Friedman, Occupational licensure. In Friedman and Friedman, *Capitalism and freedom* ([1962] Chicago: University of Chicago Press, 2002), 137–63; Lionel Jeffrey Berlant, *Profession and monopoly: A study of medicine in the United States and Great Britain* (Berkeley: University of California Press, 1975), 64–127; Charles Weller, "Free choice" as a restraint of trade, and the counterintuitive contours of competition, *Health Matrix* 3, no. 2 (1985): 3–23; Clark C. Havighurst, The doctors' trust: Self-regulation and the law, *Health Affairs* 2, no. 3 (1983): 64–76. Clark C. Havighurst, Antitrust enforcement in the medical services industry: What does it all mean? *The Milbank Quarterly* 58, no.1 (1980): 89–124.

12. Arnold S. Relman, The new medical-industrial complex, *NEJM* 303, no. 17 (1980): 963–70; Arnold S. Relman, Dealing with conflicts of interest, *NEJM* 310, no. 18 (1984): 1182–83. Also see Marc A. Rodwin, Medical commerce, physician entrepreneurialism, and conflicts of interest, *Cambridge Quarterly of Healthcare Ethics* 16, no. 4 (2007): 387–97, and five other articles on commercialism and medicine in that issue. David Mechanic, *From advocacy to allocation: The evolving American health care system* (New York: Free Press, 1986), 146; William M. Sullivan, What is left of professionalism after managed care? *Hastings Center Report* 29, no. 2 (2004): 7.

13. Steven Brint, *In an age of experts: The changing role of professionals in politics and public life* (Princeton, NJ: Princeton University Press, 1994), 202–9, 23, 7–8, 17, and 16. Brint says "professions are based on the link between tasks for which . . . market demand exists; training provided by the higher educational system . . . and a privileged access of trained workers to the market," 23.

14. Freidson, *Professionalism: The third logic*, 222; Eliot Freidson, *Professionalism reborn: Theory, prophecy, and policy* (Chicago: University of Chicago Press, 1994).

Freidson's early work revealed that professionals do not adequately regulate themselves and that "professional ideologies . . . claim . . . more for the profession's knowledge and skill, and a broader jurisdiction than can in fact be justified." Eliot Freidson, *The professions and their prospects* (Beverly Hills, CA: Sage, 1971), 17–38. See also Eliot Freidson, *Professional dominance: The social structure of medical care* (New York: Atherton, 1970); Eliot Freidson, *Doctoring together: A study of professional social control* (Chicago: University of Chicago Press, 1984).

15. William M. Sullivan, Can professionalism still be a viable ethic? *The Good Society* 13, no. 1 (2004): 15–20.

16. Kenneth J. Arrow, Social responsibility and economic efficiency, *Public Policy* 21(Summer 1973): 303–17; Kenneth J. Arrow, Uncertainty and the welfare economics of medical care, *American Economic Review* 53, no. 5 (1963): 941–73; Victor R. Fuchs, Economics, values and health care reform, *American Economic Review* 86,

no. 1 (1996): 17. Fuchs adds that physicians "must be . . . held to certain standards of behavior different from those assumed by models of market competition or government regulation."

17. Eliot Freidson, *Professionalism: The third logic*, see especially Introduction, 1–17; ch. 8, The assault on professionalism, 179–96; ch. 9 The soul of professionalism, 197–222; Eliot Freidson, *Professionalism reborn: Theory, prophecy, and policy* (Chicago: University of Chicago Press, 1994).

18. Hughes, *Sociological eye*; Ezra N. Suleiman, *Elites in French society* (Princeton, NJ: Princeton University Press, 1978); Dubar et Tripier, *Sociologie des professions*, 21–35.

19. Magali Sarfatti Larson, *The rise of professionalism* (Berkeley: University of California Press, 1977); Eliot Freidson, Occupational autonomy and labor market shelters. In *Varieties of work*, ed. P. L. Steward and M. G. Cantor, 39–54 (Beverly Hills, CA: Sage, 1983).

20. Guidelines themselves may reflect conflicts of interest. Darshak Sanghavi, Plenty of guidelines, but where's the evidence? *New York Times*, 9 December 2008.

21. Egenia Delcheva, Dinva Balabanova, and Martin McKee, Under-the-counter payments for health care: Evidence from Bulgaria, *Health Policy* 42, no. 2 (1997): 89–100.

22. Donna Evleth, The ordre des medecins and the Jews in Vichy France, 1940–1944, *French History* 20, no. 2 (2006): 204–24; Michael R. Marrus, Robert O. Paxton, and Stanley Hoffmann, *Vichy France and the Jews* (Stanford, CA: Stanford University Press, 1995).

23. George J. Annas and Michael A. Grodin, *The Nazi doctors and the Nuremberg code: Human rights in human experimentation* (New York: Oxford University Press, 1995); Mark G. Field, Structured strain in the role of the Soviet physician, *American Journal of Sociology* 58, no. 5 (1953): 493–502; George J. Annas, Hunger strikes at Guantanamo: Medical ethics and human rights in a legal black hole, *NEJM* 355, no. 13 (2006): 1377–82.

24. Since 1976, the Hyde Amendment has prohibited the use of federal funds for abortions under the Medicaid program except in cases of rape or incest.

25. Freidson, *Doctoring together*, 263; Charles Bosk, *Forgive and remember: Managing medical failure* (Chicago: University of Chicago Press, 1979); Carl J. Ameringer, *State medical boards and the politics of public protection* (Baltimore, MD: Johns Hopkins University Press, 1999).

26. Prescrire English, http://english.prescrire.org/en/; Prescrire French, http://www.prescrire.org/fr/

27. Formindep, http://www.formindep.org/

28. http://www.nofreelunch.org/.

29. http://www.healthyskepticism.org/.

30. ABIM Foundation, ACP-ASIM Foundation, and European Federation of Internal Medicine, Medical professionalism in the new millennium: A physician charter, *Annals of Internal Medicine* 136, no. 3 (2002): 242.

31. Russell L. Gruen, Steven D. Pearson, and Troyen A. Brennan, Physician-citizens: Public roles and professional organizations, *JAMA* 291, no. 1 (2004): 94–98. The Open Society Institute, Program on Medicine as a Profession was one of the leaders: see http://www.soros.org/initiatives/map. Its work continues through the Institute on Medicine as a Profession at Columbia University: http://www.imapny.org/.

32. Freidson, *Professionalism: The third logic*, 222. For some examples, see also Deborah Stone, The Samaritan rebellion, ch. 4 in *The Samaritan's dilemma: Should government help your neighbor?* (New York: Nation Books, 2008), 137–74.

33. Global Lawyers and Physicians for Human Rights, http://www.globallawyer-sandphysicians.org/.

34. David Mechanic, Managed care and the imperative for a new professional ethic, *Health Affairs* 19, no. 5 (2000): 100–11.

35. David Mechanic, Rethinking medical professionalism: The role of information technology and practice innovation, *Milbank Quarterly* 86, no. 2 (2008): 368–88.

36. Several organizations that are not physician directed or physician membership organizations help counter conflicts of interest in medicine. Among others, these include in the United States, The Public Citizen Health Research Group, http://www.citizen.org/hrg/ and Center for Science in the Public Interest, http://www.citizen.org/hrg/; in France, Fondation Sciences Citoyennes, http://sciencescitoyennes.org/

APPENDIX

1. Marc A. Rodwin, The organized American medical profession's response to financial conflicts of interest: 1890–1992, *Milbank Quarterly* 70, no. 4 (1992): 703–41.

2. William L. Burdick, *The principles of Roman law and their relation to modern law* (Rochester, NY: Lawyers Co-operative, 1938): *fideicommissa*, 619–25; fiduciary sale, 379–83. See also William W. Buckland, *Equity in Roman law* ([1911]; Buffalo, NY: William S. Hein, 1983).

3. Jean-Jacques Rousseau, *The social contract* ([1762]; Mineola, NY: Dover, 2003), 168; Elisabeth Zoller, *Introduction to public law: A comparative study* (Koninklijke Bill: Martinus Nijhoff, 2008): 1–21.

4. La loi n. 83–634 du 13 juillet 1983 portant droits et obligations des fonctionnaires (dite loi Le Pors), article 25 alinéa 2. See also Lionel Benaiche, *Expertise en Santé Publique et Principe de Précaution*, Report for the Ministry of Justice and the Ministry of the Economy, Finance, and Industry, 12 August 2004. The terms *conflit d'intérêts* and *intérêts contradictoires* are used in French public law and public administration; however, the French also speak of *désintéressement* (impartiality) as an ideal and *ingérence* (inappropriate meddling in commerce). Serge Salon and Jean-Charles

Savignac, *La Fonction Publique* (Paris: Dalloz-Sirey, 2009), 233–42; John A. Rohr, Ethical issues in French public administration: A comparative study, *Public Administration Review* 51, no. 4 (1991): 283–97

5. Loi du 24 juillet 1966. See also Dominique Schmidt, *Les conflits d'intérêts dans la société anonyme* (Paris: Joly, 1999).

6. For the history, see Claude Witz, *La fiducie en droit privé Français* (Paris: Economica, 1981), 4. For recent developments, see François Barrière, La fiducie, *Recueil Dalloz* 20 (2007): 1346–74; J. de Guillenchmidt, Présentation de l'avant-projet de loi relative a la fiducie (colloque du 5 avril 1990); Christian Larroumet, *La Fiducie inspirée du trust* (Paris: Recueil Dalloz, 1990): chron. 119–121; Madeleine Cantin-Cumyn, *L'avant Projet de loi relatif a la fiducie, un point de vue civiliste d'outre-atlantique* (Paris: Recueil Dalloz, 1992): 117–121; Article 2001, Code Civil, Loi No 2007–211 du 19 février 2007 (JO 21 février, p. 3052).

7. Buckland, *Equity in Roman law.*

8. Percy H. Winfield, *The chief sources of English legal history* (New York: Burt Franklin, 1925), 54–70; Burdick, *Principles of Roman law and their relation to modern law*, 56–86; Henry Maine, *Ancient law: Its connection with the early history of society and its relation to modern ideas* (Boston: Beacon Press, 1932).

9. William W. Buckland and Arnold McNair, *Roman law and common law: A comparison in outline* (Cambridge: Cambridge University Press, 1952), 176–79.

10. K.W. Swart, *Sale of offices in the seventeenth century* (The Hague: Martinus Nijhoff, 1949).

11. See Mabry E. Rogers and Stephen B. Young, Public office as a public trust: A suggestion that impeachment for high crimes and misdemeanors implies a fiduciary standard, *Georgetown Law Journal* 63, no. 5 (1975): 1025–49; John Locke, *Second treatise on civil government* (Indianapolis, IN: Hackett, 1980), Section 131: "But though men, when they enter into society, give up the equality, liberty, and executive power they had in the state of nature, into the hands of the society, to be so far disposed of by the legislative, as the good of the society shall require; yet it being only with an intention in every one the better to preserve himself, his liberty and property; . . . the power of the society, or legislative constituted by them, can never be supposed to extend farther, than the common good; . . . and so whoever has the legislative or supreme power of any common-wealth, is bound to govern by established standing laws, promulgated and known to the people, and not by extemporary decrees; by indifferent and upright judges, who are to decide controversies by those laws; . . . And all this to be directed to no other end, but the peace, safety, and public good of the people."

12. Commercial Code, Article 254–3; Masafumi Nakahigashi, Shōhō Kaisei Shōwa 25/Shōwa 26 [The 1950–51 Amendments to /the Commercial Code]; Hideki Kanda and Curtis J. Milhaupt, Reconsidering legal transplants: Directors' fiduciary duty in Japanese corporate law, *American Journal of Comparative Law* 51, no. 4 (2003): 887–901. Article 265, self-dealing; Article 269, compensation; Article 264, competition. See also Commerce Act, Duty of Loyalty Section 265, Prohibition on bribes,

§ 486–493. Chizu Nakajima, *Conflicts of interest and duty: A comparative analysis in Anglo-Japanese law* (The Hague: Kluwer Law International, 1999).

13. Civil Codes Sections, 108, 57. Section 57 also deals with obligation of directors of corporations.

14. Japan's Criminal Code § 197–98 prohibits public employees from accepting bribes. The Commerce Act Section 265 established a duty of loyalty and § 486–493 prohibits executives in investor-owned corporations from accepting bribes that jeopardize the corporate interest. Criminal Codes §.247 (breach of fiduciary obligations) § 197–98 (bribes and gifts); The Lawyers Act § 26.

15. For transparency in France, see Adam Gopnik, Private domain, *New Yorker*, 13 November 1995, 74–80; C. Raj Kumar, Corruption in Japan: Institutionalizing the right to information, transparency and the right to corruption-free governance, *New England Journal of International and Comparative Law*, 10, no. 1 (2004): 1–30.

16. Burdick, *Roman law*, 457–61.

17. For a comparison of mandate contracts to common law agency and fiduciary law, see Wendell H. Holmes and Symeon C. Symedonides, Representation, mandate, and agency: A commentary on Louisiana's new law, *Tulane Law Review* 73, no. 4 (1999): 1087–159.

18. Japanese Civil Code Section 100, Mandate, Part 1643–1565; Section 11, Bailment; Section 12, Partnership; Agency, 3–108.

Bibliography

ABBREVIATIONS

JAMA   *Journal of the American Medical Association*
NEJM   *New England Journal of Medicine*

Abe, Maratoshi. 1985. Japan's clinic physicians and their behavior. *Social Science and Medicine* 20 (4): 333–40.

Abraham, Jennifer Campbell, and Susan Mickler. 1983. The role of social pressure, attention to the stimulus and self-doubt in conformity. *European Journal of Social Psychology* 13 (3): 217–33.

Abramson, John. 2004. *Overdo$ed America: The broken promise of American medicine.* New York: Harper.

Adams, Samuel Hopkins. 1905. *The great American fraud.* New York: P. F. Collier and Son.

Adams, Thomas McStay. 1990. *Bureaucrats and beggars: French social policy in the age of the Enlightenment.* New York: Oxford University Press.

Als-Nielsen, Bodil, Wendong Chen, Christian Glund, et al. 2003. Association of funding and conclusions in randomized drug trials: A reflection of treatment effect or adverse events? *JAMA* 290 (7): 921–28.

Altman, Stuart H., and Marc A. Rodwin. 1988. Halfway competitive markets and ineffective regulation: The American health care system. *Journal of Health Politics, Policy and Law* 13 (2): 323–39.

American Board of Internal Medicine (ABIM) Foundation, American College of Physicians (ACP), American Society of Internal Medicine (ASIM) Foundation, and European Federation of Internal Medicine. 2002. Medical professionalism in the new millennium: A physician charter. *Annals of Internal Medicine* 136 (3): 243–46.

American College of Surgeons (ACS). 1959. Position of American College of Surgeons on proration of insurance payments. *Bulletin of the American College of Surgeons* 44 (1): 5–8.

American Medical Association (AMA). 1900. Secret nostrums and the journal. *JAMA* 34 (22): 1420.

American Medical Association (AMA). 1902. Association News. *JAMA* 38 (25): 1661.

American Medical Association (AMA). 1907. Hospital and dispensary abuse. *JAMA* 48 (7): 613–15. Reprinted 2007, *JAMA* 297 (6): 651.

American Medical Association (AMA). 1907. Medical economics: Contract practice. *JAMA* 49 (24): 2028–29.

American Medical Association (AMA). 1925. Hospital service in the United States. *JAMA* 84 (13): 961–67.

American Medical Association (AMA). 1933. Medical economics: Private group practice. *JAMA* 100 (21): 1693–99.

American Medical Association (AMA). 1986. Report of the Council on Ethical and Judicial Affairs, A(I-86): Conflicts of interest.

American Medical Association (AMA), Bureau of Economics. 1934. The insurance principle in the practice of medicine. *JAMA* 102 (19): 1612–18.

American Medical Association (AMA), Bureau of Medical Economics. 1934. *A critical analysis of sickness insurance.* Chicago: AMA.

American Medical Association (AMA), Council on Judicial Affairs (CEJA). 1991. Conflicts of interest: Physician ownership of medical facilities, Report C (I-91).

American Medical Association, Council on Pharmacy and Chemistry. 1905. Report of the Council. *JAMA* 40:265–66.

American Medical Association, Council on Pharmacy and Chemistry. 1905. The secret nostrum vs. the ethical proprietary preparation. *JAMA* 40 (8): 718–19.

American Medical Association (AMA), Council on Pharmacy and Chemistry. 1955. New program of operation for evaluation of drugs. *JAMA* 158 (13): 1170–72.

American Medical Association (AMA), House of Delegates. 1903. *Principles of medical ethics.* Available at http://www.ama-assn.org/ama1/pub/upload/mm/43/1903principlesofethi.pdf (accessed 10 November 2009).

American Medical Association (AMA), House of Delegates. 1934. Sickness insurance problems in the United States. *JAMA* 102 (26): 2200–2201.

American Medical Association (AMA), House of Delegates. 1989. Physicians' involvement in commercial ventures: Status report. *Proceedings* (December): 131–32.

American Medical Association (AMA), House of Delegates. 1942–present. *Proceedings.*

American Medical Association (AMA), Organization Section, 1942. *JAMA* 111 (1): 59–60.

Ameringer, Carl F. 1999. *State medical boards and the politics of public protection.* Baltimore, MD: Johns Hopkins University Press.

Ameringer, Carl F. 2008. *The health care revolution: From medical monopoly to market competition.* Berkeley: University of California Press.

Andersen, Morten, Jakob Kragstrup, and Jens Sondergaard. 2006. How conducting a clinical trial affects physicians' guideline adherence and drug preferences. *JAMA* 295 (23): 2759–64.

Anderson, Odin W., Patricia Collette, and Jacob J. Feldman. 1963. *Changes in family medical expenditures and voluntary health insurance: A five-year resurvey.* Cambridge, MA: Harvard University Press.

Angel, Marcia. 2004. *The truth about drug companies: How they deceive us and what to do about it.* New York: Random House.

Annas, George J. 1974. The hospital: A human rights wasteland. *Civil Liberties Review* 1 (4): 9–29.

Annas, George J. 1975. *The rights of hospital patients.* New York: Avon.

Annas, George J. 2006. Hunger strikes at Guantanamo: Medical ethics and human rights in a legal black hole. *NEJM* 355 (13): 1377–82.

Annas, George J. 2009. Globalized clinical trials and informed consent. *NEJM* 360 (20): 2050–53.

Annas, George J., and Michael A. Grodin. 1995. *The Nazi doctors and the Nuremburg Code: Human rights in human experimentation.* New York: Oxford University Press.

Aoki, I. 1988. Shōki iryō-riyō kumiai no shōsō, *Han-Nan Rōnshū* [Evolution of early state of medical co-operatives society, *Social Science*] 24 (1988): 1–18, 41–55 (in Japanese).

Applebaum, Leon. 1961. The development of voluntary health insurance in the United States. *Journal of Risk and Insurance* 28 (3): 25–33.

Appelbaum, Paul S., Charles W. Lidz, and Alan Meisel. 1987. *Informed consent: Legal theory and clinical practice.* New York: Oxford University Press.

Arai, Ko. 2006. Reforming hospital costing practices in Japan: An implementation study. *Financial Accountability & Management* 22 (4): 425–51.

Arrow, Kenneth J. 1963. Uncertainty and the welfare economics of medical care. *American Economic Review* 53 (5): 941–73.

Arrow, Kenneth J. 1973. Social responsibility and economic efficiency. *Public Policy* 21 (Summer): 303–17.

Audere, Y., et G. Delteil. 1994. *La médecine malade de l'argent.* Paris: Edition de l'Atelier.

Baker, Tom. 2005. *The medical malpractice myth.* Chicago: University of Chicago Press.

Barber, Bernard. 1963. Some problems in the sociology of the professions. *Daedalus* 92 (43): 669–88.

Barth, Caroline, and Richard Vargas. 2001. *Quand l'ordre règne: L'ordre des médecins en question.* Paris: Mango Document.

Bazzoli, Gloria J., Stephen M. Shortell, Nicole Dubbs, et al. 1999. A taxonomy of health networks and systems: Bringing order out of chaos. *Health Services Research* 33 (3): 1683–717.

Bekelman, Justin E., Yan Li, and Cary P. Gross. 2003. Scope and impact of financial conflicts of interest in biomedical research: A systematic review. *JAMA* 289 (4): 454–65.

Benaiche, Lionel. 2004. *Expertise en santé publique et principe de précaution.* Report for the Ministry of Justice and the Ministry of the Economy, Finance, and Industry. 12 August.

Béraud, Claude. 1992. Le rapport Béraud. *Le Concours Médical* 114, no. 30 (3 October): 2616–2724.

Berlant, Jeffrey Lionel. 1975. *Profession and monopoly: A study of medicine in the United States and Great Britain.* Berkeley: University of California Press.

Berman-Sandler, Leatrice. 2004. Independent medical review: Expanding legal remedies to achieve managed care accountability. *Annals of Health Law* 13 (1): 233–302.

Bevan, Arthur Dean. 1928. Cooperation in medical education and medical services: Functions of the medical profession, of the university and of the public. *JAMA* 90 (15): 1173–77.

Bickman, Leonard. 1974. The social power of a uniform. *Journal of Applied Social Psychology* 4 (1): 47–61.

Blau, Peter M. 1964. *Exchange and power in social life.* New York: John Wiley.

Blum, John. 1993. Evaluation of medical staff using fiscal factors: Economic credentialing. *Journal of Health and Hospital Law* 26 (3): 65–72, 82.

Blumenthal, David. 1994. The vital role of professionalism in health care reform. *Health Affairs* 13 (1): 252–56.

Bodenheimer, Thomas. 2000. Uneasy alliance: Clinical investigators and the pharmaceutical industry. *NEJM* 342 (20): 1539–42.

Bosk, Charles L. 1979. *Forgive and remember: Managing medical failure.* Chicago: University of Chicago Press.

Bosk, Charles L. 2006. Avoiding conventional understandings: The enduring legacy of Eliot Friedson. *Sociology of Health & Illness* 28 (5): 637–53.

Bourgeois, Léon. 1896. *Solidarité.* Paris: Armand Colin.

Bowman, John G. 1919. General hospitals of 100 or more beds. *Bulletin of the American College of Surgeons* 5 (1): 66–69.

Bowman, Marjorie A. 1986. The impact of drug company funding on the content of continuing medical education. *Mobius* 6 (1): 66–69.

Bowman, Marjorie A., and David L. Pearle. 1988. Changes in drug prescribing patterns related to commercial company funding of continuing medical education. *Journal of Continuing Education in the Health Professions* 8 (1): 13–20.

Brennan, Troyen A. 1994. Buying editorials. *NEJM* 331 (10): 673–75.

Brint, Steven. 1994. *In an age of experts: The changing role of professionals in politics and public life.* Princeton, NJ: Princeton University Press.

Brockliss, Laurence, and Colin Jones. 1997. *The medical world of early modern France.* New York: Oxford University Press.

Brown, Lawrence D. 1983. *Politics and health care organization: HMOs as federal policy.* Washington, DC: Brookings Institution.

Brown, Lawrence D., and Elizabeth Eagan. 2004. The paradoxical politics of provider reempowerment. *Journal of Health Politics, Policy and Law* 29 (6): 1045–72.

Buchmueller, Thomas C., and Agnès Couffinhal. 2004. Private health insurance in France. Organization for Economic Cooperation and Development (OECD), Health Working Papers, No. 12. ESLSA/ELSA/WD/HEA(2004)3. Available at http://www.oecd.org/dataoecd/35/11/30455292.pdf (accessed 10 November 2009).

Buckland, William W. [1911] 1983. *Equity in Roman law.* London: University of London Press; reprint Buffalo, NY: William S. Hein.

Buckland, William W., and Arnold McNair. [1936] 1952. *Roman law and common law: A comparison in outline.* Cambridge: Cambridge University Press.

Burdick, William L. 1938. *The principles of Roman law and their relation to modern law.* Rochester, NY: Lawyers Co-operative.

Burrows, James G. 1977. *Organized medicine in the Progressive era: The move toward monopoly.* Baltimore, MD: Johns Hopkins University Press.

Cain, Daylian M., George Loewenstein, and Don A. Moore. 2005. The dirt on coming clean: Perverse effects of disclosing conflicts of interest. *Journal of Legal Studies* 34 (1): 1–23.

Calabro, Sheryl. 2004. Breaking the shield of the learned intermediary doctrine: Placing the blame where it belongs. *Cardozo Law Review* 25 (6): 2241–16.

Campbell, Eric, Russell Gruen, James Mountford, et al. 2007. A national survey of physician-industry relationships. *NEJM* 356 (17): 1742–50.

Campbell, John Creighton, and Naoki Ikegami. 1998. *The art of balance in health policy: Maintaining Japan's low-cost, egalitarian system.* New York: Cambridge University Press.

Cantin-Cumyn, Madeleine. 1992. *L'avant projet de loi relatif a la fiducie: un point de vue civiliste d'outre-atlantique.* Paris: Recueil Dalloz, 117–21.

Carlson, Robert. 1999. Is there a physician union in your future? *Family Practice Management* 6 (1): 21–25.

Carr-Saunders, Alexander Morris, and P. A. Wilson. 1933. *The Professions.* Oxford: Clarendon Press.

Casalino, Lawrence P. 1992. Balancing incentives: How should physicians be reimbursed? *JAMA* 267 (3): 403.

Catrice-Lorey, Antoinette. 1982. *La dynamique interne de la sécurité sociale, du système de pouvoir à la fonction personnelle.* Paris: Economica.

Chadalat, Jean-François. 2003. *La répartition des interventions entre les assurances maladies obligatoires et complémentaires en matière de dépense de santé.* Paris: Commission des comptes de la sécurité sociale.

Champy, Florent. 2009. *La Sociologie des professions.* Paris: Presses Universitaires France.

Chase-Lubitz, Jeffrey F. 1987. The corporate practice of medicine doctrine: An anachronism in the modern health care industry. *Vanderbilt Law Review* 40 (2): 445–88.

Chatriot, Alain. 2002. *La démocratie sociale à la française: L'expérience du conseil national économique 1924–1940.* Paris: Éditions la Découverte.

Chevit, P. 1978. L'ordre des médecins. Thèse de Médecine, Faculté de Médecine de St. Antoine, Paris.

Chino, Tetsurō. 2007. An economic analysis of institutions and regulations in the Japanese healthcare system. *Government Auditing Review* 14 (March): 13–25.

Choudhry, Niteesh K., Henry Thomas Stelfox, and Allan S. Detsky. 2002. Relationships between authors of clinical practice guidelines and the pharmaceutical industry. *JAMA* 287 (5): 612–17.

Chren, Margaret M., and C. Seth Landefeld. 1994. Physicians' behavior and their interactions with drug companies: A controlled study of physicians who requested additions to a hospital drug formulary. *JAMA* 271 (9): 684–89.

Cialdini, Robert B. 1993. *Influence: Science and practice.* New York: HarperCollins.

Cibrié, Paul. 1954. *Syndicalisme médical.* Paris: Confédération des Syndicat Médicaux Français.

Clapesattle, Helen. 1941. *The doctors Mayo.* Minneapolis: University of Minnesota Press.

Cohen, Deborah, and Philip Carter. 2010. WHO and the pandemic flu "conspiracies." *British Medical Journal* 340 (7759): 1274–79.

Colby, Mark A. 2004. *The Japan healthcare debate: Diverse perspectives.* Folkestone: Global Oriental.

Commission on Financing Hospital Care. 1955. Prepayment and community. In *Financing of hospital care in the United States*, vol. 2, ed. Harry Becker. New York: Blakiston.

Committee on Cost of Medical Care. 1932. Medical care for the American people: Final report. Reprinted in U.S. DHEW, Public Health Service. 1970. Health Services and Mental Health Administration, Community Health Services. Washington, DC: Government Printing Office.

Corteze, Nathan. 2008. International health care convergence: The benefits and burdens of market-driven standardization. *Wisconsin International Law Journal* 26 (3): 646–704.

Cosgrove, Lisa, Sheldon Krimsky, Manisha Vijayaraghavan, et al. 2006. Financial ties between DSM-IV panel members and the pharmaceutical industry. *Psychotherapy and Psychosomatics* 75 (3): 154–60.

Couffinhal, Agnès, and Valérie Paris. 2001. Utilization fees imposed to public heath care system users in France. Available at http://www.irdes.eu/EspaceAnglais/Publications/OtherPubs/UtilisationFeesImposedFrance.pdf (accessed 10 November 2009).

Couffinhal, Agnès, and Valérie Paris. 2003. Cost sharing in France. Working Paper. Available at http://www.irdes.fr/english/wp/CostSharing.pdf (accessed 10 November 2009).

Council for the Promotion of Regulatory Reform (CPRR). 2004. First report on the promotion of regulatory reform and the opening up of government-driven markets for entry into the private sector. 24 December. Available at http://www8.cao.go.jp/kisei-kaikaku/old/publication/2004/1224/item041224_02e.pdf (accessed 1 September 2010).

Cunningham, Robert III, and Robert Cunningham, Jr. 1997. *The Blues: A history of the Blue Cross and Blue Shield system.* DeKalb: Northern Illinois University Press.

Dana, Jason, and George Loewenstein. 2003. A social science perspective on gifts to physicians from industry. *JAMA* 290 (2): 252–55.

Davis, Loyal. 1960. *Fellowship of surgeons: A history of the American College of Surgeons.* Springfield, IL: Charles C. Thomas.

De Kervasdoué, Jean. 1980. La politique d'État en matière d'hospitalisation privée (1962–1978), analyse des conséquences contradictoires. *Les Annales Economiques* 16:25–56.

De Kervasdoué, Jean, ed. 2000. *Le carnet de santé de la France 2000.* Paris: Mutualité Française/Editions Dunod.

De Kervasdoué, Jean, ed. 2003. *Le carnet de santé de la France 2003.* Paris: Mutualité Française/Editions Dunod.

De Kervasdoué, Jean, ed. 2009. *Le carnet de santé de la France 2009: Economie, droit et politiques de santé.* Paris: Dunod.

De Kervasdoué, Jean. 2009. *Très chèr santé.* Paris: Perrin.

De Kervasdoué, Jean, et Rémi Pellet, eds. 2002. *Le carnet de santé de la France 2000–2002.* Paris: Editions Dunod.

De Kervasdoué, Jean, et Rémi Pellet, eds. 2006. *Le carnet de santé de la France 2006: Economie, droit et politiques de sante.* Paris: Dunod.

De Kervasdoue, Jean, et Henri Picheral, eds. 2004. *Le carnet de santé de la France 2004: Santé et territoire.* Paris: Editions Dunod.

Delaunay, Paul. 1906. *Le monde médical Parisien au dix-huitième siècle.* Paris: Jules Rousset.

Delaunea, Paul. 1935. *La vie médicale aux XVIIe et XVIIIe siècles.* Paris: Hippocrate.

Delcheva, Eugenia, Dinva Balabanova, and Martin McKee. 1997. Under-the-counter payments for health care: Evidence from Bulgaria. *Health Policy* 42 (2): 89–100.

Desrosieres, Alain. 1977. Éléments pour l'histoire des nomenclatures professionnelles. In *Pour une histoire de la statistique,* Tome 1, INEE.

Desrosieres, Alain, and Laurent Théveont. 2002. *Les catégories socio-professionnelles.* Paris: La Découverte.

Dorsey, E. Ray, Jason de Roulet, Joel P. Thompson, et al. 2010. Funding of US biomedical research, 2003–2008. *JAMA* 30(2): 137–43.

Dossier Special. 2007. La fiducie. *Recueil Dalloz* 20: 1346–74.

Douglas, Paul. 1932. The French social insurance act. *Annals of the American Academy of Political and Social Science* 164 (1): 211–48.

Dowling, Harry F. 1970. *Medicines for man: The development, regulation and use of prescription drugs.* New York: Alfred A. Knopf.

Dowling, Harry F. 1970. The American Medical Association's policy on drugs in recent decades. In *Safeguarding the public: Historical aspects of medicinal drug control,* ed. J. B. Blake, 123–31. Baltimore, MD: Johns Hopkins University Press.

Downing, W. L., and Paul R. Hawley. 1952. Two physicians speak their minds on fee-splitting. *Bulletin of the American College of Surgeons* 37 (4): 388–90, 392–93.

Dreyfus, Michel. 1988. *La mutualité: Une histoire maintenant accessible.* Paris: Mutualité Française.

Dryer, Owen. 2004. Journal rejects article after objections from marketing department. *British Medical Journal* 328 (7434): 244.

Dubar, Claude, et Pierre Tripier. 1998. *Sociologie des professions.* Paris: Armand Colin.

Dupeyroux, Jean-Jacques, Michel Borgetto, et Robert Lafore. 2008. *Droit de la sécurité sociale.* 16ème ed. Paris: Dalloz.

Duriez, M., P. Lancry, D. Lequet-Slama, et S. Sandier. 1999. *Le système de santé en France.* Paris: Presses Universitaires de France.

Durkheim, Émile. 2008 [1912]. *The elementary forms of religious life.* Translated by Joseph Ward Swain. Mineola, NY: Dover Publications, Inc.

Durkeim, Émile. 2008 [1893]. *The division of labor in society.* Translated by George Simpson. New York: Free Press.

Dutton, Paul V. 2002. *Origins of the welfare state: The struggle for social reform in France, 1914–1947.* New York: Cambridge University Press.

Dutton, Paul V. 2004. La médecine libérale rencontre le médecin syndicaliste (1920–1930). *Bulletin de l'Histoire de la Sécurité Sociale* 49:79–98.

Dutton, Paul V. 2007. *Differential diagnoses: A comparative history of health care problems and solutions in the United States and France.* Ithaca, NY: Cornell University Press.

Ehrenreich, Barbara, and Jon Ehrenreich. 1970. *The American health empire.* New York: Random House.

Ellis, R. P., and Thomas G. McGuire. 1986. Provider behavior under prospective payment. *Journal of Health Economics* 5 (2):129–51.

English Regulatory Information Task Force, Japan Pharmaceutical Manufacturers Association. 2008. *Pharmaceutical administration and regulations in Japan,* 166–67. Available at http://www.jpma.or.jp/english/ or http://www.nihs.go.jp/English/index.htpl (accessed 10 November 2009).

Europe stratégie analyse financière (EUROSTAF). 1996. *Les cliniques privées: Perspectives stratégiques et financières.* Paris: EUROSTAF.

Evans, C. L. 1912. Sic vos non vobis. *Journal of the Missouri State Medical Association* 8 (April): 405–6.

Evleth, Donna. 2006. The ordre des medecins and the Jews in Vichy France, 1940–1944. *French History* 20 (2): 204–24.

Evleth, Donna. 2009. La bataille pour l'ordre des médecins, *1944–1950 Le Mouvement Social* 229 (Octobre–décembre): 61–77.

Faden, Ruth R., and Thomas L. Beauchamp. 1986. *A theory and history of informed consent.* New York: Oxford University Press.

Falit, Benjamin. 2007. Curbing industry sponsors' incentive to design post-approval trials that are suboptimal for informing prescribers but more likely than optimal designs to yield favorable results. *Seton Hall Law Review* 37 (4):969–1049.

Falk, Isadore Sydney. 1936. *Security against sickness: A study of health insurance.* Garden City, NY: Doubleday, Doran.

Federation of Pharmaceutical Manufacturer Associations of Japan. 1976. *Code of practices for the promotion of ethical drugs.* Tokyo: Federation of Pharmaceutical Manufacturer Associations of Japan.

Fein, Rashi, 1986. *Medical care, medical cost: The search for a national health insurance policy.* Cambridge, MA: Harvard University Press.

Feldman, Eric A. 1994. Legal transplants, organ transplants: The Japanese experience. *Social and Legal Studies: An International Journal* 3 (1):71–91.

Feldman, Eric. 2000. Blood justice: Courts, conflict, and compensation in Japan, France, and the United States. *Law and Society Review* 34 (3):651–702.

Feldman, Eric. 2000. *The ritual of rights in Japan: Law, society, and health policy.* New York: Cambridge University Press.

Feldman, Eric. 2009. Suing doctors in Japan: Structure, culture, and the rise of malpractice litigation. In *Fault lines: Tort law as cultural practice,* ed. M. McCann and D. Engel, 211–32. Stanford, CA: Stanford University Press.

Ferber, Robert, and Hugh G. Wales. 1958. The effectiveness of pharmaceutical promotion. *University of Illinois Bureau of Economic and Business Research Bulletin* No. 83.

Ferrer, Jose M. 1975. How are the costs of continuing medical education to be defrayed? *Bulletin of the New York Academy of Medicine* 5 (6):785–88.

Festinger, Leon. 1950. Informal social communication. *Psychology Review* 57 (5): 271–82.

Field, Mark G. 1953. Structured strain in the role of the Soviet physician. *American Journal of Sociology* 58 (5): 493–502.

Finkelstein, Stan, and Peter Temin. 2008. *Reasonable Rx: Solving the drug price crisis.* Upper Saddle River, NJ: FT Press.

Fishbein, Morris. 1934. *Sickness insurance and sickness costs.* Chicago: AMA

Fishbein, Morris. 1947. *A history of the American Medical Association: 1847 to 1947.* Philadelphia: W.B. Saunders.

Flanagin, Annette, Lisa A. Carey, Phil B. Fontanarosa, et al. 1998. Prevalence of articles with honorary authors and ghost authors in peer-reviewed medical journals. *JAMA* 280 (3): 222–24.

Flexner, Abraham. 1910. *Medical education in the United States and Canada.* New York: Carnegie Foundation for the Advancement of Teaching.

Flexner, Abraham. 1911. Medical colleges: The duty of the state to suppress bad ones and to support good ones. *The World's Work* 21:1438–42.

Fligstein, Neil. 2001. *The architecture of markets.* Princeton, NJ: Princeton University Press.

Frangos, John. 1997. *From housing the poor to healing the sick: The changing institution of Paris hospitals under the old regime and revolution.* Madison, WI: Associated University Presses.

Frankford, David M. 1989. Creating and dividing the fruits of collective economic activity: Referrals among health care providers. *Columbia Law Review* 89 (8): 1861–938.

Freidson, Eliot. 1970. *Professional dominance: The social structure of medical care.* New York: Atherton.

Freidson, Eliot. 1973. Professions and the occupational principle. In *The Professions and their prospects,* ed. Eliot Freidson, 19–38. Beverly Hills, CA: Sage. Reprinted 2001 in Freidson, *Professionalism reborn,* 61–74.

Freidson, Eliot. 1983. Occupational autonomy and labor market shelters. In *Varieties of work,* ed. P. L. Steward and M. G. Cantor, 39–54. Beverly Hills, CA: Sage.

Freidson, Eliot. 1984. *Doctoring together: A study of professional social control.* Chicago: University of Chicago Press.

Freidson, Eliot. 1988. *Professional powers: A study of institutionalization of formal knowledge.* Chicago: University of Chicago Press.

Freidson, Eliot. 2001. *Professionalism: The third logic.* Chicago: University of Chicago Press.

Freidson, Eliot. 2001. *Professionalism reborn: Theory, prophecy, and policy.* Chicago: University of Chicago Press.

Friedman, Lawrence M. 1965. Freedom of contract and occupational licensing 1890–1910: A legal and social study. *California Law Review* 53 (1): 487–534.

Friedman, Milton, and Simon Kuznets. 1945. *Income from independent professional medical practice.* New York: National Bureau of Economic Research.

Fuchs, Victor R. 1996. Economics, values and health care reform. *American Economic Review* 86 (1): 1–24.

Fuji, Ryoji. 2009. The reform of health care system and complementary health insurance in France. *The Japanese Journal of Social Security Policy* 8 (2): 57–67.

Fukuhara, Shunichi, Chikao Yamazaki, Yasuaki Hayashino, et al. 2007. The organization and financing of end-stage renal disease. *International Journal of Health Care Finance and Economics* 7 (2): 217–31.

Funk, Edwin. 1967. Yesterday, today and tomorrow in drug advertising. *Drug Advertising, Pharmaceutical Marketing and Media* 2 (March): 13–16.

Fuse, Shouichi. 1979. *Ishi no rekisi* [*History* of doctors —its Japanese characteristics]. (Tokyo: *Chūō Kōronsha,* 1979).

Gabel, Jon. 1997. Ten ways HMOs have changed during the 1990s. *Health Affairs* 16 (3): 134–45.

Gaffin, Ben. 1961. Report on a study of advertising and the American physician, part 1. Based on Ben Gaffin and Associates. 1956. *Fond du Lac study: An intensive study of the marketing of five new ethical pharmaceutical products in a single market, resulting in some theory of scientific marketing and service programs for action.* Chicago: AMA. Reprinted in U.S. Senate, Hearing, Subcommittee on Antitrust and Monopoly. *Drug industry antirust act* (1961–1962), pt. 1, 490–529.

Gagnon, Marc-André, and Joel Lexchin. 2008. The cost of pushing ills: A new estimate of pharmaceutical promotion expenditures in the United States. *PLoS Medicine* 5 (1). Available at http://www.plosmedicine.org/article/info:doi/10.1371/journal.pmed.0050001 (accessed 10 November 2009).

Gallant, Henry C. 1955. *Histoire politique de la sécurité sociale française 1945–1952.* Paris: Cahiers de la Fondation Nationale des Sciences Politiques.

Garai, Pierre R. 1964. Advertising and promotion of drugs. In *Drugs in our society,* ed. P. Talalay, 189–202. Baltimore, MD: Johns Hopkins University Press.

Gawande, Atul. 2009. The cost conundrum. *New Yorker,* 1 June, 36–44.

Gibbons, Robert, Frank J. Landry, Denise Blouch, et al. 1998. A comparison of physicians and patients' attitudes toward pharmaceutical industry gifts. *Journal of General Internal Medicine* 13 (3): 151–54.

Gilb, Corinne Lathrop. 1976. *Hidden hierarchies: The professions and government.* Westport, CT: Greenwood Press.

Ginzberg, Eli, ed. 1991. *Health service research: Key to health policy.* Cambridge, MA: Harvard University Press.

Glasser, Stephen, Maribel Salas, and Elizabeth Delzell. 2007. Importance and challenges of studying marketed drugs: What is a phase IV study? Common clinical research designs, registries, and self-reporting system. *Journal of Clinical Pharmacology* 47 (9): 1074–86.

Gold, Marsha R., and Ingrid Reeves. 1987. Preliminary results of the GHAA-BC/BS survey of physician incentives in health maintenance organizations (HMOs). *Research Briefs* 1 (November): 1–15.

Gold, Marsha, Timothy Lake, and Robert Hurley. 2001. Provider organizations at risk: A profile of major risk bearing intermediaries, 1999. *Health Affairs* 20 (2): 175–85.

Goldsmith, Jeff. 1981. *Can hospitals survive? The new competitive health care market.* Homewood, IL: Dow Jones-Irwin.

Goode, William J. 1969. The theoretical limits of professionalization. In *The semiprofessions and their organizations*, ed. Amitai Etzioni, 266–313. New York: Free Press.

Gopnik, Adam. 1995. Private domain. *New Yorker*, 13 November, 74–80.

Gordon, Andrew. 1985. *The evolution of labor relations in Japan: Heavy industry 1853–1955.* Cambridge, MA: Council on East Asian Studies, Harvard University.

Graunder, T. M. 1980. On the readability of surgical consent forms. *NEJM* 302 (16): 900–902.

Gray, Bradford H., and Marilyn J. Fields, eds. 1989. *Controlling costs and changing patient care: The role of utilization management.* Washington, DC: National Academy Press.

Greene, Jeremy A. 2007. Pharmaceutical marketing research and the prescribing physician. *Annals of Internal Medicine* 146 (10): 742–47.

Greene, Jeremy A., and Scott H. Podolsky. 2009. Keeping modern in medicine: Pharmaceutical promotion and physician education in postwar America. *Bulletin of the History of Medicine* 83 (2): 331–77.

Greer, Scott L. 2008. *Becoming European: How France, Germany, Spain and the UK engage with European Union health policy.* London: the Nuffield Trust. http://www.nuffieldtrust.org.uk/ecomm/files/Becoming-European-191108.pdf (accessed, 12 May 2010).

Greer, Scott L. 2009. *The politics of European Union health policies.* Maidenhead, Berks, England: Open University Press.

Greenwood, Ernest. 1957. Attributes of a profession. *Social Work* 2 (3): 45–55.

Grossman, J. M., and B. C. Strunk. 2004. For-profit conversions and merger trends among Blue Cross Blue Shield health plans: Issue brief. Center for Studying Health System Change 76 (January): 1–6.

Gruen, Russell L., Steven D. Pearson, and Troyen A. Brennan. 2004. The physician citizens: Public roles and professional organizations. *JAMA* 291 (1): 94–98.

Guillaume, Pierre. 1995. La préhistoire de l'Ordre des médecins. In *L'exercice médical dans la société: Hier, aujourd'hui, demain. Contributions au colloque organisé par l'Ordre national des médecins les 29 et 30 Septembre 1995 à Paris*, 273–84. Paris: Masson.

Guillaume, Pierre. 1996. *Le rôle social du médecin depuis deux siècles: 1800–1945*. Paris: Association pour l'Etude de l'histoire de la Sécurité Sociale.

Guillaume, Pierre. 2000. *Mutualistes et médecins: Conflits et convergences, XIXe-XXe siècles*. Paris: Editions de l'Atelier/Editions Ouvrières.

Haayer, Flora. 1982. Rational prescribing and sources of information. *Social Science and Medicine* 16 (23): 2017–23.

Hafferty, Frederic W., and John B McKinlay,.eds. 1993. *The changing medical profession: An international perspective*. New York: Oxford University Press.

Hager, Mary, Sue Russell and Suzanne W. Fletcher. 2009. *Continuing education in the health professions: Improving healthcare through lifelong learning*. New York: Josiah Macy, Jr. Foundation. Available at www.joshiahmacyfoundation.org.

Hall, Mark A. 1988. Institutional control of physician behavior: Legal barriers to health care cost containment. *University of Pennsylvania Law Review* 137 (2): 431–536.

Hansen, Horace R. 1958. Group health plans: A twenty-year legal review. *Minnesota Law Review* 42 (4): 527–48.

Harichaux, Michele. 1979. *La rémunération du médecin*. Paris: Economica.

Harris, Richard. 1964. *The real voice*. New York: Macmillan.

Hassenteufel, Patrick. 1997. *Les médecins face à 1'état: Une comparaison européenne*. Paris: Presses de Sciences Po.

Hatzfeld, Henri. 1963. *Le grand tournant de la médecine libérale*. Paris: Les Éditions Ouvrières.

Hatzfeld, Henri. 1971. *Du paupérisme à la sécurité sociale, 1850–1940*. Paris: Armand Colin.

Havighurst, Clark C. 1983. The doctors' trust: Self-regulation and the law. *Health Affairs* 2 (3): 64–76.

Havighurst, Clark C. 1980. Antitrust enforcement in the medical services industry: What does it all mean? *The Milbank Quarterly* 58 (1): 89–124.

Havlicek, Penny L., Ann Eiler, and Ondria T. Neblett. 1993. *Medical groups in the United States: A survey of practice characteristics*. Chicago: AMA.

Haward, J. E. S. 1959. Solidarity: The social history of an idea in 19th century France. *International Review of Social History* 4: 261–64.

Haward, J. E. S. 1961. The official social philosophy of the French third republic: Léon Bourgeois and Solidarism. *International Review of Social History* 6:19–48.

Hawkins, Norman G. 1959. The detailman and preference behavior. *Southwestern Social Science Quarterly* 40:213–24.

Hawley, Paul R. 1952. American College of Surgeons restates principles of financial relations. *Bulletin of the American College of Surgeons* 37 (3): 233–36.

Health Care Advisory Board. 1989. *Physician bonding*, vol. 2. *Perfecting the physician network*. Washington, DC: Advisory Board Company.

Hellinger, Fred. J. 1996. The impact of financial incentives on physician behavior in managed care plans: A review of the evidence. *Medical Care Research and Review* 53 (3): 294.

Henderson, L. E., R. L. Sensenich, and Ernest E. Irons. 1949. Medicine in Japan: A report to General Douglas MacArthur, SCAP. *JAMA* 139 (18): 1277–83.

Herzlich, Claudine. 1982. The evolution of relations between French physicians and the state from 1880 to 1980. *Sociology of Health and Illness* 4 (3): 241–53.

Hibbard, Judith H., Paul Slovic, and Jacquelyn J. Jewett. 1997. Informing consumer decisions in health care: Implications from decision-making research. *Milbank Quarterly* 75 (3): 395.

Higuchi, Norio. 1999. *Fuideyusharii (shinnin) no jidai: Shintaku to keiyaku [The age of fiduciaries: Trusts and contracts]*. Tokyo: Yuhikaku.

Hildreth, Martha L. 1987. *Doctors, bureaucrats, and public health in France, 1888–1902.* New York: Garland.

Hildreth, Martha L. 1987. Medical rivalries and medical politics in France: The physicians' union movement and the medical assistance law of 1893. *Journal of the History of Medicine and the Allied Sciences* 42 (1): 5–29.

Hillman, Allan L., W. Pete Welch, and Mark V. Pauly. 1992. Contractual arrangements between HMOs and primary care physicians: Three-tiered HMOs and risk pools. *Medical Care* 30 (2): 136–48.

Himmelstein, David U., Elizabeth Warren, Deborah Thorne, et al. 2005. Illness and injury as contributors to bankruptcy. *Health Affairs* W (5): 63–73.

Hirsh, Bernard D. 1984. *History of the judicial council of the American Medical Association.* Chicago: AMA.

Hoffer, George E. 1974. Physician-ownership in pharmacies and drug repackagers. *Inquiry* 12 (1): 26–36.

Holmes, Wendell H., and Symeon C. Symedonides. 1999. Representation, mandate, and agency: A commentary on Louisiana's new law. *Tulane Law Review* 73 (4): 1087–159.

Hoy, Elizabeth W., Richard E. Curtis, and Thomas D. Rice. 1991. Change and growth in managed care. *Health Affairs* 10 (4): 18–36.

Hughes, Everett C. 1971. *The sociological eye.* Chicago: Aldine.

Hyman, David, and Joel V. Williamson. 1988. Fraud and abuse: Regulatory alternatives in a competitive health care era. *Loyola University of Chicago Law Journal* 19 (4): 1131–96.

Iglehardt, John K. 1988. Japan's medical system, Part I, *NEJM* 319 (12): 807–12.

Iglehardt, John K. 1988. Japan's medical system, Part II. *NEJM* 319 (17): 1166–72.

Ikegami, Naoki. 1988. Health technology development in Japan. *International Journal of Technology Assessment in Health Care* 4 (2): 239–54.

Ikegami, Naoki. 1989. Economic aspects of the doctor-patient relationship in Japan from the eighteenth century until the emergence of social insurance. In *History of the doctor-patient relationship: Proceedings of the 14th international symposium on the comparative history of medicine—East and West*, ed. Y. Kawakita, S. Sakai, and Y. Otsuka, 131–46. Tokyo: Ishiyaku EuroAmerica.

Ikegami, Naoki. 1991. Japanese health care: Low cost through regulated fees. *Health Affairs* 10 (3): 87–109.

Ikegami, Naoki. 1994. Efficiency and effectiveness in health care. *Daedalus* 123 (4): 113–25.

Ikegami, Naoki. 2006. Should providers be allowed to extra-bill for uncovered services? Debate, resolution and the sequel in Japan, *Journal of Health Politics, Policy and Law* 31 (6): 1129–49.

Ikegami, Naoki. 2009. Games policy makers and providers play: Introducing case-mix-based payment to hospital chronic care units in Japan. *Journal of Health Politics Policy and Law* 34 (3): 361–80.

Ikegami, Naoki, and John Creighton Campbell. 1995. Medical care in Japan. *NEJM* 333 (19): 1295–99.

Ikegami, Naoki, and John Creighton Campbell. 1999. Health care reform: The virtues of muddling through. *Health Affairs* 18 (3): 56–75.

Illich, Ivan. 1976. *Medical nemesis: The expropriation of health.* New York: Pantheon Books.

Immergut, Ellen M. 1992. *Health politics: Interest and institution in Western Europe.* Cambridge: Cambridge University Press.

Inoue, Mitsusada, Kazuo Kasahara, and Kota Kodama. 1975. *Japan's history.* Tokyo: Yamakawa.

Institut de Recherche et documentation en Economie de la Santé. 2004. Sickness funds reform; new governance: France Survey no. 4: 2004. *Health Policy Monitor.* International Network Health Policy and Reform Bertelsmann Stiftung Foundation. Available at http://www.healthpolicymonitor.org/index.jsp (accessed 10 November 2009).

Institut de Recherche et documentation en Economie de la Santé. 2005. Hospital payment reform survey. *Health Policy Monitor* 5. International Network Health Policy and Reform Bertelsmann Stiftung Foundation. Available at http://www.healthpolicymonitor.org/index/jsp (accessed 10 November 2009).

Institute of Medicine, Board on Health Sciences and Policy. 2009. *Conflict of interest in medical research, education, and practice,* ed. Bernard Lo and Marilyn Field. Washington, DC: National Academy of Sciences.

Irons, Ernest E. 1929. The clinical evaluation of drugs. *JAMA* 93 (20): 1523–24.

Ishikawa, Kazuhiro, Masato Yamamoto, Donald T. Kishi, et al. 2005. New prospective payment system in Japan. *American Journal of Health-System Pharmacy* 62 (15): 617–19.

Jacobson, Peter. 2002. *Strangers in the night: Law and medicine in the managed care era.* New York: Oxford University Press.

Jamison, Douglas W., and Christina Jansen. 2000. Technology transfer and economic growth. *Journal of Association of University Technology Managers* 12: 24–35.

Japan Medical Association (JMA). 1951. *Physician's ethics code.* Tokyo: JMA. Available at http://www.med.or.jp/english/02_princ.html (accessed 9 June 2009).

Japan Medical Association (JMA). 1951. *Principles of ethics.* Available at http://www.med.org.jp.english, about JMA/principles.html (accessed 9 June 2009).

Japan Medical Association (JMA). 1951. *Remuneration of doctors, ethical codes for doctors.* Tokyo: JMA.

Japan Medical Association (JMA). 2009. The JMA guidelines for physician's professional ethics 2008. *Japan Medical Association Journal* 52 (2): 75–91.

Japan Medical Association (JMA), Committee on Bioethics. 1996. Social responsibility expected of doctors: In search of good professionalism. *Journal of the Japan Medical Association* 116 (3): 243–50.

Japan Pharmaceutical Manufacturers Association (JPMA). 1984. *Fair competition rules of pharmaceutical manufacturers on gift-giving.* Tokyo: JPMA.

Japan Pharmaceutical Manufacturers Association (JPMA). 1993. *Guidelines on gift-giving to health care providers permissible under FTC rules.* Tokyo: JPMA.

Japan Pharmaceutical Manufacturers Association (JPMA). 1993. *Guidelines on remuneration for case reporting allowable under FTC rules.* Tokyo: JPMA.

Japan Pharmaceutical Manufacturers Association (JPMA). 1993. *Promotional code of pharmaceuticals.* Tokyo: JPMA.

Japan Pharmaceutical Manufacturers Association (JPMA). 2008. *Promotion code for prescription drugs.* 23 May. Tokyo: JPMA. Available at http://www.jpma.or.jp/english/issues/pdf/2007code_e.pdf (accessed 8 June 2009).

Jeong, Hyoung-Sun, and Jeremy Hurst. 2001. An assessment of the performance of the Japanese health care system. *OECD Labour Market and Social Policy Occasional Papers.* Available at http://www.oecd.org/dataoecd/35/28/34687614.pdf (accessed 10 November 2009).

Jha, Ashish K., Jonathan B. Perlin, Kenneth W. Kizer, et al. 2003. Effect of the transformation of the veterans affairs health care system on the quality of care *NEJM* 348 (22): 2218–27.

Johansen, Helle Krogh, and Peter C. Gotzche. 1999. Problems in the design and reporting of trials of antifungal agents encountered during meta-analysis. *JAMA* 282 (18): 1752–59.

Johns, Margaret Z. 2007. Informed consent: Requiring doctors to disclose off-label prescriptions and conflicts of interest. *Hastings Law Journal* 58 (5): 967–1024.

Johnston, Helen L. 1951. *Rural health cooperatives.* Public Health Bulletin No. 308. Washington, DC: Cooperative Research and Service Division, Farm Credit Administration, and Division of Medical and Hospital Resources, Public Health Service.

Joseph, John N., et al. 2009. Enforcement related to off-label marketing and use of drugs and devices: Where have we been and where are we doing? *Journal of Health & Life Sciences Law* 2 (2): 73–108.

Juppé, Alain. 1996. Discours de Alain Juppé, 15 Novembre 1995. *Droit Social* 3: 221–37.

Kanda, Hideki, and Curtis J. Milhaupt. 2003. Reconsidering legal transplants: Directors' fiduciary duty in Japanese corporate law. *American Journal of Comparative Law* 51 (4): 887–901.

Kassirer, Jerome P. 1994. The use and abuse of practice profiles. *NEJM* 330 (9): 634–36.

Kassirer, Jerome P. 2005. *On the take: How America's complicity with big business can endanger your health.* New York: Oxford University Press.

Kasza, Gregory J. 2002. War and welfare policy in Japan. *Journal of Asian Studies* 61 (2): 417–27.

Kasza, Gregory J. 2006. *One world of welfare: Japan in comparative perspective.* Ithaca, NY: Cornell University Press.

Katz, Jay. 1984. *The silent world of doctor and patient.* Baltimore, MD: Johns Hopkins University Press.

Katz, Elihu, and George Menzel. 1955. Social relations and innovation in the medical profession: the epidemiology of a new drug. *Public Opinion Quarterly* 19 (4): 337–72.

Keehan, Sean, Andrea Sisko, Christopher Truffer, et al. 2008. Health spending projections through 2017: The baby-boom generation is coming to Medicare. *Health Affairs* 27: 145–55.

Kelman, Steven. 1987. *Making public policy: A hopeful view of American government.* New York: Basic Books.

Kenpōren. 1990. *History of Japanese NHI.* Tokyo: Kenpōren.

Kenpōren. 2007. *Health insurance, long-term care insurance and health insurance societies in Japan 2007.* Tokyo: Kenpōren.

Kikuni, Kenzō. 1984. Quality assurance programs in Japan. *Japan Hospitals* 3 (July): 29–31.

Kimura, Rihito. 1991. Fiduciary relationship and the medical profession: A Japanese view. In *Ethics, trust, and the professions: Philosophical and cultural aspects,* ed. D. Pellegrino, R. M. Veatch, and J. Langan, 235–45. Washington, DC: Georgetown University Press.

Kjaergard, Lise L., and Bodil Als-Nielsen. 2002. Association between competing interests and authors' conclusions: Epidemiological study of randomized clinical trials published in the *BMJ. British Medical Journal* 325 (7358): 249–52.

Kodaka, Michio. 1986. Present status of hemodialysis in Japan. *Journal of the Japanese Society for Dialysis Therapy* 19: 1–21

Kodansha Encyclopedia of Japan. 1983. Tokyo: G. Itasaka, Kodansha America.

Kovner, Anthony R., and James R. Knickman. 2008. *Jonas and Kovner's health care delivery in the United States.* 9th ed. New York: Springer.

Kozeki, Oshamu. 1995. Consequences of fixed-payment for dialysis. *Banboo* 164 (February): 68–72. *Kyodo News,* 30 March.

Krause, E. 1996. *Death of the guilds: Professions, states, and the advance of capitalism, 1930 to the Present.* New Haven, CT: Yale University Press.

Kredel, Frederick Evert, and John Hampton Hoch. 1939. Early relation of pharmacy and medicine in the United States. *Journal of the American Pharmaceutical Association* 28 (10): 702–7.

Krimsky, Sheldon. 2003. *Science in the private interest: Has the lure of profits corrupted biomedical research?* Lanham, MD: Rowman and Littlefield.

Krimsky, Sheldon, and L. S. Rothenberg. 2001. Conflict of interest policies in science and medical journals: Editorial practices and author disclosures. *Science and Engineering Ethics* 7 (2): 205–18.

Kumar, C. Raj. 2004. Corruption in Japan: Institutionalizing the right to information, transparency and the right to corruption-free governance. *New England Journal of International and Comparative Law* 10 (1): 465–66.

Kusserow, Richard P. 1989. *Financial arrangements between physician and health care businesses: Report to Congress.* Washington, DC: Office of the Inspector General-Department of Health and Human Services (OIG-DHHS).

Kusserow, Richard P. 1990. *Ensuring appropriate use of laboratory services: A monograph.* Washington, DC: OIG-DHHS.

Kusserow, Richard P. 1992. *Promotion of prescription drugs through payment and gifts: Physicians' perspectives.* Washington, DC: OIG-DHHS.

La Berge, Ann E., and Mordechai Feingold. 1994. *French medical culture in the nineteenth century.* Amsterdam: Edition Rodopi B.V.

Lamy. 2009. Droit de la santé. Editions Lamy, Paris.

Laroque, Pierre, ed. 1983. *The social institutions of France.* London: Taylor and Francis.

Larroumet, Christian. 1990. *La fiducie inspirée du trust.* Paris: Recueil Dalloz.

Larson, Magali Sarfatti. 1977. *The rise of professionalism.* Berkeley: University of California Press.

Laubenthal, Connie. 1996. Physician's office laboratory adviser. Part 1, Physician office laboratories, history of government regulation. *Medical Laboratory Observer*

(November). Available at http://findarticles.com/p/articles/mi_m3230/is_n11_
v28/ai_18899710/ (accessed 13 November 2009).

Laufer, Joseph. 1939. Ethical and legal restrictions on contract and corporate practice
of medicine. *Law and Contemporary Problems* 6 (4): 516–27.

Law, Sylvia A. 1976. *Blue Cross: What went wrong?* New Haven, CT: Yale University Press.

Le Pen, Claude. 1999. *Les habit neufs d'Hippocrate*. Paris: Calmann-Lévy.

Le Goff, Jacques. 1980. Les métiers et l'organisation du travail dans la France
médiévale. In *La France et les français*, ed. M. François, 310–37. Gallimard.

Leake, Chauncey D. 1929. The pharmacologic evaluation of new drugs. *JAMA* 93
(21): 1632–34.

Lear, John. 1962. The unfinished story of Thalidomide. *Saturday Review of Literature*
45:35–43.

Leflar, Robert B. 1996. Informed consent and patients' rights in Japan. *Houston Law
Review* 33 (1): 1–112.

Leflar, Robert B. 2007. Law and patient safety in the United States and Japan. In
Readings in comparative health law and bioethics, ed. T. S. Jost, 124–26. Durham,
NC: Carolina Academic Press.

Leflar, Robert B. 2009. Unnatural deaths, criminal sanctions, and medical quality
improvement in Japan. *Yale Journal of Health Policy, Law and Ethics* 9 (1): 11.

Leflar, Robert B., and Futoshi Iwata. 2005. Medical error as reportable event, as tort,
as crime: A transpacific comparison. *Widener Law Review* 12 (1): 189–225.

Léonard, Jacques. 1981. *La médecine entre les savoirs et les pouvoirs: Histoire intellectuelle et politique de la médecine française au XIXème siècle* (Paris: Aubier, 1981).

Lexchin, Joel, Lisa A. Bero, Benjamin Djulbegovic, et al. 2003. Pharmaceutical industry sponsorship and research outcome and quality: Systematic review. *British
Medical Journal* 326 (7400): 1167–70.

Liebrand, Wim B., David M. Messick, and Fred J. Wolters. 1986. Why we are fairer
than others? A cross-cultural replication and extension. *Journal of Experimental
Social Psychology* 22 (6): 590–604.

Light, Donald W. 2004. Ironies of success: A new history of the American health care
"system." *Journal of Health and Social Behavior* 45 (extra issue): 1–24.

Lincoln, James, and Arne L. Kalleberg. 1985. Work organization and workforce commitment: A study of plants and employees in the U.S. and Japan. *American Sociological Review* 50 (6): 738–60.

Lock, Margaret M. 1980. *East Asian medicine in urban Japan*. Berkeley: University of
California Press.

Locke, John. [1689] 1960. *Two treatises of government*, ed. Peter Laslett. Cambridge:
Cambridge University Press.

Long, Susan Orpett. 1987. Health care providers: Technology, policy, and professional
dominance. In *Health, illness, and medical care in Japan: Cultural and social dimensions*, ed. E. Norbeck and M. Lock, 66–88. Honolulu: University of Hawaii Press.

Ludmerer, Kenneth M. 1999. *Time to heal: American medical education from the turn of
the century to the era of managed care*. New York: Oxford University Press.

Luft, Harold S. 1987. *Health maintenance organizations: Dimensions of performance*.
New Brunswick, NJ: Transaction Books.

Lydston, Frank G. 1899. The surgical commission man and surgical canvassing.
Philadelphia Medical Journal 4 (1): 837–40.

MacLeod, Gordon K., and M. Roy Schwartz. 1986. Faculty practice plans: Profile and critique. *JAMA* 256 (1): 58–62.

Maillard, Christian. 1986. *Histoire de l'hôpital de 1940 à nos jours: Comment la santé est devenue une affaire d'état.* Paris: Dunod.

Maine, Henry. 1932. *Ancient law: Its connection with the early history of society and its relation to modern ideas.* Boston: Beacon Press.

Marmor, Theodore R. 2000. *The politics of Medicare.* 2d ed. Hawthorne: Aldine de Gruyter.

Marrus, Michael R., Robert O. Paxton, and Stanley Hoffmann. 1995. *Vichy France and the Jews.* Stanford, CA: Stanford University Press.

Marshal, T. H. 1939. The recent history of professionalism in relation to social structure and social policy. *Canadian Journal of Economics and Political Science* 5 (3): 325–40.

Masuyama, Mikitaka, and John Creighton Campbell. 1996. The evolution of fee-schedule politics in Japan. In *Containing health care costs in Japan*, ed. N. Ikegami and J. C. Campbell, 265–77. Ann Arbor: University of Michigan Press.

May, Charles D. 1961. Selling drugs by educating physicians. *Journal of Medical Education* 36 (1): 1–23.

McCann, James C. 1958. Consideration of deduction and allocation of surgical fees by Blue Shield plans. *JAMA* 166 (6): 624–28.

McDonough, John. 1997. Tracking the demise of state hospital rate-setting. *Health Affairs* 16 (1): 142–49.

Mechanic, David. 1986. *From advocacy to allocation: The evolving American health care system.* New York: Free Press.

Mechanic, David. 2000. Managed care and the imperative for a new professional ethic. *Health Affairs* 19 (5): 100–11.

Mechanic, David. 2008. Rethinking medical professionalism: The role of information technology and practice innovation. *Milbank Quarterly* 86 (2): 368–88.

Medical Association of the State of Alabama. 1890. Report of the Board of Censors. *Transactions of the Medical Association of the State of Alabama.* Birmingham.

Mehlman, Maxwell J. 2006. Dishonest medical mistakes. *Vanderbilt Law Review* 59 (4): 1137–73.

Mény, Yves. 1990. *La corruption de la république.* Paris: Fayard.

Mény, Yves. 1997. France: The end of the republican ethic? In *Democracy and corruption in Europe*, ed. D. D. Porta and Y. Meny, 7–21. Paris: La Découverte.

Meyers, Harold B. 1970. The medical industrial complex. *Fortune* 81 (January), 1.

Ministry of Health, Labor, and Welfare (Japan), Central Social Insurance Medical Care Committee, Subcommittee on Price Setting. 1995. Report on pharmaceutical evaluation and price setting in foreign countries. March.

Milgram, Stanley. 1974. *Obedience to authority.* New York: Harper and Row.

Millard, Perry H. 1887. The propriety and necessity of state regulation of medical practice. *JAMA* 9 (16): 491.

Miller, Francis H. 1983. Secondary income from recommended treatment: Should fiduciary principles constrain physician behavior? In *The new health care for profit: Doctors and hospitals in a competitive environment*, ed. B. Gray, 153–69. Washington, DC: National Academies Press.

Millis, Harry Alvin. 1937. *Sickness and insurance: A study of the sickness problem and health insurance.* Chicago: University of Chicago Press.

Mitchell, Alan. 1991. The function and malfunction of mutual aid societies in nine-teenth century France. In *Medicine and charity before the welfare state*, ed. J. Barry and C. Jones, 172–89. New York: Routledge.

Mitchell, Jean M. 2007. Utilization changes following market entry by physician owned specialty hospitals. *Medical Care Research and Review* 64 (4): 395–415.

Mitchell, Jean M., and Elton Scott. 1992. Evidence of complex structure of physician joint ventures. *Yale Journal on Regulation* 9 (2): 489–520.

Mitchell, Jean M., and Jonathan H. Sunshine. 1992. Consequences of physicians' ownership of health care facilities: Joint ventures in radiation therapy. *NEJM* 327 (21): 1497–501.

Moore, Don A., Daylian M. Cain, George Loewenstein, et al. 2004. *Conflicts of interest: Challenges and solutions from law, medicine and organization settings.* Cambridge: Cambridge University Press.

Moore, Don A., and George Loewenstein. 2004. Self-interest, automaticity, and the psychology of conflict of interest. *Social Justice Research* 17 (2): 189–202.

Moore, Wilbert E. 1971. *The professions: Roles and rules.* New York: Russell Sage Foundation.

Moret-Bailly, Joël. 2001. *Les Déontologies.* Aix-en-Provence: Presses Universitaires d'Aix-Marseille.

Moret-Bailly, Joël. 2002. Règles déontologiques et fautes civiles. *Recueil Dalloz*, 2820–24.

Moret-Bailly Joël. 2002. L'accès à la justice disciplinaire. Paris: Mission de recherche droit et justice.

Moret-Bailly, Joël. 2003. L'organisation juridique des compétences des profession-nels de santé. In *Modalités et conditions d'évaluation des compétences professionnelles des métiers de la santé. Rapport au ministre de l'éducation et au ministre de la santé*, ed. Y. Matillon, 57–86. Paris: Ministre de la santé et des solidarités.

Moret-Bailly Joël. 2004. Les conflits d'intérêts des experts consultés par l'admin-istration dans le domaine sanitaire. *Revue Droit Sanitaire et Sociale* 4: 855–71.

Moret-Bailly, Joël. 2004. Déontologie. In *Dictionnaire de la justice*, ed. L. Cadiet, 326–30. Paris: Presses Universitaires de France.

Moret-Bailly, Joël. 2009. Le rôle des experts au sein des agences de sécurité sanitaire, *Annales de la Régulation*, LGDJ 2: 327–43.

Morgan, John. 1937. *A discourse upon the institution of medical schools in America.* Baltimore, MD: Johns Hopkins University Press.

Morgenthaler, Jean-Louis. 1981. La mutualité française de 1945 à 1976: De la tra-dition au modernisme. Thèse présentée pour le doctorat au troisième cycle de sociologie, Université de Nancy II.

Morone, James A. 1990. *The democratic wish: Popular participation and the limits of the American government.* New York: Basic Books.

Morrein, E. Haavi. 1990. Physician investment and self-referral: A philosophical analysis of a contentious debate. *Journal of Medicine and Philosophy* 15 (4): 425–48.

Morris, Lewis, and Julie K. Taitsman. 2009. The agenda for continuing medical edu-cation—Limiting industry's influence *NEJM:* 361 (25): 2478–82.

Muramatsu, Naoko, and Jersey Liang. 1999. Hospital length of stay in the United States and Japan: A case study of myocardial infarction patients. *International Journal of Health Services* 29 (1): 189–209.

Nagele, Robin Locke, and Elizabeth B. Bradley. 2006. Physician-owned specialty hospital and hospital conflict-of-interest policies: Healthy competition or business opportunism? In *Health Law Handbook 2006*, ed. A. G. Gosfield, 691–725. St. Paul, MN: Thompson/West.

Nakano, Yutaka, and Hiroshi Ohama. 1998. *Fee schedule made easy '98*. Tokyo: UtoBrain.

Nakajima, Chizu. 1999. *Conflicts of interest and duty: A comparative analysis in Anglo-Japanese law*. The Hague: Kluwer Law International.

National Medical Convention. 1847. Code of medical ethics. *Archives of the American Medical Association, Proceedings of the National Medical Conventions held in Philadelphia, 1846, and New York City, 1847*, 83–106. Chicago: AMA. Reprinted 1977 in *Ethics in medicine: Historical perspectives and contemporary concerns*, ed. Stanley J. Reiser, Arthur L. Dyck, and William J. Curran, 26–34. Cambridge, MA: MIT Press.

Needleman, Jack, Debora J. Chollet, and Jo Ann Lamphere. 1997. Hospital conversion trends. *Health Affairs* 6 (2): 187–95.

Niki, Ryu. 1993. Rapid increase in private multi-hospital systems in Japan. Paper presented at the Comparative Health Care Research Series, Stanford University.

Niki, Ryu. 1998. Integrated delivery systems in Japan: Brief summary of a national survey and future predictions. Paper presented at Pacific Research Center, Stanford University, 2 September.

Niki, Ryu. 1999. *Hoken iryō fukushi fukugotai I [Integrated delivery systems]*.

Office of the U.S. Trade Representative. 2004. Third report to the leader on the U.S-Japan regulatory reform and competition policy initiative. http://www.mac.doc.gov/japan-korea/deregulation/2004–06–08-japan-factsheet.pdf.

Ogawa, Sumiko, Toshihiko Segawa, Guy Carrin, et al. 2003. Scaling up community health insurance: Japan's experience with the 19th century Jyorei scheme. *Health Policy and Planning* 18 (3): 270–78.

Ohi, G., T. Hasegawa, H. Kumano, I. Kai, et al. 1986. Why are cadaveric renal transplants so hard to find in Japan? An analysis of economic and attitudinal aspects. *Health Policy* 6 (3): 269–78.

Ohnuki-Tierney, Emiko. 1984. *Illness and culture in contemporary Japan: An anthropological view*. Cambridge: Cambridge University Press.

Ohtani, Fujia. 1971. *One hundred years of health progress in Japan*. Tokyo: International Medical Foundation of Japan.

Okamoto, Etsuji. 2004. *Public health of Japan, 2004*. Tokyo: Japan Public Health Association.

Okamoto, Etsuji, and Kōzō Tatara. 2008. *Public health of Japan, 2007*. Tokyo: Japan Public Health Association.

Organization for Economic Cooperation and Development (OECD). 2004. Reviews of regulatory reform. Japan: Progress in implementing regulatory reform. No. 56, OECD Publishing. Available at http://www.oecd.org/dataoecd/56/2/32983995.pdf (accessed 10 November 2009).

Osler, William. 1906. Chauvinism in medicine. In Osler, *Aequanimitas, with other addresses to medical students, nurses and practitioners of medicine*, 277–306. 2d ed. Philadelphia: Blakiston.

Ouchi, William C. 1981. *Theory Z: How American business can meet the Japanese challenge*. Reading, MA: Addison-Wesley.

Parsons, Talcott. 1968. Professions. In *International encyclopedia of the social sciences*, ed. D. Sills, 536–47. New York: Macmillan.

Patsopoulos, Nikolaos A., John P. A. Ioannidis, and Apostolos A. Analatos. 2006. Origin and funding of the most frequently cited papers in medicine: Database analysis. *British Medical Journal* 332 (7549): 1061–64.

Pekkanen, Robert. 2003. Molding Japanese civil society: State-structured incentives and the patterning of civil society. In *The state of civil society in Japan*, ed. F. J. Schwartz and S. J. Pharr, 117–34. Cambridge: Cambridge University Press.

Pekkanen, Robert, and Karla Simon. 2002. Taxation of not-for-profit organizations and their donors in Japan: Is this tax reform or not? *International Journal of Not-for-Profit Law* 4 (2/3): 1–5.

Petit, Donald W. 1970. The physician recognition award. *JAMA* 213 (10): 1668–70.

Podolsky, Scott H., and Jeremy A. Greene. 2008. A historical perspective of pharmaceutical promotion and physician education. *JAMA* 300 (9): 1071–73.

Polton, Dominique. 2004. Recent reforms affecting private health insurance in France. *Euro Observer* 6 (1): 4–5.

Powell, Margaret, and Masahira Anesaki. 1990. *Health care in Japan*. London: Routledge.

Puckner, W. A., and Paul Nicholas Leech. 1929. The introduction of new drugs. *JAMA* 93 (21): 1627–30.

Ramsey, Mathew. 1988. *Professional and popular medicine in France, 1770–1830*. Cambridge: Cambridge University Press.

Ramsey, Matthew. 1994. Academic medicine and medical industrialism: The regulation of secret remedies in nineteenth-century France. In *French medical culture in the nineteenth century*, ed. A. La Berge and M. Feingold, 25–32. Amsterdam: Edition Rodopi B.V.

Raoux, F. 1979. Naissance de la corporation médicale 1879–1943. Thèse de médecine, Faculté de St. Antoine, Paris.

Rayack, Elton. 1967. *Professional power and American medicine: The economics of the American Medical Association*. Cleveland: World Book.

Rebecq, Geneviève. 2007. *Protection sociale*. Paris: Editions de Juris Classeur.

Reed, Louis S. 1967. Private health insurance: Coverage and financial experience, 1940–66. *Social Security Bulletin* 30 (November): 3–22.

Rehder, Robert R. 1965. Communication and opinion formation in a medical community: The significance of the detail man. *Journal of the Academy of Management* 8 (4): 282–91.

Reinhardt, Uwe E. 1996. A social contract for 21st century health care: Three-tier health care with bounty hunting. *Health Economics* 5 (6): 479–99.

Reinhardt, Uwe. 1996. Is the target-income hypothesis an economic heresy? *Medical Care Research and Review* 53 (3): 274–87.

Reinhardt, Uwe E. 2000. The economics of for-profit and not-for-profit hospitals. *Health Affairs* 19 (6): 178–86.

Relman, Arnold S. 1980. The new medical-industrial complex. *NEJM* 303 (17): 963–70.

Relman, Arnold S. 1984. Dealing with conflicts of interest. *NEJM* 310 (18): 1182–83.

Relman, Arnold S. 2001. Separating continuing medical education from pharmaceutical marketing. *JAMA* 285 (15): 2009–12.

Relman, Arnold S. 2007. *A second opinion: Rescuing America's health care*. New York: Public Affairs.

Relman, Arnold S., and Uwe E. Reinhardt. 1986. An exchange on for-profit health care. In *For-profit enterprise in health care*, ed. B. H. Gray, 209–23. Washington, DC: National Academy Press.

Reynaud. 1989. *Les règles du jeu: L'action collective et la régulation sociale.* Paris: Armand Colin.

Rice, Thomas. 2003. *The economics of health reconsidered.* 2d ed. Chicago: Health Administration Press.

Richter, Judith. 2005. *Global strategy for infant and young child feeding.* Geneva: International Baby Food Action Network.

Robinson, James C. 1999. Blended payment methods in physician organizations under managed care. *JAMA* 282 (13): 1258–63.

Robinson, James C. 2001. The end of managed care. *JAMA* 285 (20): 2622–28.

Robinson, James C. 2001. Theory and practice in the design of physician payment incentives. *Milbank Quarterly* 79 (2): 149–77.

Robinson, James C., and Lawrence Casalino. 2001. Reevaluation of capitation contracting in New York and California. *Health Affairs* 20 (4): W3–W9.

Rochaix, Maurice. 1996. *Les questions hospitalières: De la fin d l'ancien régime à nos jours.* Paris: Berger-Levrault.

Rodwin, Marc A. 1989. Physicians' conflicts of interests: The limitations of disclosure. *NEJM* 321 (20): 1405–8.

Rodwin, Marc A. 1992. The organized American medical profession's response to financial conflicts of interest: 1890–1992. *Milbank Quarterly* 70 (4): 703–41.

Rodwin, Marc A. 1993. *Medicine, money and morals: Physicians' conflicts of interest.* New York: Oxford University Press.

Rodwin, Marc A. 1994. Patient accountability and quality of care: Lessons from medical consumerism and the patients' rights, women's health and disability rights movements. *American Journal of Law and Medicine* 20 (1&2): 147–67.

Rodwin, Marc A. 1995. Strains in the fiduciary metaphor: Divided physician loyalties and obligations in a changing health care system. *American Journal of Law and Medicine* 21 (2&3): 241–57.

Rodwin, Marc A. 1995. Conflicts in Managed Care. *NEJM* 332 (9): 604–7.

Rodwin, Marc A. 1999. Backlash: Prelude to managing managed care. *Journal of Health Politics, Policy and Law* 24 (5): 1115–26.

Rodwin, Marc A. 1999. Exit and voice in American health care. *Michigan Journal of Law Reform* 32 (4): 1041–67.

Rodwin, Marc A. 2001. Consumer voice and representation in health care. *Journal of Health Law* 34 (2): 223–72.

Rodwin, Marc A. 2001. The politics of evidence-based medicine. *Journal of Health Politics and Law* 26 (2): 439–46.

Rodwin, Marc A. 2004. The dark side of a consumer driven health care system. *Frontiers of Health Care Management* 19:31–34.

Rodwin, Marc A. 2007. Medical commerce, physician entrepreneurialism, and conflicts of interest. *Cambridge Quarterly of Healthcare Ethics* 16 (4): 387–97.

Rodwin, Marc A. 2010. The metamorphosis of managed care. *Journal of Law, Medicine, & Ethics* 36 (2): 252–364.

Rodwin, Marc A. 2011. Patient appeals as policy disputes: Individual and collective action in managed care. In *Impatient voices: Patients as policy actors*, ed. B. Hoffman, N. Tomes, R. Grob, et al. New Brunswick, NJ: Rutgers University Press.

Rodwin, Marc A., and Estuji Okomoto. 2000. Physicians' conflict of interest in Japan and the United States: Lessons for the United States. *Journal of Health Politics, Policy and Law* 25 (2): 343–75.

Rodwin, Marc A., Hak Chang, and Jeffrey Clausen. 2006. Malpractice premiums and physician income: Perceptions of a crisis conflict with empirical evidence. *Health Affairs* 25 (3): 750–58.

Rodwin, Marc A., Hak J. Chang, Melissa M. Ozaeta, et al. 2008. Malpractice premiums in Massachusetts, a high-risk state: 1975 to 2005. *Health Affairs* 27 (3): 835–44.

Rodwin, Victor G. 1984. *The health planning predicament: France, Québec, England, and the United States*. Berkeley: University of California Press.

Rodwin, Victor G., and Claude Le Pen. 2004. Health care reform in France: The birth of state-led managed care. *NEJM* 351 (22): 2259–62.

Rodwin, Victor, R. J. Launois, B. Majnoni d'Intignano, and J. C. Stéphan. 1985. Les réseaux de soins coordonnés (RSC): Propositions pour une réforme profonde du système de santé. *Revue Française des Affaires Sociales* 1 (January/March): 37–61.

Roemer, Milton I., and Jay W. Friedman. 1971. *Doctors in hospitals: Medical staff organizations and hospital performance*. Baltimore, MD: Johns Hopkins University Press.

Roemer, Milton I., and Max Shain. 1959. *Hospital utilization under insurance*. Ithaca, NY: Cornell University School of Business and Public Administration.

Rogers, Mabry E., and Stephen B. Young. 1975. Public office as a public trust: A suggestion that impeachment for high crimes and misdemeanors implies a fiduciary standard. *Georgetown Law Journal* 63 (5): 1025–49.

Röhl, Wilhelm 2005. *A history of law in Japan since 1868*. Leiden: Brill.

Romains, Jules. [1925] 2000. *Knock: Ou le triomphe de la médecine: Comédie en trois actes*. Paris: Gallimard; Harley Granville-Barker, trans. 1935. *Doctor Knock: A Comedy in Three Acts*. London, Sidgwick and Jackson.

Rorem, C. Rufus. 1931. *Private group practice clinics*. Chicago: University of Chicago Press.

Rorem, C. Rufus, and Robert P. Fischelis. 1932. *The costs of medicine*. Committee on the Cost of Medical Care, No. 14. Chicago: University of Chicago Press.

Rosanvallon, Pierre. 2008. *L'état en France de 1789 à nos jours*. Paris: Seuil.

Rosen, George. 1974. *From medical police to social medicine: Essays on the history of health care*. New York: Sciences History Publications.

Rosenberg, Charles. 1974. Social class and medical care in nineteenth-century America: The rise and fall of dispensary. *Journal of the History of Medicine and the Allied Sciences* 29 (1): 32–54.

Rosner, David. 1982. *A once charitable enterprise: Hospitals and health care in Brooklyn and New York, 1885–1915*. Cambridge: Cambridge University Press.

Ross, Joseph S., Kevin P. Hill, David S. Egilman, et al. 2008. Guest authorship and ghostwriting in publications related to Rofecoxib: A case study of industry documents from Rofecoxib litigation. *JAMA* 299 (15): 1800–1812.

Roth, Julius A. 1974. Professionalism: The sociologists' decoy. *Work and Occupations* 1 (1): 6–23.

Rothman, David J. 1991. *Strangers at the bedside: A history of how law and bioethics transformed medical decision making*. New York: HarperCollins.

Rothman, David J. 1993. A century of failure: Health care reform in America. *Journal of Health Politics, Policy and Law* 18 (2): 271–86.

Rothman, David J., Walter J. McDonald, Carol D. Berkowitz, et al. 2009. Professional medical associations and their relationships with industry: A proposal for controlling conflicts of interest. *JAMA* 301 (13): 1367–72.

Rousseau, Jean-Jacques. [1762] 2003. *The social contract and discourses*, trans. G. D. H. Cole. Mineola, NY: Dover.

Rucker, T. Donald. 1972. Economic problems in drug distribution. *Inquiry* 9 (3): 43.

Rupp, Katherine. 2003. *Gift-giving in Japan: Cash, connections, cosmologies*. Stanford, CA: Stanford University Press.

Rayack, Elton. 1967. *Professional power and American medicine: The economics of the American Medical Association*. Cleveland, OH: World Book.

Sage, William M., David A. Hyman, and Warren Greenberg. 2003. Why competition law matters to health care quality. *Health Affairs* 22 (2): 31–43.

Sage, William M. 2007. Some principals require principles: Why banning "conflicts of interest" won't solve incentive problems in biomedical research, *Texas Law Review* 85 (6): 1413–64.

Salon, Serge, and Jean-Charles Savignac. 2009. *Code de la fonction publique*. Paris: Dalloz-Sirey.

Sams, Crawford F. 1998. *"Medic": The mission of an American military doctor in occupied Japan and war-torn Korea*. Armonk, NY: M.E. Sharp

Sand, R. 1948. *Vers la médecine sociale*. Liège, Belgique: Baillere.

Sandier, Simone, Valérie Paris, and Dominique Polton. 2004. *Health care systems in transition: France*. Copenhagen: European Observatory on Health Systems and Policies.

Sasamori, Norio. 1982 The present condition of the human dry dock in Japan and its outlook for the future. *Japan Hospitals* 1: 49–55.

Sawaniski, K. 1990. Follow up on dialysis patients initiated below serum creatinine level 8.0 mg/dl. *Journal of Japanese Society of Dialysis Therapy* 23: 1–10.

Schlesinger, Mark. 1997. Countervailing agency: A strategy of principled regulation under managed competition. *Milbank Quarterly* 75 (1): 35–87.

Schlesinger, Mark. 2002. A loss of faith: The sources of reduced political legitimacy for the American medical profession. *Milbank Quarterly* 80 (2): 185–235.

Schlesinger, Mark J., Bradford H. Gray, and Krista M. Perreira. 1997. Medical professionalism under managed care: The pros and cons of utilization review. *Health Affairs* 16 (1): 106–24.

Schmidt, Dominique. 1999. *Les conflits d'intérêts dans la société anonyme*. Paris: Joly.

Schwartz, Frank J., and Susan J. Pharr, eds. 2003. *The state of civil society in Japan*. Cambridge: Cambridge University Press.

Schwartz, Jerome L. 1965. Early history of prepaid medical care plans. *Bulletin of the History of Medicine* 39 (5): 450–75.

Searle, John G., L. D. Barney, Francis Boyer, et al. 1961. The pharmaceutical industry. *Journal of Medical Education* 36 (1): 24–32.

Seikyō, Iryōbukai. 1982. *Iryō seikyō no rekishi to tokuchō* [The history and characteristics of health care cooperatives]. Tokyo: Iryō Seikyō.

Sevringhaus, Elmer L. 1953. Interdependence of the medical profession and the pharmaceutical industry. *JAMA* 152 (16): 1522–25.

Sewell, William H., Jr. 1980. *Work and revolution in France: The language of labor from the old regime to 1848*. Cambridge: Cambridge University Press.

Shaw, George Bernard. [1913] 1988. Preface. *The doctor's dilemma: A tragedy*. Baltimore, MD: Penguin.

Shimm, David S. 1996. Conflicts of interest in relations between physicians and the pharmaceutical industry. In *Conflicts of interest in clinical practice and research*, ed. R. Spece, D. S. Shimm, and A. E. Buchanan, 321–57. New York: Oxford University Press.

Shoji, Arahira, and Onishi Hironari. 1999. Reform of the Japanese health insurance system. *International Social Security Review* 52 (2): 101–8.

Shyrock, Richard Harrison. 1967. *Medical licensing in America, 1650–1965*. Baltimore, MD: Johns Hopkins University Press.

Sieyès, Emmanuel Joseph. [1789] 1964. *What is the third estate?* trans. M. Blondel, ed. S. E. Finer. New York: Praeger.

Sigerist, Henry E. 1951. *A history of medicine*. New York: Oxford University Press.

Silverman, Milton, and Philip R. Lee. 1974. *Pills, profits and politics*. Berkeley: University of California Press.

Simmons, George H. 1908. The Abbott alkaloidal company—high finance and methods of working the medical profession. *JAMA* 50 (11): 895–900.

Smith, Donald H. 1997. Wishful thinking about unions. *Physician News Digest*. Available at www.physiciansnews.com/discussion/smith.html (accessed 4 September 2007).

Smith, Richard. 2006. *The trouble with medical journals*. London: Royal Society of Medicine Press Ltd.

Smith, Timothy B. 1998. The social transformation of hospitals and the rise of medical insurance in France, 1914–1944. *Historical Journal* 41 (4): 1055–87.

Smith, Timothy B. 2003. *Creating the welfare state in France: 1880–1940*. Montreal: McGill-Queen's University Press.

Snoke, Albert W. 1958. The future role of hospitals in medical care. *American Journal of Public Health* 48 (4): 468–72.

Somers, Herman Miles, and Anne Ramsay Somers. 1961. *Doctors, patients, and health insurance*. Washington, DC: Brookings Institution.

Spece, Roy, David. S. Shimm, and Alan. E. Buchanan. 1996. *Conflicts of interest in clinical practice and research*. New York: Oxford University Press.

Spingarn, Roger W., Jesse A. Berlin, and Brian L. Strom. 1996. When pharmaceutical manufacturers' employees present grand rounds, what do residents remember? *Academic Medicine* 1 (1): 86–88.

Starr, Paul. 1982. *The social transformation of American medicine*. New York: Basic Books.

Stearns, Norman S., Marjorie E. Getchell, and Robert A. Gold. 1971. *Continuing medical education in community hospitals: A manual for program development*. Boston: Massachusetts Medical Society.

Steffen, Monika. 1983. Régulation, politique et stratégies professionnelles: Médecine libérale et émergence des centres de santé. Thèse de science politique, Institut d'Etudes Politiques, Université des Sciences Sociales de Grenoble.

Steffen, Monika. 1987. The medical profession and the state in France. *Journal of Public Policy* 7 (2): 189–208.

Steffen, Monika. 1989. Privatization in French health politics: Few projects and little outcome. *International Journal of Health Services* 18 (4): 651–61.

Steffen, Monika. 2005. *Health governance in Europe: Issues, challenges, and theories.* London: Routledge.

Steffen, Monika. 2010. The French health care system: Liberal universalism. *Journal of Health Politics, Policy and Law* 35 (3): 336–69.

Steffan, Monika, and Wolfram Lamping. 2009. The "chaordic" dynamics of integration. *Social Science Quarterly* 90 (5): 1361–79.

Steinbrook, Robert. 2005. Financial conflicts of interest and the Food and Drug Administration's advisory committees. *NEJM* 353 (2): 116–18.

Steinbrook, Robert. 2006. For sale: Physicians' prescribing data. *NEJM* 354 (26): 2745–47.

Steinbrook, Robert. 2007. Financial support of continuing education in the health professions. In *Continuing education in the health professions: Improving healthcare through lifelong learning,* ed. H. M. Russell and R. S. Fletcher, 104–26. Available at www.joshiahmacyfoundation.org (accessed 10 November 2009).

Steinman, Michael A., Lisa A. Bero, Mary-Margaret Chren, et al. 2006. Narrative review: The promotion of Gabapentin: An analysis of internal industry documents. *Annals of Internal Medicine* 145 (4): 284–93.

Steinwald, Bruce, and Duncan Neuhaurser. 1970. The role of the proprietary hospital. *Law and Contemporary Problems* 35 (4): 824.

Steslicke, William E. 1973. *Doctors in politics: The political life of the Japan Medical Association.* New York: Praeger.

Steslicke, William E. 1982. Development of health insurance policy in Japan. *Journal of Health Politics, Policy and Law* 7 (1): 197–226.

Stevens, Rosemary. 1971. *American medicine and the public interest.* New Haven, CT: Yale University Press.

Stevens, Rosemary. 1989. *In sickness and in wealth: American hospitals in the twentieth century.* New York: Basic Books.

Stevez-Abe, Margarita. 2003. State-society partnership in the Japanese welfare state. In *The state of civil society in Japan,* ed. F. J. Schwartz and S. J. Pharr, 152–74. Cambridge: Cambridge University Press.

Stone, Deborah. 1980. *The limits of professional power: National health care in the Federal Republic of Germany.* Chicago: University of Chicago Press.

Stone, Deborah. 2008. The Samaritan rebellion. Ch. 4 in *The Samaritan's dilemma: Should government help your neighbor?* New York: Nation Books.

Suda, Yuko. 2006. Devolution and privatization proceed and centralized system maintained: A twisted reality faced by Japanese nonprofit organizations. *Nonprofit and Voluntary Sector Quarterly* 35 (3): 430–52.

Sugerman-Brozan, Alex, and James Woolman. 2005. Drug spending and the average wholesale price: Removing the AWP albatross from Medicaid's neck. *Pharmaceutical Law & Industry Report* 3 (35): 1–8.

Sugita, Satoru. 1989. A historical study of *Iyaku-Bungyō* [the separation of the dispensary from medical practice] in Japan. In *History of the doctor-patient relationship: Proceedings of the 14th international symposium on the comparative history of medicine—East and West*, ed. Y. Kawakita, S. Sakai, and Y. Otsuka. Tokyo: Ishiyaku EuroAmerica.

Sugita, Yoneyuki. 2007. Universal health insurance: The unfinished reform of Japan's health care system. In *Democracy in occupied Japan: The U.S. occupation and Japanese politics and society*, ed. M. E. Caprio and Y. Sugita. Routledge, London, 2007.

Suleiman, Ezra N. 1978. *Elites in French society*. Princeton, NJ: Princeton University Press.

Sullivan, William 1995. *Work and integrity: The crisis and promise of professionalism in America*. New York: HarperCollins.

Sullivan, William M. 2004. Can professionalism still be a viable ethic? *The Good Society* 13 (1): 15–20.

Sullivan, William M. 2004. What is left of professionalism after managed care? *Hastings Center Report* 29 (2): 7–13.

Supreme Commander of the Allies Powers (SCAP), General Headquarters, Social Security Mission. 1947. *Report of the social security mission*. Papers of George F. Rohlick, Library, Special Collections Dept., SUNY Albany.

Supreme Commander for the Allied Powers. 1948. *Public health and welfare in Japan, with Annex and Charts*. Tokyo: The Commander.

Swart, K. W. 1949. *Sale of offices in the seventeenth century*. The Hague: Martinus Nijhoff.

Takagi, Yasuo. 1992. Effects of per-diem payment method in geriatric care: Changes in pharmaceutical and laboratory costs and ADL of the inpatients. *Medicine and Society* 2 (1): 43–62.

Takahashi, Mutsuko. 1997. *The emergence of welfare society in Japan*. Brookfield: Ashgate.

Takahashi, Takeshi. 1974. Social security for workers. In *Workers and employers in Japan: The Japanese employment relations system*, ed. K. Okochi, B. Karsh, and S. B. Levine, 442–43. Princeton, NJ: Princeton University Press.

Takemi, Tarō. 1982. A History of the Japan Medical Association. In Takemi, *Socialized medicine in Japan: Essays, papers and addresses*. Tokyo: JMA.

Talcott, Paul David. 1999. Why the weak can win: Healthcare policies in postwar Japan. Ph.D. diss., Harvard University.

Tanti-Hardouin, Nicolas. 2005. Le système de santé: La recomposition de l'offre hospitalière. *La santé: Cahiers Français* 324: 60–64.

Tanti-Hardouin, Nicolas. 1996. *L'hospitalisation privée: Crise identitaire et mutation sectorielle*. Paris: La Documentation Française.

Tatara, Kōzō, and Estuji Okamoto. 2009. Japan: Health system review. *Health Systems in Transition* 11 (5). Available from *European Observatory on Health Systems and Policies* at http://www.euro.who.int/Document/E92927.pdf (accessed 10 November 2009).

Tawney, R. H. 1920. *The acquisitive society*. New York: Harcourt Brace.

Temin, Peter. 1980. *Taking your medicine: Drug regulation in the United States*. Cambridge. MA: Harvard University Press.

Theil, Pierre. 1943. *Le corps médical devant la médecine sociale*. Paris: Librairie Bailliere. Université de Paris X.

Thompson, Dennis F. 1993. Understanding financial conflicts of interest. *NEJM* 329 (8): 573–76.

Thouvenin, Dominique. 1982. *Le secret médical et l'information du malade*. Lyon: Presses Universitaires de Lyon.

Totten, George Oakley. 1966. *The social democratic movement in prewar Japan*. New Haven, CT: Yale University Press.

U.S. Department of Health, Education, and Welfare (HEW), Office of the Secretary, Task Force on Prescription Drugs. 1968. *The drug makers and the drug distributors*. Washington, DC: Government Printing Office.

U.S. Department of Health and Human Services (DHHS), Office of the Inspector General (OIG). 1988. *Physician drug dispensing: An overview of state regulation*. Washington, DC: DHHS.

U.S. Federal Trade Commission (FTC). 1958. *Economic report on antibiotics manufacturers*. Washington, DC: Government Printing Office.

U.S. General Accounting Office (GAO). 2003. *Specialty hospitals: Information on national market share, physician ownership and patients served*. Washington, DC: Government Printing Office.

U.S. House of Representatives. 1987. Hearing before the Committee on Energy and Commerce, Subcommittee on Health and the Environment. 1987. *Physician dispensing of drugs: Hearings on H.R. 2093*, 1st session, 21 April.

U.S. House of Representatives, Subcommittee on Health and the Environment, Committee on Energy and Commerce. 1989. *Medicare and Medicaid initiatives hearings*, 1st Session. 8 June.

U.S. House of Representatives, Subcommittee on Health, Committee on Ways and Means. 1993. *Physician ownership and referral arrangements*. 1st Session, vol. 2, 20 April.

U.S. Senate, 88th Congress. 1965. Subcommittee on Antitrust and Monopoly, Committee on the Judiciary. *Physician ownership in pharmacies and drug companies*.

U.S. Senate, 90th Congress. 1967. Subcommittee on Antitrust and Monopoly, Committee on Judiciary. *The medical restraint of trade act*.

U.S. Senate, 98th Congress. 1961–1962. Subcommittee on Antitrust and Monopoly of the Committee on the Judiciary. *Drug industry antitrust act (S. 1551)*.

U.S. Senate, Committee on the Judiciary, Subcommittee on Antitrust and Monopoly. 1961. *Administered prices. drugs*. Study of Administered Prices in the Drug Industry.

U.S. Senate, Committee on the Judiciary, Subcommittee on Antitrust and Monopoly, 1961. Pursuant to S. Res. 52 *Administered prices drugs*. 1st Session. Washington, DC: Government Printing Office.

U.S. Senate, Committee on the Judiciary, U.S. Senate, Subcommittee on Antitrust and Monopoly. 1961. *Administered prices, drugs*, Report No. 448. Washington, DC: Government Printing Office.

U.S. Senate, Committee on Labor and Human Resources. 1990. *Advertising, marketing and promotion*. December 11 and 12.

U.S. Senate, Select Committee on Small Business, Subcommittee on Monopoly 1968. *Present status of competition in the pharmaceutical industry*. Washington, DC: Government Printing Office.

U.S. Senate, Select Committee on Small Business, Subcommittee on Monopoly. 1969. *Present status of competition in the pharmaceutical industry*. Washington, DC: Government Printing Office.

U.S. Senate, Select Committee on Small Business, Subcommittee on Monopoly. 1971. *Effect of promotion and advertising of over-the-counter drugs on competition, small business, and the health and welfare of the public.* Washington, DC: Government Printing Office.

U.S. Senate, Subcommittee on Health, Committee on Labor and Public Welfare, *Examination of the pharmaceutical industry: Hearings on Section 3441 and Section 966,* Part 3, 8 March, 1974, 12, 13, 1974. Washington, DC: Government Printing Office.

Veatch, Robert M. 1991. *Patient-physician relationship. The patient as partner, part II.* Bloomington: Indiana University Press.

Vedula, S. Swaroop, Lisa Bero, Roberta W. Scherer, et al. 2009. Outcome reporting in industry-sponsored trials of gabapentin for off-label use. *NEJM* 361 (20): 1963–71.

Wagner, Tobias. 1959. *Ethical pharmaceutical promotion: The workings and philosophies of the pharmaceuticals industry.* New York: National Pharmaceutical Council.

Wassenaar, John D., and Sara L. Thran. 2003. *Physician socioeconomic statistics 2003.* Chicago: AMA.

Watkins, Michael. 2004. *The medical technology industry and Japan (A).* Cambridge, MA: Harvard Business School, Case No. 9–904–018.

Waud, Douglas.R. 1992. Pharmaceutical promotions—a free lunch? *NEJM* 327(5):351–53.

Webb, Sydney, and Beatrice Webb. 1917. Special supplement on professional associations, parts 1, 2. *New Statesmen* 9 (211) (April 21): 1–24.

Weindling, Paul. 1991. The modernization of charity in nineteenth-century France and Germany. In *Medicine and charity before the welfare state*, ed. Jonathan Barry and Colin Jones, 190–206. New York: Routledge.

Weiler, Paul C., Howard H. Hiatt, Joseph P. Newhouse, et al. 1993. *A measure of malpractice: Medical injury, malpractice litigation, and patient compensation.* Cambridge, MA: Harvard University Press.

Weller, Charles. 1985. "Free choice" as a restraint of trade, and the counterintuitive contours of competition. *Health Matrix* 3 (2): 3–23.

Wilensky, Harold L. 1964. The professionalization of everyone? *American Journal of Sociology* 70 (2): 137–58.

Williams, Greer. 1952. The Columbus five-year cure for fee-splitting. *Modern Hospital* 78 (6): 67–69, 94–95.

Wilsford, David. 1991. *Doctors and the state: The politics of health care in France and the United States.* Durham, NC: Duke University Press.

Wilsford, David. 1993. The state and medical profession in France. In *The changing medical profession: An international perspective*, ed. F. W. Hafferty and J. B. McKinlay, 124–37. New York: Oxford University Press.

Wilson, Timothy D., and Nancy Brekke. 1994. Mental contamination and mental correction: Unwanted influences on judgments and evaluations. *Psychological Bulletin* 116 (1): 117–42.

Winfield, Percy H. 1925. *The chief sources of English legal history.* Cambridge, MA: Harvard University Press.

Wing, Kenneth. 1998. *The law and American health care.* New York: Aspen Law and Business.

Witz, Claude. 1981. *La fiducie en droit privé français.* Paris: Economica.

Wocher, John C. 1994. The Japanese health care system: Planning the extinction of the private hospitals. *Japan Hospitals* 13 (July): 37–43.

Wocher, John. C. 1997. TQM/CQI efforts in Japanese hospitals—Why not? In *The effectiveness of CQI in health care: Stories from a global perspective*, ed. V. A. Kazandjian, 51–107. Milwaukee, WI: ASQ Quality Press.

Wolman, Dianne Miller, Andrea L. Kalfoglou, and Lauren LeRoy. 2000. *Medicare laboratory payment policy: Now and in the future*. Washington D.C.: National Academy Press.

Yamagami, M., and Y. Seoka. 1995. Health economics analysis on dialysis treatment. *Banboo* 163 (January): 64–68.

Yoshikawa, Aki. 1993. Doctors and hospitals in Japan. In *Japan's health system: Efficiency and effectiveness in universal care*, ed. D. I. Okimoto and A. Yoshikawa, 63–89. Washington, DC: Faulkner and Gray.

Yumiko, Nishimura, and Aki Yoshikawa. 1993. A brief history of Japan's passage to the universal health insurance system. In *Japan's health system: Efficiency and effectiveness in universal care*, ed. D. I. Okimoto and A. Yoshikawa, 11–19. Washington, DC: Falkner and Gray.

Zola, Irving Kenneth. 1972. Medicine as an institution of social control. *Social Review* 20 (487): 487–504.

Zoller, Elisabeth. 2008. *Introduction to public law: A comparative study*. Koninklijke Bill: Martinus Nijhoff.

Index

About the Author

Marc A. Rodwin is Professor of Law at Suffolk University Law School. He has been a visiting researcher at Tokyo University Law School and the French national research agency (*Centre National de Recherche Scientifique*) at *l'Institut de l'Ouest: Droit et Europe*. He was visiting professor at the University of Rennes Law School and previously was Associate Professor at the Indiana University School of Public and Environmental Affairs–Bloomington.

Rodwin is the author of *Medicine, Money and Morals: Physicians' Conflicts of Interest* (Oxford, 1993) and numerous articles on health law, policy, and ethics, heath care consumer issues, regulatory issues, and medical malpractice. He has received grants from the German Marshall Fund, the Fulbright Fellowship, the Abe Fellowship of the Social Science Research Council, and a Robert Wood Johnson Foundation Investigator Award. He holds a Ph.D. from Brandeis University, a J.D. from the University of Virginia Law School, a B.A. and an M.A. from Oxford University, and a B.A. from Brown University.